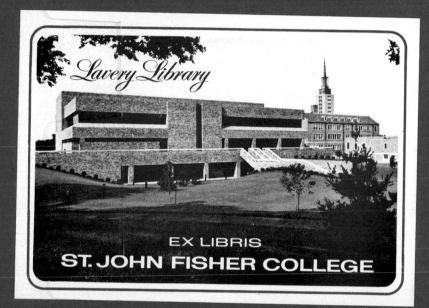

T H E
LONGEVITY FACTOR

THE NEW REALITY OF LONG CAREERS
AND HOW IT CAN LEAD TO RICHER LIVES

LYDIA BRONTË, Ph.D.

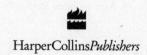

HarperCollins*Publishers*

HarperCollins books may be purchased for educational, business, or sales promotional use. For information, please write: Special Markets Department, HarperCollins Publishers, Inc., 10 East 53rd Street, New York, NY 10022.

FIRST EDITION

Designed by George J. McKeon

Library of Congress Cataloging in Publication Data

Brontë, Lydia, 1938–
  The longevity factor : the new reality of long careers and how it can lead to richer
lives / Lydia Brontë. — 1st ed.
    p.   cm.
  Includes bibliographical references and index.
  ISBN: 0-06-016755-6
  1. Aged—Employment—United States.   2. Retirees—Employment—United States.
3. Career changes—United States. 4. Aged—United States—Psychology. I.Title.
HD6280.B76 1993
331.3'98'0973—dc20   91-50447

94 95 96 ❖/HC 10 9 8 7 6 5 4 3

For the friends who were a constant source of strength:
Phyllis Collins; Francoise Gilot; Dr. Jonas Salk;
Tilak Fernando, a wellspring of inspiration;
and for Francis Lear, who made the world
safe once again for wisdom and maturity

Contents

Acknowledgments

My most profound appreciation goes to the men and women who took part in the Long Careers Study. Busy people with full and engaging lives, they graciously gave their time, their attention, and their insights to the study without any compensation other than the idea that doing so might eventually help other people. To the extent that the Long Careers Study and this book are useful, the greatest debt is owed them.

Dr. David A. Hamburg was President of Carnegie Corporation of New York and Ms. Helene Kaplan was Chair of Carnegie's Board of Trustees when I first invented the Long Careers Study. Without their faith in the value of the idea, and without Carnegie's funding of the project for its first fifteen months, the Study and this book would never have come into being.

Three other officers at Carnegie encouraged and contributed to the project in many ways, beginning in its earliest stages: Barbara D. Finberg, Carnegie's Executive Vice President; Sara Englehardt, now President of New York's Foundation Center; and Avery Russell, Carnegie's Director of Publications.

I am also grateful to Alan Pifer, now Chairman of the Southport Institute for Policy Analysis but for many years Carnegie's President. His insight into the importance of population aging for the entire society captured my imagination initially and drew me into the field of aging; his many qualities made my five years at Carnegie rich and productive ones.

Margaret Mahoney, President of the Commonwealth Fund, shared vital research information with me and introduced me to several participants who were extraordinarily rich sources of information. William Whyte, author of *The Organization Man*, served as a friend and valued adviser, critiquing ideas and constantly urging me on.

Three members of the study contributed far more than anyone could have anticipated and literally rescued both the study and me at several points. Mr. and Mrs. John L. Loeb made a substantial gift to the study at a time when an unexpected illness almost stopped my work on the project altogether. Because of their generosity the project survived, and my health has been permanently improved.

Dr. W. Edwards Deming took a keen interest in the project, adopted me into his wide circle of students and friends, and made a generous gift to the project which enabled the work to proceed far more rapidly. His encouragement was vital.

Frances Lear, founder and publisher of *Lear's* magazine, generously provided for several periods of work which were extraordinarily productive. She was a vital source of encouragement and enthusiasm in every respect.

Good luck led me to an exceptionally fine working environment. The Hon. Franklin Williams, President of the Phelps-Stokes Fund, suggested during his interview for the study that I become affiliated with their Research Institute. This invitation proved to be a godsend, enormously facilitating my work. Dr. Ronald Wells, the Institute's then-director, was tireless in his assistance. After Ambassador Williams's tragic death of lung cancer, I found in his able successor, Dr. Wilbert J. LeMelle, a good friend and wise adviser. Special thanks for their friendship and help go to Samuel Kwofie; Abu Sillah; Viola Morris; Gerald LeMelle; and Enid Gort.

The founders of the Brookdale Center on Aging of Hunter College, Dr. Rose Dobrof and Dr. Harry R. Moody, were a constant source of ideas, and enthusiasm.

The former board of the Aging Society Project—Dr. Andrew W. Achenbaum, Dr. and Mrs. James E. Birren, Dr. Harry R. Moody, Dr. Bernice Neugarten, Drs. John and Matilda Riley, and Dr. Fernando Torres-Gil—were an inexhaustible source of information, criticism, and affection.

ACKNOWLEDGMENTS

Two expert career counselors, Dr. Letitia Chamberlain of New York University and Dr. Adele Scheele, mapped career theory for me and provided vital research references.

Elizabeth Massie served as my executive assistant during the last two and a half years when the project was coming to fruition. I do not believe I could have completed the arduous task of analyzing the Long Careers Study and writing the book without her energetic and willing help. Her intelligence, perceptive comments, skill and fierce loyalty were immensely supportive in so many ways it would be impossible to describe them all. The daughter of two talented writers herself, she is a writer/researcher's dream assistant. When the book was completed, Liz left to follow her lifelong dream of becoming a film producer. She will be a wonderful success.

Bonnie Talbot, a computer genius, upgraded my system and helped integrate me into it. Katherine Emmet True, a long-time friend, threw her lot in with the Study for some eight months and contributed immensely to its progress. Laurie Maddigan gave heroic amounts of time and atttention to making sure the interview transcripts were accurate. Dr. Elizabeth Buck served as my alter ego at several stages; a brilliant administrator, her help was priceless.

Among the treasured members of my crew at various points were: Amy Bryson, Caryn Burton, Linda Gelerter, Jill Jeffries, Christina Baker Kline, Angela Orlow, Mindy Krasner, Cindy Morris, Trudie Reiss, Nancy Romeu, Jennifer Rose, Anita Sharper, and Susan Smiley. Elizabeth Riddler pulled together a digest of research at the beginning of the project; Dennis Thread was my invaluable assistant and adopted younger brother during the earliest years of work.

Many friends embellished my life and work during the period of research and writing: Nancy and Robert Bell, M.D., Dr. O. Gilbert Brim; Joan Bryan; Jeanne Beauregard; Allison Bernstein; Terri, Aneya, and Orion Brennan Fernando; Timmie Burke; Nancy Burson; Dr. Robert Butler and Myrna Lewis; Lisle Cade; Linda and Donald Cain; John Child and Julie Winter; Ellen Cousins; James Elder; Ann Fishman; Janaka Fernando; Carol Gilligan; Marifrances and the late O.B. Hardison; Irving Heisler; Arlene, Ronald, Jennifer and Joshua Kahn; Dr. Arthur D, Kirsch; Marty, Pamela, and Parker Krasney; Steven Lazarus; Dr. and Mrs. Warren Levin; John Maguire; Kyriacos and Emily Markides;

Robert Massie and Debra Karl; Suzanne Massie; Bettye Morris; Ed Morris; Mary Beth Norton; Elaine, Sarah, and David Pagels and the late Heinz Pagels; Dr. Richard Rockefeller; Nancy Anderson, and Clayton and Rebecca Rockefeller; Dr. John H. Rowe; Rakesh Sharma; Helen Shaskan; Dr. Vergil Slee; Helen Stephenson; Anita Stowell; Ingo Swann; Drs. Stanley Turesky, Gerry Otremba and their daughter Penny; and Michael and Pat York, whose splendid book, *Going Strong*, was a source of great inspiration.

Dr. Charles Seigler of Ciba-Geigy referred me to several extremely fine study participants, as did Eleanor Elliott. Marty Edelston, founder of Boardroom reports, was a source of constant aid and inspiration.

My sister Gloria Brontë Lane, Academic Director in Computing Services at the University of Arkansas Little Rock, gave me many good suggestions and referred me to a capable colleague, Tracey Schroepfer, who with Boyd Selby analyzed the survey of study participants.

The Schrimper Foundation and its president, Myles Canc, assisted the project at several important times when no other source of funding was available. The study received critical funding at several crucial points from the Dillon Family Fund, the Commonwealth Fund, the John D. and Catherine T. MacArthur Foundation, the Retirement Research Foundation, the Charles Stewart Mott Foundation, the Florence V. Burden Foundation, the H. W. Durham Foundation, and the Marpat Foundation, headed by Mrs. Jefferson Patterson. The Maurice Falk Medical Fund, the Metropolitan Life Foundation, The Travelers Foundation, The Shainberg Foundation, Ian Armof, Shelley Fraser Mickle, Arthur Ross, Sana Sabbagh, Eleanor Winthrop, and Dr. and Mrs. Irving Wright also contributed welcome support. I am grateful for the help of Adele Simmons; Trudy Cross, Robert and Nancy Ewing, Barbara Greenberg, Phil Hallen, Marilyn Hennessy, Bryan Hofland, Ph.D., Joan Koven, David Nee, Lenore Parker; and Nell Eurich, Steve Moseley and the Academy for Educational Development. Peter Libassi, formerly corporate Vice President of the Travelers Companies, was of tremendous assistance in putting me in touch with the Travelers Job Bank.

I owe a great deal to John Brockman and Katinka Matson, two of the finest literary agents in existence, and to my publicist,

Lynn Goldberg Communications. Finally, I was exceptionally lucky to be found by a real editor, Janet Goldstein, whose wonderful intelligence and gentle diplomacy are bound to carry her one day to the top of the publishing world.

Lydia Brontë, Ph.D.
New York, May 13, 1993

Prologue

This book is about the rest of your life. Specifically, it is about how long you will live and what you will be able to do with that time.

Beginning in childhood, all of us form basic assumptions about the length of our lives—assumptions on which all our other plans, expectations, dreams, and hopes are based. We form those ideas by observing the lives of those around us and by absorbing the beliefs that are current in our society.

But during the course of the twentieth century, something has happened that has almost certainly altered the pattern of your life, most likely without your realizing it. A new element has appeared that is transforming life in totally unexpected ways: the longevity factor. There has been a revolution regarding the length of time we live, and it is changing the future for every American.

If you are in your twenties, thirties, or forties, you may not yet understand how much the longevity factor will affect you. But you should begin to be aware of it now, for it will almost surely be a major influence in your own life as well as in the lives of your family and friends. In a long-lived society, how you think about your life now can make a tremendous difference in what you do for many years to come.

Unlike most revolutions, the longevity revolution took us by surprise. We didn't expect it. We didn't lay any plans for it; no one did anything deliberate to create it. We didn't even realize that such a thing was possible until it happened. In fact, if someone had suggested the possibility of radically increasing the length of time we live, we might have rejected the thought—because we would have believed it would mean radically extending old age, which wouldn't have seemed like a very good idea.

The statistics that describe this revolution may be familiar to you already. In 1900, the average life expectancy at birth for a newborn baby was roughly 47 years; in 1991, it was about 75 (72 for men and 79.2 for women). That is a net gain of 28 years. Thus, since the turn of the century, the lifetime of the ordinary American has lengthened by 60 percent, and the amount of time that we spend in adulthood has more than doubled.

One way of grasping the dramatic nature of this change has been offered by Dr. Robert N. Butler, a geriatric physician who was the first director of the National Institute on Aging and is now head of geriatric medicine at Mount Sinai Medical School in New York. Dr. Butler noted that there has been a greater increase in average life expectancy at birth during the twentieth century than there was from ancient Rome to the year 1900! A quick calculation shows that from 100 B.C. to A.D. 1900 (about two thousand years) average life expectancy at birth increased by twenty-five years—from twenty-two to forty-seven—an average rate of one and a half years per century if it increased at an even rate (we don't know whether it grew evenly, but that assumption is always involved in averages of this kind). Yet from 1900 to 1990, average life expectancy grew more than it did in the previous two thousand years; it gained by twenty-eight years, an increase twenty-three times greater than the average for any previous century.[1]

Carrying this example one step further, demographer Samuel Preston in a 1984 *Scientific American* article gave an even more startling estimate. He asserted that two-thirds of the increase in average life expectancy from prehistoric times to the present has taken place in the twentieth century.[2] Regardless of which estimate you prefer, it is a phenomenon truly unprecedented in human history—one whose meaning for the future of humankind we have not even begun to explore.

The cause of this tremendous expansion of the length of life, which I have chosen to call the "longevity factor," is still for the most part a mystery. The most distinguished biological scientists

in the field of aging say that at present, although we have bits and
pieces of information, there is simply not enough data to give a
valid scientific explanation of why the increase in longevity has
occurred. It may have been created by a very few changes in lifestyle and health practices; or it may be the by-product of developments in many different fields of knowledge—an unintended consequence of actions taken for totally different reasons. For the
moment, we just do not know.

What we do know, however, is that this transformation of our
lifetimes is really taking place. It is not a figment of our collective
imaginations, nor a result of interpreting data differently, not a
trend dreamed up by Madison Avenue. It is real. And what it
means is that you may live a great deal longer than you expect.

You may find that your adult life will be twice as long as you
think it is going to be. If you have had reasonably good health
habits, by the time you celebrate your sixtieth birthday, instead
of being on the downward slope of old age you may have two
or three decades of productive adult time ahead of you—time
that is not much different in quality from what you experience at
age sixty.

If you are not aware of this trend, you may make decisions
that essentially foreshorten your own opportunities. You could
reach fifty and think your most creative or productive years are
behind you (they aren't); or you could think that you'll be old at
sixty-five (you probably won't be).

We have been conditioned to believe that adult life follows an
invariable pattern, with old age and retirement in the sixties and a
downhill slide after that. Even if that model of adult life was valid
during much of the twentieth century, it is no longer accurate. On
the threshold of the twenty-first century, the emerging model is
very different. And it may become even more different as we cross
into the new millennium. If important scientific discoveries are
made that can reduce the incidence of the most common health
problems for people over sixty-five and maintain vitality even
later in life, we may see average life expectancies climb even
higher—close to the century mark, or perhaps even beyond it.

We do not yet know, and cannot know, what the length of the
twenty-first-century lifetime will be. But we can be nearly certain
that the average lifetime in the next century will be longer than
ours are now, barring unexpected catastrophes such as a tremendous expansion of the AIDS virus. (Indeed, it is both sad and

ironic that at this point, when life is longer than at any other time
in human history, this new disease has appeared to tragically foreshorten life for so many talented people.)

We are all potential beneficiaries of this trend toward longer
lifetimes. This book was written to let you know that you may
have a great deal more time ahead of you than you think, and
that this is not a fearful prospect, not an expansion of old age,
but a profound and unexpected opportunity. It is an opportunity
that you can use to its fullest if you take account of it now. The
longevity factor, whatever its causes, may well have given you the
greatest gift of your life—the gift of time.

PART I

LONGEVITY, AGING, AND THE LONG CAREERS STUDY

Pioneers in Time

Dr. W. Edwards Deming rises to his feet, leaning forward slightly against the long table placed before him on the stage. As he stands, the six hundred people seated in the vast conference room fall silent. Deming lifts his head and his eyes sweep the long rows of workshop participants. His voice booms into the microphone: "Why are we here?" The silence becomes complete: no one moves. There is a moment's pause. "Who knows why we are here?" Deming thunders. The audience, made up of chief executive officers, corporate managers, and quality control staff, waits for the answer, poised as breathlessly as if they were one person. After a long moment, Deming's face breaks suddenly into a conspiratorial grin. "To have fun!" he roars, and the room explodes with laughter and relief. The participants in the workshop know that they have found more than a master teacher; they have found a friend and a powerful ally in their struggle to bring their companies back to the peak of productivity, which is their goal.

For the next four days, these six hundred men and women, each of whom has paid a $600 fee to attend Deming's workshop, will work intensively from eight o'clock in the morning until late at night, building an understanding of Deming's management method under his direction and that of his staff associates. Dr. W. Edwards Deming invented and brought to Japan after World War II a quality control method that eventually helped make Japan the most powerful manufacturing country in the world. Now he is trying to teach his method to American companies, who are at last ready, even desperate, to learn it. When he leaves Philadelphia, where this seminar is being held, Deming will continue his normal schedule, flying each week to a different city to hold seminars and workshops; consulting every other week with either General Motors or Ford; and training young managers and other staff to develop quality control programs in their own companies. Every Friday he returns to his home in Washington, D.C., to catch up on his correspondence and get ready for the following week. Every Sunday night, from September to May, he flies to New York City to teach a Monday morning course at Columbia University and a Monday afternoon course at the New York University Business School.

In October 1992, while he was in Detroit to give another four-day seminar, Dr. W. Edwards Deming celebrated a very important event: his ninety-second birthday.

At 7:30 A.M. in Chicago, Shirley Brussell parks her car, crosses the street to 180 North Wabash, and takes the elevator to the eighth-floor offices of Operation Able. Today the agency is running its twelfth annual Job Fair in the McCormick Center Hotel—an event that will draw more than four thousand Chicagoans before the day is over. The demand for what the agency offers has been so great that Able has lowered its age threshold, from the normal fifty-five to forty-five, because so many people in their forties have been hit by corporate downsizing and want the kind of access to jobs that Able can provide. This morning, before Brussell formally opens the fair, she wants to put in a few rare quiet moments at her desk.

Fifteen years ago, Shirley Brussell was part of a volunteer group that wanted to create an employment counseling service for older people. The group wrote a proposal for the Chicago Community Trust, which was accepted. Brussell—who had worked for several years until she got married and then spent twenty years raising a family—was asked to head the project. Since Operation Able opened its doors in 1977, with $47,000 in funding and a three-person staff, Brussell has built it into an organization with a $4 million yearly budget and 345 employees. It offers twenty-five different programs and has thirty-five affiliated agencies in the Chicago area, including ten agencies of its own. In the first six months of 1991, it received 9,597 telephone inquiries from job seekers, and it listed 3,307 jobs registered by employers.

Brussell's brainchild has benefited more areas than just Chicago. Operation Able has served as a model for the creation of seven other Ables, as well as four developing "baby Ables" in other American cities.

Shirley Brussell started her real career at the age of fifty-six. Now she is seventy-two and, by anyone's standards, a stunning success.

A few blocks north, at about the same time that Shirley Brussell is parking her car, stockbroker Samuel Allen Williams strides into his office at Prescott, Ball and Turben and turns on his computer screen to get the morning news. Stockbrokers have access to a continuous flow of the latest events, virtually as they happen, running across their computer terminals; this helps them in predicting the market's movements. This constant stream of world news is one aspect that Sam Williams likes best about his work—it creates the sense of being connected to what is happening at all times. Williams, who became a broker thirty-five years ago after a successful first career as a business owner, manages some two hundred accounts—a small but select number, worth millions of dollars. Williams has never advertised. All his clients have come to him by word of mouth, and some have made fortunes under his direction.

Promptly at 9:00 A.M. Williams's phone begins to ring, and it will keep ringing steadily all day. At 4:00 P.M., Williams will put on his coat and catch a bus back to the apartment he shares with his wife, Carol.

Williams is tall, well built, and attractive; he is fit and healthy, though he doesn't exercise. He is also a U.S. Army veteran—from World War I. Although one would judge from Sam Williams's appearance that he is about seventy, he was in fact born on January 18, 1899. In September 1992, he is more than halfway through his ninety-third year.

Pauline Trigere stands in a spotlight in the darkened dining hall of the Fashion Institute of Technology, her dress a glowing column of gold brocaded obi silk that shimmers like a flame in the brilliant light. Except for the sweeping pattern of the silk, the gown is utterly simple: pure straight line, high neck, long sleeves. Trigere brought the fabric back from a trip to Japan after World War II. Like its owner, the silk has worn well: its color and sparkle are as fresh as if the delicate web had been woven this year. Trigere bows her head to acknowledge the crowd around her, which has risen to its feet to applaud a retrospective showing of fashions from Trigere's fifty years as an American designer—the first to celebrate a golden jubilee.

The gala evening, which was held to benefit six AIDS organizations, drew more than six hundred people and raised over $200,000. Many of the dresses featured in the show had been lovingly kept by their owners for three or four decades, yet they are so contemporary in design that they could just as easily have been part of a new collection.

Pauline Trigere is an embodiment of the American dream. She came to the United States in 1937, passing through, as she thought, on her way to South America with her family. When they stopped over for a few days in New York and Trigere saw bathing suits in the window of Saks Fifth Avenue in December, she was enthralled. She knew that this place, which had the audacity to advertise beachwear when it was freezing cold, was where she wanted to stay.

The morning after her gala, Trigere will turn her attention back to the business at hand: her next collection. Pauline Trigere is in her seventies; every new season is an opportunity to build on, and to surpass, what she has done before.

On a sound stage in Los Angeles, actor John Forsythe is doing a run-through of a scene for his new television series, "The Powers That Be," a satire on American political life in the 1990s. Forsythe, a handsome, charismatic man with silver hair, plays a senator whose life and campaign encapsulate all of the misadventures American viewers have been acquainted with in the turbulent recent history of American politics.

Forsythe, an actor with a long and distinguished career on stage and in film, became a household word overnight in the 1970s with the first episodes of the television series "Dynasty." A sensation when it first aired, "Dynasty" kept millions of Americans enthralled with its high-powered portrayal of the life and business dealings of Forsythe's hard-driving but attractive character, Denver oil magnate Blake Carrington; Blake's angelic wife,

Krystle, played by Linda Evans; and Blake's dragon-lady ex-wife, played by Joan Collins.

One of the greatest accomplishments of the series was that it depicted mature adults whose lives were eventful, glamorous, and exciting—and the stars who played the roles were the same ages as their characters.

"Dynasty" was a milestone in breaking age barriers in television, an industry that until then had refused to acknowledge that women over forty and men over fifty could be attractive, interesting, and, yes, sexy. John Forsythe, who became a sex symbol for millions of women in the viewing audience, was in his sixties, had been happily married for many years, and was a grandfather.

After more than a decade, "Dynasty" went off the air, a victim of poor scripts and network ratings wars. But its fans longed for more. Thus, to formally resolve the show's plot lines, a two-hour miniseries was made and aired in the fall of 1991. Afterward, the producers of "The Powers That Be," searching for the perfect actor to play Senator Powers, tapped Forsythe for the role.

So far, the reviews have been raves. Forsythe has a dazzling comic sense—a talent that made his earlier TV series, "Bachelor Father," a major success from 1957 to 1962 but that was submerged for many years by producers who cast him in serious roles only. And with news headlines every day about the peccadilloes and foibles of American politicians, it looks as if Senator Powers is in for a long, tumultuous, and entertaining television life.

North of San Diego, the flat, white sand beaches suddenly spring into a series of cliffs, straining upward against the sky until they replace the beaches altogether. Near the edge of these cliffs is located one of the nation's best-known examples of modern architecture, the Salk Institute, its design a collaboration between the great architect Louis Kahn and polio vaccine discoverer Dr. Jonas Salk. The institute's parallel white-concrete office and laboratory buildings flank a long open plaza that seems to disappear into the Pacific Ocean and the limitless horizon beyond. It is a symbol of human imagination and, more than that, an embodiment of Salk's creativity, which always seems to seek out the most distant, most tantalizing horizon.

In his office overlooking the Pacific, Salk is meeting with a scientist who belongs to the network of researchers helping to test

Salk's AIDS vaccine. Dr. Salk became interested in the AIDS virus in 1982, drawn into its study by calls from researchers who wanted his advice about their own work on the baffling illness. Two years later, he himself began serious work on AIDS. Since 1987 Salk has been testing a vaccine whose basis is so original that he first called it an "immunotherapeutic." In general, vaccines prevent infection in the uninfected, but Salk reasoned that it would be easier and more efficient to find a way to stop the virus's progress in people already infected with AIDS than to try to immunize the many millions of people who do not have the disease. If the onset of physical symptoms could be arrested and the transmission of the virus to others stopped, the AIDS epidemic would be halted—and the lives of many people already infected could be saved.

Although the scientific community was skeptical at first, experiments have shown that Salk's concept is valid. Now he is going through the arduous process of steering the vaccine through further trials in order to obtain approval for wider distribution. The process of testing new drugs has grown far more bureaucratic in the thirty-seven years since Salk's polio vaccine was declared safe and effective. Although the delays are undoubtedly frustrating, Salk meets each obstacle with vigor and intelligence, encouraging researchers such as the one in his office now (who is roughly half Salk's age) to continue with their work despite the obstacles.

Dr. Jonas Salk's polio vaccine was introduced to the world in 1955, when he was forty-one. Now he is seventy-nine.

Frances Lear has just won a bet. It was for only five dollars, so what counts isn't the money but the sense of vindication, almost of personal triumph. An adopted child who was emotionally abused by her mother and sexually abused by her stepfather, Lear has had a long-standing interest in alleviating the cruelty of child abuse. She recently published a special issue of *Lear's* magazine on the subject of incest, including the announcement of a pathbreaking study of abusive fathers, which she helped to fund at the University of New Hampshire Family Violence Research Lab. Her circulation manager had argued vehemently against the issue, envisioning the magazines lying unsold on thousands of newsstands all over the country. Lear went ahead despite his dire predictions and bet him five dollars that the issue would sell. She won, and big: newsstands all over the country sold out of the issue, and letters poured in from readers. In addition, Lear's has filled requests for 25,000 reprints, a quantity that is unheard of in the magazine industry.

Frances Lear is a slender woman, elegant and intense, with a distinctive halo of curly, silver-white hair and a decisiveness that identifies her as someone to be reckoned with. Her brainchild, Lear's, is a kind of miracle. She created it out of a single brilliant idea, one that she conceived and then nurtured for years: there ought to be a publication for women over forty, for the woman "who wasn't born yesterday." At the age of sixty-two, when her marriage to producer Norman Lear ended in divorce, Lear moved to New York. With no prior experience in magazine publishing, she established one of the most original and successful new periodicals of the decade. Now she runs the magazine from her spacious, busy office and uses it as a voice for a multitude of issues.

Frances Lear began her real career at an age when many people take retirement. She is now sixty-eight, and she has the kind of plans for her future that we associate with people in their thirties.

A few weeks before her seventy-first birthday, while on vacation in the Napa Valley, Liz Carpenter got the surprise of her life: she discovered she was about to be a mother again—not of just one child but of three teenagers.

Carpenter, a journalist and public relations executive, had become nationally famous as Ladybird Johnson's press secretary during Lyndon Johnson's presidency. Since leaving political life, her dazzling sense of humor and her way with words have enabled her to continue earning her living as a writer and public speaker, flying all over the country to fill a wide variety of engagements. In July she had taken part with other celebrities in a conference program in Wichita, dressing up in a café singer's outfit with a hot-pink feather boa to give her own rendition of a song written especially for her: "I'm a Hot Tomato with a Lot of Sauce."

Now her seventy-nine-year-old brother has called to tell her that his health has suddenly disintegrated and he may be dying. Will she take in his three teenage children from his second marriage? With that telephone call, Carpenter has joined the millions of American grandparents who are raising their grandchildren or their nieces and nephews. "I may be the oldest member of the Austin, Texas, PTA," Carpenter says, "but I'm not the only one over sixty by any means. There's an entire generation now that's being raised by people other than their biological parents. It's been a revelation to me."

By the standards most of us are familiar with, these people may seem exceptional. Each is outstanding in some respect, though they are very different from each other. Some have had more than one career. Some of them are world famous, whereas others are known chiefly to their colleagues, friends, and neighbors. But in their longevity and their lifestyles they are remarkably similar. What they have in common is one of the most extraordinary developments of the twentieth century—or any other, for that matter. They are members of the first generation of human beings in history to live in large numbers into the decades previously called "old age" and to retain the physical vitality, interests, abilities, achievements, and lifestyles that we usually associate with younger people.

In the United States, people over the age of sixty-five number some thirty-one million, an amount that equals the combined populations of New Jersey, New York State, and Massachusetts. Most of us probably believe that a large percentage of the population over sixty-five is ill and either partly or wholly disabled; media presentations about older people have consistently dealt mostly with the illnesses and problems of this age group. But the sick and frail make up only 15 percent of all people over sixty. The remaining 85 percent of these older Americans—some 25,811,950, nearly the equivalent of the combined populations of New York and New Jersey—are vital and active.[1]

The U.S. Bureau of Labor Statistics states that there are 3.5 million people over sixty-five employed in the civilian labor force. Millions of others in this age group are engaged in income-earning work or volunteer activity that does not fit the bureau's definitions. Yet you may have been conditioned to believe that all older people are frail, ill, and dependent; you may not be aware of how many people over sixty-five are healthy and active and how many of these people you actually know.

These "new older Americans" are all around us. They live in every town and city, although they are not always recognizable because so many of them look younger than they are. For the most part, they did not expect to live such long lifetimes nor to remain active so long. What's more, as far as we know, they haven't done anything unusual to achieve their healthy longevity. They are the beneficiaries of a remarkable change that has occurred during this century. Without intending to take on the role of adventurers, they have become pioneers in time—people whose long lifetimes are redefining our ideas of what adult life is now and what it may become in the future.

The people who are profiled at the beginning of this chapter are the forerunners of what many Americans under sixty-five can expect in their own futures: a lifetime that reaches close to the century mark (or even beyond) and remains active and fulfilling for much or all of that time. Although the causes of this development are still mysterious, there is no question that it is real. The people taking part in it are all around us. You probably know a number of them yourself.

Perhaps the most radical change that has accompanied this trend is that many of these new older people are continuing to work beyond the age of sixty-five, into their seventies, eighties, and nineties; even, in a few cases, beyond their one-hundredth birthdays. This represents a startling departure from the concept of retirement as it has existed since the passage of the Social Security Act in 1935. For more than half a century, retirement has been the pot of gold at the end of the rainbow of adult life, a welcome and well-earned rest after a lifetime of hard work. It has been synonymous with a leisurely lifestyle and the abandonment of any connection with work.

We have grown accustomed to a road map of adulthood that begins in the early twenties, plunging into work and career building during the twenties and thirties; winds its way through the high points and crises of middle age between thirty-five and fifty; and then heads for the golf course of retirement somewhere between sixty and sixty-five. Now that road map is out of date. Middle age no longer ends at fifty, and old age no longer begins at sixty-five. What once was a comfortably predictable future has shifted, like the image in a kaleidoscope, into a pattern we no longer recognize.

In 1987 I set out to examine what this revolution in longevity means for individual Americans. I was especially interested in how longer lifetimes are changing the new older generation's participation in work and productive activity (regardless of whether that activity was paid) because of the ferment that has surrounded the issue of work for older people in recent years: age discrimination suits, the congressional elimination of mandatory retirement for most occupations, the corporate trend toward early retirement.

In the course of this research project, called the Long Careers Study, I interviewed 150 people between the ages of 65 and 101 who continued working after age sixty-five. All of them continued to work by choice, not from economic necessity; some found the additional income useful, but because of social security money it was not a crucial factor. I asked them to tell me their life stories: where they grew up, what their education was like, how they chose their work, how their goals and aspirations evolved, why they changed or did not change jobs at various points, and why they remained active, despite the prevailing pattern during most of their adult lives of retirement by age sixty-five. I asked them about their health, their exercise patterns, and their lifestyles. I also interviewed a number of experts on aging, some of whom participated in the study itself, to assess the physical and social components of this new longevity.

A high percentage of the participants were outstanding individuals whose life stories were worthy of formal biographies. (Indeed, some of them have already been subjects of published works.) The brief life histories in this book serve to illustrate specific career patterns, using certain aspects of individual careers to characterize long and often complex sequences of jobs and career choices. It was not always possible or appropriate to include all the details of a participant's career.

Part of the stimulus for the Long Careers Study and for this book came from my own recognition several years ago that I had been thinking about my own life with far too short a horizon. That experience was a very powerful one. In a curious way, it mirrored some of the changes in longevity that have taken place during this century.

Longevity is a subject that had never interested me before, because I come from a notoriously short-lived family. Three of my nineteenth-century cousins—Charlotte, Emily, and Anne Brontë— were famous both for their literary achievements and for the exceptionally short lives they and their brother, Branwell, led. Anne died at twenty-nine, a year after her first novel, *Agnes Grey*, appeared in print; Emily died at the age of thirty, only one year after the publication of her only novel, *Wuthering Heights;* Branwell died in the same year that Emily passed away, at the age of thirty-one. Only Charlotte lived to the relatively ripe age of thirty-nine and had a chance to publish two other novels after the appearance of her first, *Jane Eyre.* The two children who were said to be the most gifted in the family, Maria and Elizabeth, died at eleven and ten, respectively, so we will never know what their literary output might have been.

In the twentieth century—more than a hundred years later and thousands of miles from Haworth, England—my father's generation followed a very similar pattern. Of five siblings, one died in early childhood; three (including my father) died at around the age of fifty, not an old age for their time and place, by any means; and one lived into her early sixties, older than the others but still not a particularly long life. The ages were older than those of the earlier Brontë siblings, but the pattern was the same.

The upshot of this was that during most of my life I had believed, almost without thinking about it, that I would probably die around the age of fifty. Physically I resembled my father's side of the family more than my mother's, and it simply did not seem logical to imagine that I would do a great deal better than the rest of the Brontës in terms of my longevity.

I didn't find the possibility particularly upsetting. When you are in your twenties and thirties, fifty seems so remote that it might as well belong to a different century. The prospect affected my life only in certain odd ways, none of them troublesome. For example, although I took good care of my health, I did so merely in the interest of current, day-to-day functioning; I didn't worry about what the consequences of my health habits would be forty or fifty years in the future. Nor did I spend any time being concerned about income after retirement, since I didn't expect to live to be old enough to retire, or about who would take care of me in my old age, since I didn't expect to have one!

In 1982 I began working with Alan Pifer, former president of the Carnegie Corporation of New York, to explore how population aging would affect our society as a whole. Alan had had the brilliant insight that our view of aging was too narrow; we should be concerned with the impact of aging upon our whole society, on every institution. Our research became a full-scale Carnegie Corporation study, which we called the Aging Society Project.

About six months after I began work on the study, I was poring over population statistics one day, examining the increases in life expectancy during this century and brainstorming about what they might mean. Suddenly my mind clicked onto an idea that had never occurred to me before: if life expectancy had increased so dramatically, for such large numbers of people, then I, too, could easily live to be a great deal older than I expected. If I lived to be eighty, my adult life would be twice as long as I had been anticipating. And if I lived to be ninety or one hundred, my entire life span would be roughly doubled!

The idea hit me with a sense of shock. Without realizing it, I had been planning my whole life on the basis of how long I expected to be alive. So, if my estimate was mistaken, all the rest of my ideas were off target. I saw myself waking up on my fiftieth birthday—still alive, contrary to all my expectations—confronting a tremendous void of unplanned time ahead and wondering what on earth to do next!

The message of this book is aimed in part at the millions of Americans who are currently under sixty-five. Something very similar has happened to everyone in our society during the twentieth century: the average length of time we spend as adults has doubled. Extraordinarily large numbers of people will have twenty, thirty, or even forty years more of active life than they expected, and it will be time that is part of normal adulthood rather than of old age. A smaller number will live for twice as long as the total average life expectancy at birth in the year 1900—that is, to ninety-five or beyond. During this century there has been a phenomenal, unexpected, and largely unexplained lengthening of the amount of time we live. In its magnitude it is without precedent in human experience.

This transformation of the life course will almost certainly have a powerful impact on your own life. You may not wake up at fifty and wonder what to do next, but you could very easily do so at sixty-five. You won't automatically be "old" when you reach sixty-five, and you won't necessarily be ready to "retire" at that age. In fact, you may not get old physically until much, much later than sixty-five—or you may live into your eighties or nineties without becoming physically old at all.

In addition to having this longer life, you will probably remain active until a much older age than you expect. The younger you are now, the longer the potential lifetime that lies ahead of you. If you are now in your thirties or forties, you are likely to have the longest, most active lifetime of all. Depending on the scientific advances that may be made during the next three or four decades, the chances are good that you might live to be a hundred years old—and that most of your long life will be usefully spent.

The people described at the beginning of this chapter are a few of those who took part in the Long Careers Study, which was intended, first of all, as a glimpse into the possible future for those of us who are younger than sixty-five today. The thirtysomething, fortysomething, and fiftysomething generations are a large group, embracing almost all of the baby boomers and most of the prewar, Depression-era babies as well.

As the century nears its close, this tremendous increase in longevity has created a curious paradox for Americans under sixty-five. We live in a time-starved society, in which work and family life have expanded to fill more than the available twenty-four hours a day. All of us yearn to have more time. Our longing for it is so intense that recent years have seen many younger professionals in these age brackets dropping out of the corporate sweepstakes, "downshifting" into slower lifestyles, slower-paced jobs, smaller communities. Polls show that leisure time decreased significantly during the decades between 1960 and 1990, and that many Americans would accept salary cuts in order to have extra time to spend on family, friends, personal pursuits, and just plain shedding stress.

But even though we feel time bankrupt, we are still not prepared to have the extra time we long for added to the end of our lives. When we can barely manage the task of keeping afloat in the present, it is disconcerting or even frightening to look down the road and see twenty or thirty more years of unexpected life ahead, where once the familiar prospect of old age and retirement stood sentinel at age sixty-five. It is even more unsettling to think—as most people unfortunately do—that the additional time we have gained may be spent in poor health.

The longer horizon ahead is not the only feature that makes us anxious. The ground beneath our feet in the present is also shaking and shifting. The era of corporate downsizing has brought on a flood of early retirements, at ages as young as fifty. Retirement has conventionally been a phenomenon of old age; paradoxically, now that life lasts longer and longer, retirement seems to be arriving earlier and earlier, while the prime period of work leaves less time for family and leisure than it did before.

The result is a stress counselor's dream: an early adulthood lived in a pressure cooker, without adequate time for the essentials of everyday life; the prospect of early retirement or job loss at increasingly younger ages, which should be times of peak career satisfaction, not of uprooting and resettlement; and an old age that has expanded to fill up the rest of our longer lives. These are prospects that do not make any of us happy. In a time of widespread change and transition, those of us in the younger decades often feel that we are falling overboard in the middle of a vast uncharted ocean, without a life jacket.

The people who took part in the Long Careers Study have passed through all of this territory already, and their experiences are profoundly instructive. What emerges from their life stories is a view of the long lifetime different than what we might expect: an affirmation of the increasing richness of experience over time, of a deeper sense of identity, of a greater self-confidence and creative potential that can grow rather than diminish with maturity. It is obvious that, seen through the eyes of the study participants, chronological age markers (like sixty-five), which have held so much power in the past, are really culturally created—a norm that was accurate only for a particular place and time. And because all of the study participants are successful, whether they are well known or not, it is both fascinating and helpful to see the ways in which their lives and careers have been shaped.

The second audience for whom this book was written is the pioneer generation itself—the people over sixty-five who are rewriting our definitions of adulthood in their everyday lives. They are the real pathfinders, threading their way through the underbrush of life's unexplored terrain, marking trails that the rest of us can follow.

Although it is both admirable and useful, trailblazing is not an easy process. Exploration is not for sissies, to paraphrase Art Linkletter's quip about old age.[2] There are few models to tell you what to do when you are still healthy, energetic, and eager to keep going, before you are suddenly deemed—according to a society that judges you purely on your chronological age—"too old."

Moreover, there is very little professional advice available for individuals who want to stay active in this new period of life. Most career counselors in the past have traditionally worked with high school and college students. As a result, until fairly recently there were almost no sources of professional guidance for adults of any age who wanted to change careers or to start new ones. If your career has involved working in organizations instead of working independently, your prospects may be limited; there are few institutional connections available for older people. Many institutions and organizations have age ceilings, even for volunteer work or board membership, that operate without regard to an individual's abilities or functioning capability.

These limitations are frustrating for people who run up against them. The over-sixty-five generation of today must carve out its own footholds, a process often filled with uncertainties and frustration—all the more so because these people did not expect to have to reinvent their lives. Over and over again, people whom I told about the study echoed this point, either about themselves or their parents. One forty-year-old photographer's assistant told me that his seventy-seven-year-old father keeps getting asked when he's going to retire and always replies with a mixture of humor and frustration, "How can I retire, when I still don't know what I want to be when I grow up?" An older woman whom I met briefly at a luncheon exclaimed, as she questioned me about the study: "Here I am, at my age, having to decide all over again what to do with my life—a question I thought got settled years ago and never expected to have to ask again! What do I do now?"

Many of us who are currently under sixty-five also thought our lives would be put on track in our twenties or thirties and wouldn't have to be revised much after that. Now we are discovering that that isn't true. I am convinced, after five years of work on the Long Careers Study, that this is not an individual phenomenon, and it isn't limited to any one age group. It is a change in the structure of adult life in our society directly related to the increase in longevity. Although other factors have helped to cause this change (the roller coaster ride of the economy and the restructuring of the work force are just two such factors), the real issue is that we have moved from one model of adulthood to another, very different, one—from a short-term model based on a set of predictable stages ("predictable crises of adult life," as Gail Sheehy subtitled her 1976 book, *Passages*)[3] to a long-term model with no fixed stages, based on continuous growth and evolution.

*   *   *

What we have learned about aging as a result of the past two decades of research in the social and natural sciences is very different from what we know about stereotypes generally present in our society. Consequently, some background about how the aging process really affects human beings is necessary in order to appreciate fully the information drawn from the Long Careers Study. Aging, quite bluntly, is not what we believe it to be. Most of the myths that have been so widely publicized are just that: myths. Although it may seem like an almost incredible statement the first time you hear it, chronological age in itself does not have any inevitable or specific meaning. In every society, "oldness" is culturally and socially determined. *The Longevity Factor* has been structured with this in mind.

Chapter 2 is about the transformation of life as a result of the longevity factor—what it is and what it means. In chapter 3, I probe the areas of creativity and peak mental performance in relation to aging. Although we have long believed that our mental ability and creative powers inevitably wane as we grow older, the most recent scientific research shows very clearly that this is not true. Chapter 4 deals with the subject of physical aging and reexamines the "downhill slide" model of the aging process, which is being revised by contemporary research.

Chapter 5 begins the description of the Long Careers Study itself. In the following four chapters, different types of career patterns are identified: the Homesteaders, who stayed with one job or career throughout their lives in what was considered the ideal career pattern earlier in the twentieth century; the Transformers, who made one major career change; the Explorers, who made a number of shifts; and a handful of people who had multiple-track careers, who consistently were active in more than one field or subject throughout their work lives.

The third edition of the book, "Breaking the Boundaries," contains sections on some of the revisions older people themselves are making in the life course.

In chapter 10, "Long Growth Curves and Late Bloomers," I describe the experience of a large percentage of participants who had career peaks much later in life than we believe normally happens, or who began their careers much later than we are accustomed to. Chapter 11, "Retirers and Returners," discusses the participants who actually did retire and either went back to paid work or created volunteer careers for themselves. In some cases, these post-retirement careers were more distinguished and satisfying than the person's original primary career. Chapter 12 describes the career patterns of the women in the study, whose accounts of their careers were so different from the standard picture of women's careers in this century that they revised the history of the women's movement for us.

The last section of the book, "Growing and Growing Older," summarizes many of the useful examples and lessons provided by the experiences of the Long Careers Study participants. Chapter 13 presents a discussion of the responsibilities of the later years of life, and how some participants were drawn into philanthropy and volunteerism. Chapter 14 examines our culture's conflicting messages about retirement and offers suggestions from the participants for those considering or facing retirement. Chapter 15 reviews important information about staying healthy while growing older. Finally, chapter 16 uses the lessons of the participants' careers to develop useful ideas about career management for everyone, young and old, including how to structure your own career, when and how to change directions, and how to maintain job satisfaction.

The Long Careers Study is not, and was not intended to be, definitive. An exploratory expedition can only draw the first sketch of the terrain; it is a guide that can be used by those who follow, to map the new territory in greater detail. It is a first step in understanding major changes in adult life that are still in process and have not yet been widely recognized or examined because they are so new.

The participants, and their long-lived compatriots throughout the country, are living proof that it is possible to continue being creative and productive in the years beyond sixty-five, and that age in itself does not determine a human being's value. They also provide clear contradictions to many of our negative beliefs about what particular chronological ages mean. In the end, although I neither expected it nor sought it (and though, in our materialistic and technologically dominated society, inspiration has perhaps gone out of style), the sum total of the study participants' experience is inspiring.

2

The Longevity Factor

One reason why we haven't yet understood the meaning of certain extraordinary changes in human life is that our view of aging is based largely on a misunderstanding.

As strange as it may seem, the idea that we become old at sixty-five is purely arbitrary. There is no biological imperative that clicks in when you pass your sixty-fifth birthday. The use of this number in the United States as the threshold of old age comes from its selection in 1935 by the authors of the Social Security Act as the eligibility age for receiving Social Security benefits. Most of us believe that this age was actually taken from pension legislation proposed for the German civil service by Prime Minister Otto von Bismarck in the nineteenth century. However, according to the foremost historian of social security, University of Michigan professor W. Andrew Achenbaum, Bismarck at first selected an even older age—seventy—as the retirement level for civil servants, and it was adopted in 1889. In 1916, a quarter of a century later, the age of eligibility was amended downward to sixty-five.[1]

Bismarck's choices did not rest on any expertise in aging. At the time, the average life expectancy in Germany was an age in the early forties, and Bismarck did not want to pay more pension benefits than were absolutely necessary. Seventy was an age so advanced that he thought virtually no one would reach it. Evidently, he was right; that perceived injustice was one reason for the downward revision of the law to age sixty-five—which was still a rather high limit though not as impossible as seventy. So the selection of age seventy and later of sixty-five had little to do with biology but had a direct relationship to politics and greed.

Economic decisions of Bismarck's kind were not beyond our own politicians, although ours were decidedly more modest. At the time when the Social Security legislation was passed, average life expectancy in the United States was sixty-two.

In fact, what is defined as old age in any given time and place is a product of three very different factors, all specific to that particular time and place: average life expectancy, living conditions, and cultural definitions.[2] During most of human history, these have combined to produce a much earlier beginning for old age than age sixty-five.

In Roman times, when average life expectancy was about twenty-two, "old age" must have begun in the mid-twenties. Although a few people did live into their fifties and even beyond, such longevity was very rare. The length of life remained brief, and the onset of old age continued to occur early, for people who lived during the first six hundred years of the Christian Era. By the medieval period and the early Renaissance, lifetimes had lengthened somewhat: male life expectancy in thirteenth-century England was around thirty-four for aristocratic men, once adulthood was reached. (Peasants lived far shorter lives, but we have no way of making accurate estimates.)

The first settlers of the United States were themselves relatively long-lived, perhaps because only the hardiest survived the rigors of the trip to the New World. Death rates for infants and children were high, but the average life expectancy in the Massachusetts colonies in the seventeenth century is estimated to have been somewhere between forty-four and fifty-two. Once men and women succeeded in reaching the age of twenty-one, more than half of them could expect to live into their sixties. However, this standard did not apply to any other region of the colonies at the time (life expectancies were far shorter in the hot, humid southern states), and it would not be matched again in the United States until 1909.

At the time of the American Revolution, full adulthood came early in life. Most of the eighteenth-century Founding Fathers were mature men, but they were very young by our standards.

Thomas Jefferson was thirty-three when he wrote the Declaration of Independence. In 1776 James Monroe was eighteen; James Madison, twenty-five. John Adams at forty-one and George Washington at forty-four were already on their way to old age when the Revolution began; Washington was already beginning to think of retirement (using this mood as an indicator, he can be compared with a man in his early sixties today). Given an average life expectancy of close to forty in revolutionary times and seventy-five today, Benjamin Franklin at his death, eighty-four, can be compared with a one hundred-fifty-year-old man in our society.

During the nineteenth century, average life expectancies hovered in the late thirties and early forties, increasing gradually. Notions about when old age began changed at a similarly slow pace. In 1900, men were still considered old at around forty, and decrepit by the age of fifty. Ninety-two-year-old Dr. Irving Wright, a cardiologist, told me during his interview for the Long Careers Study that when he was a medical student in the early 1920s, he had gotten a lucky break by being invited to accompany an "elderly gentlemen of fifty-four" on a trip to Europe. When I pointed out to him that by current standards the "elderly gentleman" was pretty young—roughly half of Dr. Wright's age at the time—he chuckled with amusement. There was really no contradiction, Dr. Wright replied; back then, fifty-four *was* elderly! A fifty-four-year-old in 1920 might very well need a younger companion for such a trip.

There is also a gender factor in considering old age. Until quite recently, the standards for what was old have been consistently different for men and women: old age for women was about ten years earlier than old age for men. Around 1900, a woman was past her prime at the age of thirty and was considered by many to have crossed the threshold of old age; by forty, a woman was firmly established in old age.

Such definitions continued to be drawn more tightly for women even after the passage of the Social Security Act. Dr. John Riley, a sociologist who worked in Washington in the 1930s, recalled being told at the time by a friend who worked in a government personnel office that the government's definition of an "older woman" was "any woman over thirty-five." Louise Brown, still a crackerjack secretary in 1991 at the age of seventy-nine, recalled being turned away from a YWCA residence in the 1940s because she was over thirty-five and therefore an "older woman." In the 1930s and 1940s, the introduction to the radio serial "Helen Trent" posed the question, "Can a woman find love after thirty-five?" The assumption was that if she did, it was a real stroke of luck—because she was so old! Many women (and men) were so reluctant to pass the age of thirty-nine, the last step before forty, that they lied about their age, permanently fixing it at thirty-nine—a birthday that comedian Jack Benny claimed as his own perennial age, with great success.

By 1948, when Arthur Miller wrote *Death of a Salesman*, old age for men had been boosted up to the early sixties. Willy Loman's age in the play is sixty-three, and he is described in negative terms: washed up, worn out, too old to "cut the mustard." Because of the powerful impact of the play, Willy Loman became for millions of Americans a symbol of the old man whose life has not fulfilled his expectations, struggling desperately to keep control of his life.

It is an interesting sidelight that Arthur Miller himself does not regard Willy as a symbol of the hopelessness of old age and did not intend for him to be taken as such. In an interview that Miller gave for the Long Careers Study, he said that Willy both is and isn't a symbol of aging, "because unlike a lot of old people, he's not old. He goes down, ironically, fighting, with the illusion that he's going to win something. So he's fighting to the very last minute."

Regardless of his chronological age or society's attitude toward him, Miller thinks of Willy as young. "This is probably not typical," Miller continued. "A lot of the old ones that I know are embittered and feel that it's all worth very little, that life is a mystery that they don't have the energy anymore even to think about. But Willy's not that way; he's got the vigor of a very young man. Spiritually, he's very young. That's the irony of it. He's still going to go out and knock 'em dead, to the end. That's the way it should be played." Miller's comments suggest that Willy's ultimate defeat is not due to his own resignation to aging but rather to the perceptions of the world around him, which has decided that he is too old to be useful any more. Seen in this perspective, Willy Loman is more a victim of age bias than of aging.[3] (At seventy-seven, Miller himself is wiry and energetic, a man who looks years younger than his real age. His creative instincts are as powerful as ever. As this book goes to press he is preparing a new play, *The Ride Down Mount Morgan,* for its American debut.

Past the midpoint of the twentieth century, old age has again moved further away in chronological time. Earlier definitions of life stages and of the socially acceptable times for certain activities—marriage, childbearing, retirement—were familiar and widely recognized. As the life course has lengthened, new stages have crystallized and the distinctions between the old life periods have blurred. The noted sociologist Dr. Bernice Neugarten remarks that the concept of middle age itself is a recent invention, one that developed as family size shrank to fewer children spaced closer together, leaving the longer-lived parents in an empty nest at much younger ages than had been true before.[4]

In 1974 Neugarten coined the term *young-old* to describe people in the mature years who were not physiologically old. What had been considered "old age," is "old-old" in Neugarten's terminology—the physically frail, especially people who need special service or care. Neugarten's original idea was to use *young-old* and *old-old* to identify functional age rather than chronological age. But as the expressions were absorbed into general usage, they were translated into chronological terms in the popular mind, contrary to Neugarten's intention.

The shifts in popular perception of when the various life stages occur are demonstrated in a study undertaken by Neugarten and her associates. In the early 1960s, a group of middle-class, middle-aged people were asked their opinions on the best ages for various life events and how old people are at various life stages. Twenty years later, in the 1980s, the study was repeated. "Consensus had dropped regarding every item of the questionnaire," Neugarten and coauthor Dr. Dail Neugarten wrote. "In the first study, 'a young man' was said to be a man between eighteen and twenty-two. In the repeat study, 'a young man' was anywhere from eighteen to forty." What is extraordinary about this is that in the public mind "youth" appears to have expanded from a period lasting roughly four years to a period of about twenty-two years—more than five times longer!

There is evidence that in the 1970s the upper limits of the popular definition of "young" had risen to age thirty—but at that point it stopped there. "The most distressing fear in early adult-hood is that there is no life after youth," psychologist Daniel Levinson wrote in 1976 in his study of male life stages, *Seasons of a Man's Life*. "Young adults often feel that to pass 30 is to be 'over the hill,' and they are given little beyond hollow clichés to provide a fuller sense of the actual problems and possibilities of adult life at different ages."

But since the 1970s, the word *young* has moved up to charac-terize people in their thirties and even their forties—a description that would have been unthinkable earlier in the twentieth century, when the forties were considered part of old age. For example, the cover of *Newsweek* magazine following the 1992 Democratic National Convention carried the caption "Young Guns" superim-posed on a photograph of Gov. Bill Clinton and Sen. Al Gore. Both men are solidly in their middle forties (a few years older than the elderly George Washington in 1776).

In an unconscious effort to acknowledge the changes we have been experiencing, we have shifted upward the everyday usage of words describing the traditional age categories—*youth, middle age, old age*. But despite these signs of changing perceptions, our restrictive concepts of what particular ages mean are still very much in place.

A SECOND MIDDLE AGE

Most Americans probably believe that the increase in longevity means that we'll all spend much more time being old, based on our long-standing assumption that this period officially begins at the fixed chronological age of sixty-five. If you add from ten to thirty years to this age, then the calculation appears very straight-forward: we have many more years of old age to look forward to, instead of the five to ten we might otherwise have expected. Since old age is the period we find least attractive, this is definitely not an appealing prospect.

Fortunately for us, what is really happening is something very different. As lifetimes have grown longer, the process of physical aging has gradually and rather mysteriously been slowed down. We are not only living longer, we are entering physiological old age later in life. In effect, there has been a postponement of the physical aging process, and most of us are feeling its effect to some degree.

This postponement of old age is responsible for the most surprising effect of the longevity factor. The extra twenty or thirty years of life we have gained have really been added to the middle of life—the prime of adulthood—rather than to its end. It is youth and middle age that have been expanded, not old age. Like a rubber band pulled by giant hands, as the life course has stretched, its whole length has stretched, not just one end or the other.

The result of the longevity factor is not just a simple addition of time to the end of our lives. Instead, it is a transformation of the entire life course, especially of adulthood. The period between what was formerly the end of middle age (roughly, fifty) and what is now the beginning of real, physical old age (at some point after seventy-five) is a new stage in adult life—one that has never existed before as a generalized experience for large numbers of people.

It is as if we had created a slightly longer, second, middle age (from fifty to seventy-five) immediately following the first middle age (from thirty-five to fifty). In lifetimes that may reach close to one hundred years for many of us, especially the baby boomers, this new stage occupies the third quarter of life.

This extension of the period of vitality in the middle of adult life is astonishing. It radically alters many of our existing beliefs about the life course and the aging process. Many things we have thought inevitable may not really be inevitable at all.

Take what it means to reach the age of fifty. The conventional perspective is that this is the beginning of a long, downhill slide. A fiftieth birthday is usually treated as if it is a highly significant point in life: the end of life's potential.

It's easy to find evidence on the most elementary everyday level that this idea is very much alive in the American consciousness. For example, as this book was in preparation, NBC news correspondent Tom Brokaw celebrated his fiftieth birthday with a good-bye-to-my-youth article in the *New York Times* Sunday magazine. He characterized being fifty as "sort of an irritation," a "chronic low-level virus" whose impact was to make him feel that he was over the hill for good. For two pages he lamented the presence of aches and pains, the loss of his freedom and spontaneity, and a feeling that now he'd been been excluded from commercial advertising, which is youth oriented. He even reflected on the fact that if he were to have an affair with an older woman, she would be sixty! At the end of the article, Brokaw rouses himself out of his depression and takes it all back, spurred on by the cheery encouragement of his teenage daughter. He closes with a paragraph of praise for his wonderful marriage, his rewarding work, and his life in general. But this short, chipper closing doesn't sound convincing. The reader is left with the feeling that Tom Brokaw really does think fifty is the end of the best part of his life, and that he hates the idea.

Many of the Long Careers Study participants referred to this belief as a view they had discarded, because their experience contradicted it. "When I was fifty," seventy-seven-year-old Washington psychotherapist Evelyn Nef told me, "I thought my life was over. I was recently widowed; my job had been phased out because of my husband's death; and I was moving to a new city to start all over again. Little did I know that the best years of my life were still ahead of me."

In the interviews conducted for the Long Careers Study, many of the participants described a sequence of experiences very different from the stereotypes we might expect. In their early fifties, these people felt that they were just beginning to come into their own. They had accomplished or were nearing the end of most of the family tasks of early adulthood—marriage, childrearing, and putting children through college. They had served their apprenticeship at work; they knew how to get things done and had a firm grasp of the basics of their job or profession. With these major tasks accomplished, they were beginning to reach out for greater creativity in their work, for broader impact, for solutions that hadn't yet been found. In short, they were poised for flight. Their real stage of professional development bore no resemblance to the conventional idea of what people do at age fifty.

Because this isn't the image that our culture normally associates with turning fifty, one can ask whether these experiences are atypical or perhaps even rare. In a scientific sense, no one knows, because that question hasn't been definitively asked or answered yet. But four years of interviews with long-lived people suggest to me that our conventional picture of what happens at the older ages is not accurate. Because the stereotypes have been solidly planted, and because in the past we have focused almost exclusively on the negative aspects of aging—illness, frailty, the need for health care and nursing home care—we simply have not seen the positive shifts that have taken place, even though they have been occurring right in front of us. We can hope that in the future more research will be devoted to the positive aspects of aging, and that more answers will emerge.

WHAT CAUSED THE LONGEVITY REVOLUTION?

What caused the longevity revolution? The simple answer at present is: we don't really know. It appears to be a complex phenomenon, not attributable to one single cause. We do know that all the industrialized countries have experienced similar expansions of life expectancy during this century, whereas in developing nations life expectancy rates resemble our rates from the last century. An increase in longevity appears to be a byproduct of the lifestyle changes growing out of modern, technologically advanced society.

The life expectancies in a few countries are longer than that in the United States. For many years, Sweden had the highest life expectancy rate in the world, followed closely by Japan; now Japan has overtaken and surpassed Sweden. Germany and Great Britain also have longer average life expectancies at birth than does the United States. As Third World countries begin the process of economic development, and as living conditions improve, their average life expectancies will also begin to lengthen. Speculation about the reason for this touches a number of factors.

Modern medical technology: In industrialized countries as well as in developing nations, part of this increase can be explained by advances in medical care and sanitation, which have led to dramatic improvements in the survival rates of infants. In the United States, about half of the increase in average life expectancy during this century is a result of this improvement in children's survival rates. In many families of the early 1900s, one or more children died in childhood, often during the first two or three years of life. The experiences of the Long Careers Study participants reflected this. A number of them had lost either a brother or a sister at young ages. Some families fared even worse. For instance, former *Town and Country* editor Frank Zachary, seventy-eight, lost both of his brothers in childhood; and although eighty-eight-year-old Elizabeth Burns, a member of the Travelers Insurance Company Job Bank in Hartford, Connecticut, was one of nine children, only four survived to adulthood. In the early 1900s the death of a child was a commonplace occurrence, so much so that death was associated more with childhood and young adulthood than with old age—an idea that seems very strange to us now.

But the increase in adult longevity over the course of the twentieth century also contributed dramatically to the rise in average life expectancy. This longevity may arise in part from medical procedures, developed since 1950, to save adult lives: vaccines, antibiotics, surgical innovations, and new techniques for treating heart disease, cancer, and other potentially fatal conditions. These advances may explain why some people live longer than they once might have. However, they do not explain why such large numbers of people remain physically young and active later in life.

Easier work: One study participant, Peter Drucker, the internationally known management expert, believes that the change in the nature of work that has occurred during the twentieth century is a major contributor to the longevity factor. "Not so very long ago," Drucker reflected, "most people at forty-five were physically broken. Have you ever read *Giants in the Earth,*. . . [about] the American frontier, by Rölvaag? Those South Dakota farmers at age forty-five were very old." Both men and women were worn down by the demands of frontier work, which required physically strenuous labor; women had the additional hazards of frequent childbearing.

In the twentieth century, Drucker believes, work itself is far less demanding, both physically and emotionally, than it ever was. We have moved from a society in which the majority of jobs required hard physical labor—manufacturing, farming, and service jobs such as blacksmithing and heavy household work—to a society in which most jobs involve no physical labor at all. The result may be far less wear on the physical body and increased vitality later in life.

Pension plans: Norman Cousins, who spent the last ten years of his life designing and participating in medical research on the mind–body connection, told me during several long conversations about his work that he believed that the Social Security legislation itself might have had a positive effect on increased longevity. The existence of an assured income beyond age sixty-five frees millions of people from the stress of constant worry about financial survival in their older years. Although this is only hypothetical, Cousins added, such an effect would be consistent with the existing research on stress and the immune system. Constant anxiety about financial survival would flood the body with a toxic mixture of hormones intended for fight or flight. Over long periods of time this internal toxicity could contribute to a shortened life span.

Better human relationships: Epidemiologist Dr. Leonard Sagan, in his book *The Health of Nations,* proposed the theory that much of our increased longevity may be due to better contemporary nurturing of the young—the greater emotional closeness of mothers to infants and children—and to more constructive relationships among adults. Such constructive and supportive behavior could strengthen the will to live, as well as reinforce the immune system.[5]

Heredity: Some experts have suggested that heredity has played an important role in lengthening life expectancies. But heredity is clearly not the only important element. If all of us simply repeated the life spans of our parents, life expectancies would not have grown longer, they would have stayed the same. Most of the Long Careers Study participants have lived longer than their parents did—some, a great deal longer.

Nutrition is better now in some respects than it was in 1900. We have more fresh food year-round and a greater variety of food in general; therefore we have a more plentiful constant supply of vitamins, minerals, and other nutrients. But in some respects contemporary diets may also be worse: our food is highly processed, and many natural nutrients are removed during this processing. Chemical preservatives, unknown earlier in the century, are now added to many foodstuffs; we don't know how many of them are hazardous or in what way.

Environmental factors similarly are better now in some respects and worse in others. We have better housing, better sanitation, and better transportation. Our streets are paved, and we are not constantly exposed to dust and manure from horse traffic, as town and city dwellers were at the beginning of this century. Water pollution existed in the early part of this century as it does now, but it came mostly from human waste rather than industrial sewage, and it produced epidemics of infectious diseases like typhoid, typhus, and cholera. These diseases killed quickly, whereas modern pollution produces increases in birth defects and in long-term illnesses like cancer. Now our air is full of chemical pollutants, our water has numerous additives, and the ground in some localities is filled with buried hazardous waste that can invade underground water sources.

THE SWEDISH STUDIES OF DR. ALVAR SVANBORG

The most compelling scientific documentation of the lengthening of the adult prime comes from an extraordinary longitudinal study created by a Swedish geriatrician, Dr. Alvar Svanborg. It is the most detailed and extensive study ever undertaken of the physiological process of aging in the years beyond age seventy. Because the Swedish standard of living is similar to that in the United States, and because the increase in longevity is proceeding at a similar rate in both countries (slightly faster in Sweden), the Svanborg study has implications for the United States, as well as for other industrialized countries.[6]

Svanborg, a tall, limber man in his early seventies, with a shock of silver hair, an easy smile, and penetrating blue eyes, was for many years on the medical school faculty at the University of Gothenburg. Because retirement at age sixty-five was mandatory at the university until recently, when Svanborg reached his sixty-fifth birthday in 1988 he decided to begin another phase of his career in the United States. He accepted an appointment as professor of geriatrics at the University of Illinois at Chicago, where he is now head of the geriatric medicine program and is designing research on older Americans.

The Svanborg study was initiated in the late 1960s when Svanborg decided that not enough was known about the many physical changes that take place as people grow older. Both physicians and the general public had a great many assumptions about how health changes with age and what kind of physical condition older people are in. But for the most part those assumptions had never been tested. Are all old people ill? Is there such a thing as healthy aging? How frequently do abnormal conditions and severe illnesses occur among older people? Does illness progress differently in older people than in younger people? Do older people react differently to drugs? Can older people change physically and mentally? For example, can they be strengthened by exercise? Can they learn at the same rate of speed as when they were younger? Or are physical weakness and mental slowing inevitable accompaniments of aging?

Such information would be useful, Svanborg thought, first to understand illness and to treat it, and also eventually to find out how to maintain good health longer. Perhaps it would even help us learn how to avoid some illnesses altogether.

Svanborg designed a complex study, employing medical, biological, and psychological tests, which would involve successive groups of seventy-year-olds at five-year intervals. The people selected will participate in the study for the rest of their lives. The first group, consisting of twelve hundred seventy-year-olds (roughly 30 percent of the seventy-year-olds in Gothenburg), started the program in 1971–72. In 1976–77 a second group of about the same size entered the study, and the first group was retested. In 1981–82 a third group entered, and the first and second groups were tested again. The study is highly interdisciplinary; staff members include, in addition to physicians, a range of specialists in other fields, such as architecture, dentistry, psychology, sociology, and history.

Originally, Svanborg and his colleagues thought that they would find more frail and chronically ill people in the two younger groups—the second and third groups—than in the first, oldest group, because the two younger groups contained more people who had received sophisticated medical treatment with antibiotics, pacemakers, beta blockers, and surgical procedures. It seemed reasonable to expect that these people would be in worse condition and that they might deteriorate more rapidly than the people in the first group, who had survived without such interventions and therefore might be hardier.

The team found that it was true that a larger percentage of the two later groups had had such treatment. However, the tests showed that vitality and health were better, on average, in the second group and even better in the third group! To the researchers' surprise, it appears that these life-prolonging techniques may have a generally positive impact on overall health and vitality rather than a negative one. "In short," Svanborg says, "our comparisons show that people are 'putting off' aging and staying healthy longer than previous generations did." He goes on to say that in the second and third groups the period of severe illness and frailty at the end of life generally is occurring increasingly later in life.

With the third group, an intervention program was added whose aim is to see whether specific changes in routine or lifestyle can help the participants improve their health more than they normally would, or keep it in good condition even later in life. Svanborg's goal, he says, is "to maintain or improve the physical and mental functions of older people, or to delay the development of handicaps through measures which aid well-being, raise the quality of life in a subjective sense, and reduce the need for social and medical services."

The study's collaborating psychologist, Dr. Stig Berg, has also found that most measurable aspects of intelligence and memory remain virtually unchanged well into the seventies and eighties, as long as people remain healthy. (An American psychologist from Pennsylvania State University, Dr. K. Werner Schaie, who has been studying a five-hundred-person group in Seattle for the past thirty years, has obtained similar results in his own research, which will be discussed in chapter 3.) The older people in the study perform intellectually at the same levels, roughly, as those of young adults. Svanborg notes that the people in the study "seem progressively to be delaying their intellectual aging and to be performing better. We do not know how long this extension of intelligence will continue, and it would be exciting to study it through future generations."

In short, the conclusion that Svanborg's group draws about aging is that "our functional abilities are maintained to higher degrees and later in life than we previously thought." In the study participants, Svanborg says, "the reserve capacity for most nervous functions was so large that no measurable fall in function—for example, of intelligence or memory—occurred until late in life, and then foremost among those who suffered disease." He also says that, in general, sensible physical activity (within reason—i.e., exercise or activity at a level that isn't so strenuous that it would cause injury) has had beneficial effects for the study group participants.

There are a few negative changes from group to group that have surfaced during the twenty years of the Svanborg study. On the whole, however, the negative changes are few and the positive changes are numerous. One negative difference is that skeletal stability is decreasing from group to group; the second and third groups are more prone to bone injuries than is the first group. (The research team does not know why this is the case.) A second is that bereavement occuring after the death of a spouse has a very negative impact on health in the period immediately following the loss. Svanborg found that the death rate increases 48 percent for men and 22 percent for women in the three months following the loss of a spouse, and that the rate of physical aging also accelerates. A third negative change confirms results of earlier studies both in Sweden and the United States showing that physical reaction time is slower in older people than it is in younger people.

The Svanborg study's most substantial evidence of the trend toward longer lifetimes is that additional life expectancy after age seventy is increasing markedly, especially for women. In addition, the death rate from age-related causes between seventy and eighty has decreased noticeably.

Finally, the Svanborg study results indicate that lifestyle changes have a much larger impact on health and aging than we had previously thought. This in itself is a finding with major importance for everyone. Our destiny isn't unalterably written in our genes. What we do does make a difference—in some cases a huge difference. In particular, Svanborg says, excessive smoking and drinking are extremely negative influences, affecting both the length of time an individual lives and his or her state of health. For smokers and drinkers, a number of manifestations of aging come earlier—and, to the research team's surprise, the most negative results come from smoking.

HOW FAR WILL THE LONGEVITY REVOLUTION GO?

As life expectancies have risen since 1900, statistical predictions of how much they will increase have also gone up. Some scientists and demographers have suggested that average life expectancies could rise to as high as 100, 120, or 140 years during the next century, and these researchers generally view this possibility as a very negative one. Some years ago, Dr. Joshua Lederberg, then the president of Rockefeller University in New York City, gave a speech at Hahneman Hospital in Philadelphia in which he predicted that average life expectancy might rise to 140 or 150 as a result of scientific interventions, but that the additional 50–70 years would be years of decrepitude. In such a case the entire society might be crippled by the overwhelming task of providing institutional care for some people for as long as 40 or 50 years, a prospect Lederberg finds horrendous. This is the most extreme (and the most pessimistic) of such projections, but it is a good example of how longevity has been regarded by many scientists.

Dr. Alvar Svanborg speculates that because the oldest person on record who was fully documented lived to the age of 115, there may be a kind of natural term to the potential length of human life, at roughly that age. But he acknowledges that that is just a speculation on his part. We don't really know; and at the moment, we don't have any way of constructing more accurate guesses.

None of these predictions takes into account, however, the possibility of more radical scientific breakthroughs with more positive results in the modification of the aging process. If we were to discover the physical mechanism through which aging works—what Dr. John H. Rowe, head of the MacArthur Foundation Research Network on Aging, calls the "gero-gene"—we might develop the capacity to slow down the aging process even further, or perhaps simply turn it off. As this book is being written, a number of scientists scattered throughout the country have made striking laboratory advances in controlling the length of life in other species; some of these techniques may yield knowledge that can someday be applied to human beings.

One of the most suggestive lines of research involves fruit flies. Prof. Michael R. Rose of the University of California at Irvine has extended the life span of fruit flies more than 85 percent by genetically increasing their ability to destroy free radicals, toxic molecular by-products of oxygen metabolism that destroy DNA and are thought to hasten aging. A human equivalent of these long-lived insects would be 135–140 years old. Another researcher, Prof. Thomas E. Johnson of the University of Colorado at Boulder, discovered that by chemically manipulating a single gene of the roundworm he was able to increase that species' life span by 70 percent.[7]

Moreover, research on simpler species has yielded results indicating that the progression of aging is not as invariable as we have thought. Dr. James R. Carey of the University of California at Davis and Dr. James R. Curtsinger of the University of Wisconsin have reported that in their large research populations of fruit flies, some flies actually had an increased life expectancy once they got beyond a certain age, and they lived to very advanced ages. This contradicts the long-held concept that there is a "biological clock" that controls aging and is invariable beyond a certain minimal point.[8]

Some research has also concentrated on the question of not just prolonging life but maintaining functioning. Among the most intriguing experiments are those of Dr. Richard Cutler at the Gerontological Research Center of the National Institute on Aging. Cutler has restored normal functioning in old gerbils that have had strokes by giving them PBN, a substance that combats free radicals and appears to rejuvenate the brain. The treated gerbils run mazes as well as young gerbils do. The PBN gerbils also live longer on the average than untreated gerbils do.

These experiments on physical mechanisms of aging will have to be replicated successfully by other scientists, and their applicability to human life for the moment remains unknown. Yet it is possible that at some time in the future a discovery might be made that could extend not just life itself but also the period of vitality much further than we now expect. Developments of this kind, however, would present us with societal restructuring that make today's adjustments look trivial by comparison.

Practically all of our society's institutions and systems are designed with chronological age as a major reference point. Just imagine a society in which a scientific discovery like those above has been developed into a product that is safe and effective for human beings and is widely available—resulting in an increase of average total life expectancy to somewhere around 125 years (we could just as easily use 150, but it might be less believable for most readers than a conservative 125). Because average life expectancy is a median number, there would also be people who lived to be older, as well as those who did not live that long. In such a society, 115-year-olds might be the physical and mental equivalent of today's 75-year-olds, who are themselves more like 50-year-olds were at the start of this century. In other words, there would be as many active, healthy 115-year-olds as there are 75-year-olds today. The conventional life pattern—of high school and college in the late teens and early twenties, work from the early twenties to the early or mid-sixties, and than retirement— would be completely inappropriate in such a long-lived society. People would have time for many more careers per lifetime than they do now. They might choose to renew their education periodically, perhaps every twenty or thirty years and certainly every half-century. Institutions of higher education would inaugurate new programs for returning adults, who would have a broader background of general knowledge but might be preparing to change careers after spending several decades in the work force. Existing families would easily span five or six generations, and the generally recognized stages of adult life in such a long-lived society might be quite different.

The concept of living so long is hard to grasp, because our culture is structured around the idea that people grow old and withdraw from an active life by age sixty-five. Our ideas about age are a complicated mixture of prejudice and customs, expectations and legislation. It has been disruptive in certain respects simply to find that we have added twenty to thirty years to what used to be the normal adult lifetime—how disruptive would it be to add sixty, seventy, or even more? If the immune system could be maintained at high levels throughout life, and the mechanisms that cause cardiovascular disease, cancer, and Alzheimer's could be blocked, who knows how long we might live? What would be the possibilities for growth and learning inherent in, say, a 150- or 200-year life span? Looking at it retrospectively, a person with a 200-year life span who was born in 1800 would still be alive in the 1990s and would be able to give us detailed recollections of the early nineteenth century—of the Gold Rush, the settling of the West, the Civil War, the Industrial Revolution in the United States, and many other events. Will a 200-year-old born in 1950 live through a corresponding number of changes during his or her lifetime, and would the changes be as dramatic as in the past?

If average life expectancy were to lengthen radically, we would have to redesign totally many of our notions of how things are done and who does them. It would have seemed inconceivable in 1900 that average life expectancy could almost double before the end of this century, just as it now seems impossible that average life expectancy might reach or exceed the hundred-year mark within a few years. But in the twentieth century, as we have all seen, the impossible has become possible more than once.

3

Creativity and Peak Mental Performance

One reason Americans resist so vigorously the idea of growing older is that we have been led to believe that old age is the end of accomplishment. A workaholic nation from the very beginning, we dislike enormously the prospect of losing our creativity, our drive, and our sense of effectiveness. In the past we have assumed that this kind of deterioration was the natural consequence of aging.

The origin of these ideas is hard to tease out of a tangled thicket of popular opinion and scientific theories on the subject, which stretches back to the nineteenth century. But the ideas themselves are unquestionably present in our culture. They exert a powerful impact both on society's customs and on the lives of individuals.

These negative stereotypes of maturity can be stated fairly succinctly. Moreover, our beliefs about the decline of creativity parallel our negative concepts of physical functioning in the older years, which will be discussed in the next chapter.

First, we tend to believe that there is a particular chronological period (roughly between the ages of thirty and forty-five) when creativity is at its peak, and that afterward creativity declines, in something like a biological rhythm. Second, we have a companion belief that mental ability, too, inevitably declines beyond a certain age, and that the brain itself loses millions of cells every year once we go beyond early adulthood.

Evidence of these ideas is found everywhere in our society, and we use such concepts matter-of-factly as reference points for everyday experience. However, both of these ideas are false. Based on scientific studies from the past four decades, we know that they are illegitimate, inaccurate beliefs about adult functioning. In fact, as it turns out, these beliefs are based on research that was distorted by the communication process or by existing cultural biases about aging.

During the past twenty years, we have learned more about the life course and the process of aging than has ever been known before. Moreover, we have gained a much greater sense of the variety and complexity of the aging process from the emergence of this extended, or second, middle age and from the presence of so many healthy, active older people. These developments have given us the ability for the first time to separate what is factual from what is culturally imposed—to distinguish the reality from the mythology. In many respects, the reality is different from anything that our previous knowledge prepared us for.

It is worth noting at the outset that a process of selective perception often operates when we think about aging, on both the collective and the individual levels. For example, we suddenly notice negative things we've always done and assume they are signs of aging. Dr. James E. Birren, a psychologist who in the 1960s founded the first major center in the United States for the study of aging (the Andrus Center for Gerontology at the University of Southern California), points out that there are behaviors that normally occur in all of us—like becoming distracted or forgetting about something—which we then explain to ourselves in one way or another. Our explanations are likely to change as we get older because we have so many negative ideas about aging. If I am in my thirties or forties and forget something, I am likely to be annoyed at having forgotten it and will be determined to be more vigilant in the future. But if I am in my sixties, I may interpret the forgetting as part of the inevitable onset of old age and tell myself that I've forgotten it because I'm getting old. Birren has seen this phenomenon in people who have been chronically absentminded throughout their lives and who then begin to interpret their absentmindedness as a sign of old age once they're past midlife.

TV commentator Hugh Downs tells a similar story about his father. "My dad, when he was eighty-one or so, had mislaid a checkbook. He said, 'Damn it, I'm getting old.' I jumped on him and said, 'Don't talk like that, because I remember you when you were thirty, and you forgot more then than you do now.'" Downs recalls that his father was "kind of a forgetful guy, but when you are thirty you don't think about your age. At eighty you do think about your age. That's the prejudiced pressure that society puts on you." The belief that aging brings a loss of memory is so entrenched that we can distort our perception of reality to fit the belief.

CAN WE STILL BE CREATIVE?

THE DEBATE ON AGE AND ACHIEVEMENT

The notion that people become less creative as they age had a powerful public airing soon after the turn of the twentieth century. In the autumn of 1904, Sir William Osler, a distinguished physician on the faculty of Johns Hopkins University, decided to leave the United States at the age of fifty-six and move to England to accept the post of regius professor of medicine at Oxford. Osler, born and educated in Canada, was one of the two or three most famous physicians in the United States at the time and a genuinely distinguished scientist; he had taught at McGill and the University of Pennsylvania before going to Johns Hopkins in 1889. On February 22, 1905, Osler delivered a valedictory address in Baltimore, which was well attended by an audience eager to hear the pearls of intellect that the great man wished to leave with them.

Osler's talk was entitled "The Fixed Period," after the title of an Anthony Trollope novel referring to the useful years of a man's life. He began by saying that he thought American education was in jeopardy because college and university professors were all growing older. Then he explained this statement, using "two fixed ideas well known to my friends, harmless obsessions with which I sometimes bore them."

The first of Osler's ideas on aging concerns "the comparative uselessness of men above forty years of age." Osler contended that world history confirms this view, and that if the work of all men over forty were subtracted from "the sum of human achievement in action, in science, in art, in literature," though we would lose some great treasures, their loss would make very little difference to us. It is hard to name a great conquest of the mind, Osler continued, that wasn't made by "a man on whose back the sun was still shining. The effective, moving, vitalizing work of the world is done between the ages of twenty-five and forty—those fifteen golden years of plenty, the. . . constructive period, in which there is always a balance in the mental bank and the credit is still good."

Osler went on to say that his "second fixed idea is the uselessness of men above sixty years of age, and the incalculable benefit it would be in commercial, political and in professional life, if, as a matter of course, men stopped work at this age." Osler then referred his listeners to Trollope's "charming" novel, which discussed what he believed to be the practical advantages of forcing men to stop work at the age of sixty. In fact, Osler continued, "the plot hinges upon the admirable scheme of a college into which at sixty, men retired for a year of contemplation before a peaceful departure by chloroform." The benefits of such a scheme, Osler said, must be evident to anyone who, like himself, was moving upward in age and had considered the "calamities which may befall men during the seventh and eighth decades."

This was an outrageous proposition, and Osler's audience, I am happy to say, was shocked and offended. While age discrimination had grown rapidly during the last years of the nineteenth century, no one was yet prepared to advocate chloroform for everybody on their sixty-first birthday—not even just for college professors. Osler may have intended his speech to be taken humorously, but if so, he seriously miscalculated. It is worth pointing out that Osler himself did not take his own advice; he would retain his post at Oxford for fourteen years, until he was seventy.[1]

Owing to Osler's reputation, the ideas he stated in 1905 regarding retirement (particularly for teachers) were widely circulated. Andrew Carnegie had sold his business the previous year in order to concentrate on philanthropy; he read Osler's speech and the following year formed the Carnegie Foundation for the Advancement of Teaching, charged with creating a retirement plan for American college teachers. From this emerged the Teachers Insurance and Annuity Association/College Retirement Equities Fund [TIAA-CREF], which today provides pension plans to almost all American colleges and universities.

A debate about the productivity of older people had been simmering beneath the surface just as the nineteenth century neared its end. Osler's speech brought the subject to public attention in an extremely vivid way. As scholars and researchers began to take on Osler's thesis, pro and con, both sides acquired strong, vocal advocates. One school held that creative ability is the province of the young and is strongest in the twenties and thirties; the other side advocated that creativity is a human trait that is present throughout the life course and is undiminished or even increased by chronological age. The proponents of these two opposing views still vie for our attention today. Osler's argument has been one of the chief influences shaping American attitudes toward older people during the twentieth century, and until the distortions and mistaken assumptions that it generated are openly refuted, it will continue to have a powerful negative impact on the lives of millions of Americans.

Many popular beliefs in our society are born from professional dialogues of this sort. The process works like this: A researcher has a point of view that he believes in emphatically and which he airs in one or more professional arenas—sometimes orally, sometimes in writing. His view is discussed and debated among the professionals in his field; eventually, it is communicated to the public at large. Once his view becomes widely accepted, it takes on the appearance of fact (whether it is factual or not). Professionals who have accepted the viewpoint then have something to lose if it is proven false, so attempts to revise or contradict it are met with doubt, resistance, and counterattack.

The public may never know the origins of the ideas that reach them and which thus have an impact on their lives. But we are deeply influenced by these ideas, all the same. If the general belief in a society is that chronological age brings a loss of creativity and an inevitable decline, then whatever the facts may be, many individuals will be denied the opportunity to use their abilities, without regard to how well they function or to the amount of useful knowledge they may possess—in other words, for no other reason than their chronological age.

* * *

In the next skirmish, the first volley was fired by a professor of psychology at Columbia University, Robert S. Woodworth. Following in Osler's footsteps, Woodworth voiced an extremely negative opinion about the potential of older people. The book in which Woodworth's view was published, his *Psychology: A Study of Mental Life,* became a widely used textbook. Echoing Osler, Woodworth stated the following:

Seldom does a very old person get outside the limits of his previous habits. Few great inventions, artistic or practical, have emanated from really old persons, and comparatively few even from the middle-aged. . . . The period from twenty years up to forty seems to be the most favorable for inventiveness.

Woodworth's gauntlet was taken up by another psychologist, who published a rebuttal in the *American Journal of Psychology* in 1928 under the fictitious name of Helen Nelson. (To this day no one knows Nelson's true identity nor the educational institution from which she wrote.) In her article, Nelson lists a number of persons whose accomplishments were made at least in part after the age of forty and then asserts that "in the case of these great names at least, invention of the highest order, far from beginning to decay at 40, seems to be at very prime or just ready to begin."

Nelson's list is an impressive one: dozens of writers, sculptors, scientists, composers, and philosophers who produced extraordinary works and all of whom ranged in age from forty to the late eighties and early nineties. In short, Nelson's article makes it clear that individuals older than forty—and in many cases older than sixty—have made tremendous contributions in all areas of human activity, accomplishments that cannot be dismissed nor ignored.

Such a challenge to established opinion could not be left unanswered. The subject was next taken up by Harvey Lehman, a psychologist and a professor at the University of Ohio. Lehman tells us that he set out to see if Woodworth was correct, designing a research project that ultimately took him twenty years to complete. In that era, before the advent of the Xerox machine, the electric typewriter, the word processor, and the computer, most research took a great deal longer than it does now. All recording and tabulating had to be done by hand, and for a project such as this it could quite literally occupy decades. Lehman's book, *Age*

and Achievement, was published in 1953 with a foreword by
Lewis Terman, the distinguished Stanford psychologist who developed the Stanford-Binet intelligence test (and who was, inciden-
tally, the graduate school adviser of Long Careers Study participant John W. Gardner).

For decades to come, *Age and Achievement* would shape public opinion and professional debate about the relationship of age
to ability. Lehman analyzed the professional contributions of people in six different fields in which creativity could be quantita-
tively measured to some degree: science, medicine and surgery,
philosophy, music, art, and literature. In each field, he located a
reference work that listed the achievements of a number of professionals throughout their careers. He then cross-checked these
lists with professionals from other universities to achieve a kind
of consensus as to the importance of these individuals and their
achievements. Since he believed it was impossible to evaluate
accurately the production of people who were still alive—a common belief among researchers during the first half of this century—he eliminated any living individuals from his lists and
worked with names of only those who had died. Finally, he
attempted to correct his information for length of life, adjusting it
to take into account the unequal numbers of persons still alive at
successive age levels.

Lehman begins his work with the study of chemists. His calculations indicated that the age range of their most intense contribution—the peak of their creativity—was between thirty and
thirty-four. However, there were only slight differences in the
rates of contribution between the three age groups of thirty to
thirty-four, thirty-five to thirty-nine and forty to forty-four.

He goes on to make similar calculations about a large number
of other occupations, with roughly similar results, and concludes
that while there are slight differences from one field to another,
the end result is the same: the peak of professional contribution
comes in every instance between the ages of thirty and forty-five,
in most cases between thirty and thirty-four.

Lehman's choice of words is an important issue. The "peak"
that he wrote about was really only a slightly higher point in an
almost uniformly high plateau. But that is not what most of us
think of when we hear the word *peak*—it conjures up an image of
something a great deal higher than the surrounding territory. For
example, Pikes Peak is a very high mountain, not just a bump in

an almost level playing field. Lehman's choice of words grew out of a bias in his own perspective, and it created similar distortions in the minds of his readers.

Lehman goes to great pains, at various points in his book, to assert that he had attempted to do only one thing in the project: "to set forth the relationship between chronological age and outstanding performance." In his preface he itemizes the things he did not intend to do, including discussing the advantages of hiring young men or the disadvantages of hiring old ones. The fact that outstanding creative performance tended to occur at these younger ages did not mean, he said, that there were not some outstanding performances at older ages, or that older people could not perform "adequately and well" (as contrasted with "outstandingly well").

To a contemporary reader, Lehman's virtuous protests seem disingenuous, like the alibis of an angel-faced child caught with his hand in the cookie jar. The structure of the book gives a very different message than the one Lehman says he intended, one that its readers discerned very clearly. *Age and Achievement* was widely understood to provide documentation for precisely the idea that Lehman says he did not mean to convey: that older people are less capable and less creative than younger people. Such an interpretation is easy to understand, given what Lehman measured, the assumptions he made about it, and the words he used to communicate it.[2]

In 1976, nearly a quarter of a century after Lehman's work, Canadian scholar John A. B. McLeish published his refutation.[3] *The Ulyssean Adult* grew out of McLeish's seminars on the contemporary adult and adult learning, given at three different universities over a span of seven years. His students ranged in age between twenty and sixty, with the majority in their thirties and early forties.

McLeish says of his students:

Most of them were emotionally opposed to Harvey Lehman's thesis in *Age and Achievement* that the peak of creative production occurs during the 30s. Without substantial evidence to contradict this, the seminar groups felt in their bones that this thesis was wrong. To them, Lehman had not sufficiently taken into account the whole domain of what one anthropologist calls "the beautiful creature, man."

Now, a "feeling in the bones" is not scientific evidence. It may or may not prove to have correspondences in the external world. McLeish's work was not quantitative, so it did not have much impact on the debate among social and natural scientists. McLeish could not adequately refute Lehman on numerical grounds—that is, on Lehman's home territory—but he had something to go on that Lehman did not have: a far more sophisticated understanding of the nature of prejudice.

In the years between the publications of Lehman's book and McLeish's, social scientists had learned a great deal about prejudice, in part from the civil rights movement in the United States and later from the women's movement. McLeish saw a shadow hiding behind this seemingly innocent protestation of scientific objectivity: he understood that prejudice, rather than scientific rationality, had been at work. McLeish described his own book in this way:

[T]he central and major motive of this book, is that many regenerative and creative powers which are unused form part of the equipment of man throughout his life. . . that great numbers of adults in the later years are inhibited from accomplishments which would glorify those years because they have succumbed to modern myths and negative social conventions about the decline and fall of creativity.

McLeish had also had a number of conversations with men and women in their fifties and sixties who believed (often contrary to their own experience) that they were in a period of inevitable decline characterized by a "withering of the brain cells" or a "daily loss of neurons." They had been influenced by a widespread belief that

not only can you not teach old dogs new tricks, but they do not perform even the tricks they know nearly so well as in younger adulthood. This is also, when all is said and done, a passive or at best a reactive philosophy of the later years. Life is conceived as happening to oneself as a reactor, rather than of oneself acting influentially and decisively upon life.

Old age, McLeish says, is the ultimate stigma. He sees it as a kind of role-play passed on from the present generation of older people to younger people in the community, who are always "silently observing" older people in their roles and relationships.

The "Ulyssean adult" is McLeish's name for the older adult who, like Ulysses did, sets out on new voyages in his later years, leaving the reign of his little kingdom of Ithaca to his son, Telemachus. This final odyssey was mentioned only briefly in Homer, but even this fragmentary reference interested later authors; it is elaborated both in Dante's *Inferno* and in a famous poem by Tennyson.

The qualities McLeish sees as most characteristic of the Ulyssean adult are a governing sense of quest and a fundamental creativity. He dubs Ulyssean One "the man or woman who begins new creative enterprises, small or large, in later life. The other, which might be called Ulyssean Two, is the older adult who does not strike out on new paths and creative territories but who remains creatively productive within his or her own familiar arena of life and work from later middle age into the very late years." The two categories are descriptive types, not a ranking of any kind.

McLeish gives numerous examples of such individuals: Edith Hamilton, a classics professor at Bryn Mawr, retired to a peaceful country life and began writing her stories of Greek and Roman mythology at the urging of friends, who had been fascinated by endless hours of storytelling; the novelist Lou Andreas-Salomé, who began studying with Sigmund Freud at age fifty and became a practicing psychotherapist at age sixty; Cyrus Eaton, a business tycoon who in his seventies founded the Pugwash Conference, bringing together leaders from the West and from Iron Curtain countries; Arturo Toscanini, who continued to conduct superbly into his eighties; Pablo Casals and Pablo Picasso, both of whom remained active artistically until their deaths in their nineties; and on and on.

McLeish also contrasts the behavior of the Ulyssean adult— who is outgoing, interested in the world, and deeply engaged with other people—with the conventional image of the older adult as someone involved in a process of disengaging from society. While there are undoubtedly people who do disengage, it is not by any means an inevitable movement; it is equally likely that people will continue moving toward life instead of withdrawing from it.

During the two decades when McLeish was marshaling his batallions of older achievers, other researchers were grappling more directly with Lehman's work. In the mid-1950s and early 1960s, psychologist Wayne Dennis analyzed more carefully Lehman's calculations and showed that despite his protestations to the contrary, Lehman had not accounted adequately for shorter life spans prior to the twentieth century or for increasing longevity.[4] If almost everyone in a society dies before the age of forty, then it stands to reason that the greatest number of contributions will be made by younger people.

Meanwhile, a gifted young Columbia University sociologist named Harriet Zuckerman was building her own case against Lehman's conclusions. While working toward her doctorate in sociology in the early 1960s, Zuckerman became interested in the relationship of age to science. She had chosen as her dissertation topic the question of whether scientists do their best work alone or in groups, and she settled on Nobel laureates as the subjects of her interviews. The project evolved into a detailed study of Nobel laureates in the sciences in the United States, a subject directly related to the question of age and achievement. Her book, *Scientific Elite: Nobel Laureates in the United States,* was published in 1977 and contains significant refutations of Lehman's work.

Because of the pervasive notion that scientists are most creative in their twenties and that they "burn out" beyond this decade, science provides a particularly intriguing realm for research of this kind. Certainly there have been very famous cases of scientists who did path-breaking research in their twenties: Isaac Newton was twenty-four when he began his work on universal gravitation; Charles Darwin was twenty-two when he made his historic voyage on the *Beagle;* and, more recently, James Dewey Watson was twenty-five when he did his research on the structure of DNA.

But Zuckerman found that the median age was higher for Nobel Prize–winning scientists than for laureates in nonscientific fields, "neither group being nearly so young as the ideological accent on youth would have us believe," she notes. The median age at which the scientists won their awards was 39.9; for the nonscience laureates, the median age was 37.6. In other words, scientists who win Nobel Prizes are in general two years older than nonscientists when they win the prize. As Zuckerman reminds us, a median age is a halfway mark: half the group is younger than that mark, and half is older. That means there were just as many people who made outstanding contributions past the age of forty as there were who did so before they were forty.

Zuckerman found that among scientists it was not the young who turn up disproportionately often among laureates but rather the middle aged (forty to forty-four years old).

"The data that I've looked at," Zuckerman remarked, "all suggest a somewhat different pattern [than the conventional notion]: people who are very creative start early and continue well past the forties and fifties. It doesn't shut off. And the second set of findings is that you don't get a marked fall-off in [the older years]. What you get is a gradual decline . . . a trailing off in that late period."[5]

More recently, psychologist Dean Keith Simonton of the University of California at Davis has also been exploring the subject of creativity and aging. His findings have generated new insights into how creativity changes over the life span. Using records and data on creative people over time, he has constructed a more precise schema of how creativity expresses itself.[6]

First, Simonton says, there is the problem of the group versus the individual. The curve that shows a peak before the age of fifty and a decline afterward is accurate for the group, but it matches only about 10 percent of individual curves. There are people who peak at the end of their careers and late in life, whereas others peak at the beginning or the middle.

Second, although there is a gradual decline in creativity during the period between middle age and the eighties, Simonton says, it is a mild decline, not a sharp falling off. In fact, it is far more gradual than the steep rise at the beginning of a career; even at its lowest point in late life, it is still far higher than it was in the early years of creative activity. And, it is a decline in the *number* of products, not in their quality. In other words, an eighty-year-old may produce only half of what he or she did at forty, but the eighty-year-old's production may be equal to or greater than that of a twenty-five-year-old and far higher in quality.

Third, at the level of the individual, there are tremendous variations, both in creativity and in its pattern throughout a lifetime. For example, there are one-book authors, and there are other writers who never run out of ideas. In terms of lifetime productivity, some people experience a decline; others have little or no decline; and some keep climbing even at late ages. Simonton points out that there are many authors and composers who have produced their greatest works after the age of sixty. For example, *Don Quixote* was completed in Cervantes's sixty-eighth year, and

Titian's "Christ Crowned with Thorns" was painted when the artist was almost eighty. Goethe was placing the finishing touches on his *Faust* when he died at eighty-three. Verdi completed his opera *Falstaff* in his early eighties. There have been important scientific contributors as well: Laplace's *Celestial Mechanics* was completed when the astronomer was seventy-nine; the naturalist Humboldt finished his *Kosmos* when he was eighty-nine; the chemist Chevreul, who began to study gerontology in his nineties, published his last scientific paper two years after he celebrated his hundredth birthday. There are some people, Simonton says, who never run out of steam. People can produce masterpieces up until the day they die.

Fourth, there are huge differences across disciplines. In fields like scholarship, where an accumulation of essential knowledge or expertise takes place over time, the curve does not decline but continues to rise. And this is only one of many patterns found in various fields.

Fifth, in talking about productivity in careers, we may be talking about *career age* rather than chronological age. There are stages of career involvement and mastery that are completely distinct from chronological age: a progression from student to apprentice to mature practitioner to master. One way by which some of the people Simonton studied rejuvenated themselves in middle or late life was to change careers, giving themselves a new cluster of interests and a different field for their creativity.

Simonton's overall conclusion from his research is that creativity does not necessarily decline as we grow older. As long as they remain healthy, most people will probably experience no decline in creative ability. If you have been creative, you are most likely to remain creative, regardless of your age; it is part of your basic makeup. And in the relatively small number of cases where decline occurs, it is likely to be a very gradual decline in the number of things you create, not in their quality.

CAN WE STILL THINK?

THE CASE OF THE DYING BRAIN CELLS

John McLeish noted that his students feared they were suffering from "a withering of the brain cells" or a "daily loss of neurons."

The case of the dying brain cells is related to, but separate from, the debate on age and achievement. It is one of the most widely disseminated notions about aging, and it has been understood by the public to mean that in early adulthood we begin the steady process of losing a percentage of the physical mass of the organ of mental function: the brain. While the myth acknowledges that we start out with and retain millions and millions of brain cells— many more than we apparently make use of—the prospect of losing so many of them in what appears to be a highly physical "brain drain" is nevertheless understandably frightening.

This idea, too, is a distortion. It stems from a major misinterpretation of the findings of some extremely complex neurological research, whose real meaning is still not precisely determined. It is a prime example of how assumptions attach themselves to scientific research in such a way as to appear to be the proper conclusions drawn from the research, when in reality they are not.

The concept of brain cell loss goes back initially to anatomical studies performed in the mid-1800s by Robert Boyd, a physiologist who began weighing the brains of cadavers of all ages, trying to see whether there were differences in weight and mass according to age. This rather gruesome activity could not, of course, track the brain weight of one individual over a lifetime; so the most effective manner of comparison was not available to the study from the very beginning.[7]

Boyd and three later researchers—Raymond Pearl in 1906 and Appel and Appel in 1942—made estimates from the brain weights of different age groups and found what all of them thought was a steady decline in weight with advancing age.[8] But it was not a large decline: roughly 11 percent from early adulthood to age eighty, or an average of about 1 percent for every six years. However, since we don't know at what pace the decline took place, or how, this average is really a metaphor, not a scientific fact. We have no idea what that reduction amounts to; we don't know whether cells are lost from the same areas in all individuals or from different ones. Nor do we know why this cell loss takes place. We do know that the brain has ways of redistributing functions if there is loss or injury, so there is no evidence that this normal cell loss affects functioning. In fact, surprising though it may seem, size does not seem to be directly related to brain functioning.

As a coincidental example, one member of the Long Careers Study group who is a scientist and a university teacher included in one of his interviews an account of an event that he found fascinating because it was so unusual. A year or two before the study, one of his students received medical treatment for an unrelated condition and discovered by accident that she had been born with only one hemisphere of the brain—literally, with only half a brain. Neither she nor her parents had known about this before. The girl functioned absolutely normally; in fact, the scientist said, she was quite bright. Nevertheless, despite her lifelong record of far better than average intelligence and functioning, the girl was profoundly shocked and upset. She and her family went through a traumatic period of adjustment to this discovery. Even though she had been regarded as perfectly normal for close to twenty-five years, she found it highly unsettling to discover that she only had half of a physical brain.

I include this story simply as a confirmation that sheer weight isn't everything where the brain is concerned, nor is the number of cells the whole story. An 11 percent loss (up to age eighty, remember) does not necessarily mean that there would be an effect on function. We don't know exactly what it means, but we do know that you can lose a certain number of brain cells without, as it were, losing any of your marbles. Based on our current state of knowledge, functioning is the only valid measure.

In the 1950s and 1960s, scientists progressed from weighing brains to counting the number of cells in the various regions, in an effort to map which functions are handled by which part of the brain. One of the most distinguished physicians still engaged in this type of research is Dr. Harold Brody, chair of the department of anatomical sciences at the State University of New York at Buffalo School of Medicine and Biochemical Sciences. Brody's research was widely published, and it showed that, with advancing age, there are decreasing numbers of cells in certain regions of the brain—but not by any means in every region.[9]

In his publications, Dr. Brody himself drew no conclusions about the cause of the phenomenon he discovered, or its effect on functioning. In fact, Brody stated that the decrease in the number of cells may have no effect on functioning at all. "There is no reason to conclude," Brody wrote, "that although cells may be lost, there is a related change in functions especially since we do not know what numbers of cells must exist for optimum function or even for marginal function."

However, for some unknown reason Brody's disclaimer was ignored. Shortly after the appearance of one of Brody's more important articles, a neurologist named B. D. Burns took Brody's data, along with some other information, and attempted to calculate how many brain cells are lost per year, per day, per hour. It was a calculation that Brody says is meaningless, because we don't know how the loss of cells occurs, nor at what rate it proceeds, nor what it means! Nevertheless, journalists and the public assumed that it meant that vital functions are being steadily lost along with the loss in cells. The notion has been with us ever since.

Brody found himself saddled with a misinterpretation of his research which he has never been able to rectify. To add to his frustration, the misinterpretation has even influenced people who ought to know better—other distinguished scientists, colleagues in his own department. Brody says that his predecessor as chairman of the anatomy department, who "was one of the most careful people in the world" about the accuracy of his language, used to give an annual lecture on blood formation to the medical students. He would close the lecture by telling them that during the lecture, each of them had lost so-and-so many blood cells but that those would be replaced, whereas they had also lost a large number of irreplaceable brain cells, as Professor Brody had shown, and that was what they really should be concerned about!

If the missing brain cells don't cause us to lose functions, what do they mean? Brody thinks that one possible answer is that the phenomenon is part of a process of eliminating duplication. Nature, he says, has a number of fail-safe systems. All organs have a reserve of unused cells, and for something as important as the brain, the reserve may be particularly large. The embryo produces 65 percent more brain cells than the newborn actually has. An adult, once he or she is fully grown, may also have more brain cells than necessary. After the human being reaches physical adulthood, there may occur, in all organ systems, a process of paring down similar to the one that occurred in an earlier stage as the embryo became a newborn. If so, it probably occurs in the brain as well as in other organs. Redundant cells are eliminated and the structure is made more compact; other nerve cells then grow and branch to pick up the connections formerly made by the eliminated cells, in a process that has been observed to go on continuously even at very old ages.

Brody quotes Dr. Alex Comfort's analogy of the work of a sculptor, who takes a block of wood or stone, pares away the excess, and gives a shape to the remaining material.[10] That metaphor, he believes, may be closer to the truth of the brain's structure. But Brody reminds us that he still does not know for certain. Research by other brain scientists suggests that Brody's guess may be correct, that the decrease in cells may be an elimination of redundancy accompanied by an increase in connections between cells. Paul Coleman, a neuroanatomist at the University of Rochester, has built up a fascinating body of research on these developmental changes in the brain. In a 1979 article in *Science* coauthored with Stephen J. Buell, Coleman described how they had compared the neurons of a group of people who died at about eighty with those from a group who died at about fifty and a third group who died from Alzheimer's disease. To the authors' surprise, they found that the neurons of the normal eighty-year-olds had many more interconnections than those of the normal fifty-year-olds.[11]

It is the number of connections between cells, not the number of cells themselves, that is crucial to learning and intelligence. The implications are that the mind may continue to improve its ability to process information and to use that information in complex ways throughout adulthood.

In another remarkable bit of research, University of California at Berkeley neuroanatomist Marian Diamond created a now-famous experiment in which she put mother and baby rats in an enriched environment—a large cage with several other rat families and a number of interesting toys (blocks, tubes, etc.), which both adults and offspring could explore.[12] The thickness of the rats' cortex and the weight of their brains increased measurably in the enriched environment—a change that became apparent after only four days. When Diamond put elderly rats in the same enriched environment, she found that the old rats' brains increased in size and weight at the same rate as those of younger rats. However, the very oldest rats needed some private time away from the enriched community pen; if they spent all their time in the enriched environment, they tended to die at an age equivalent to that of a human at ninety, whereas elderly rats in ordinary cages lived beyond that point.

Diamond then conducted a series of interviews with older people who were extremely active after the age of eighty-eight. "I found that the people who use their brains don't lose them," she said. "It was that simple. They kept healthy bodies. They drank milk and ate an egg a day. . . . Other denominators were activity, and love of life; and love of others and being loved. Love is very basic," she said.

Although the brain is the seat of consciousness and mental activity, the brain itself is not the mind. One is a physical organ, the other is a property of consciousness that expresses itself through the physical organ. While neurologists and anatomists were probing the question of how the brain changes with aging, psychologists were exploring how the processes of how thinking might change.

Dr. K. Warner Schaie, a psychologist at Pennsylvania State University, has spent over thirty years studying the development of mental processes in a group of adult residents of the Seattle, Washington, area. The Seattle Longitudinal Study is one of the most important psychological studies related to aging. This is partly because of the size of the group—originally it numbered five hundred people—and partly because the participants were randomly chosen. Moreover, from its inception, the group comprised a wide range of ages, including people from twenty-five to eighty-one. Finally, Schaie and a colleague, Prof. Sherry Willis, have followed the group for an unusually long period of time.[13]

The members of the Seattle study have been assessed every seven years on five measures of psychological competence, called "primary mental abilities": the ability to (1) comprehend words (verbal meaning); (2) mentally rotate objects in two-dimensional space (spatial orientation); (3) infer rules from information that contains a regular progression (inductive reasoning); (4) manipulate numbers, as shown by simple addition; and (5) recall words according to a lexical rule (word fluency).

If the group of Schaie's participants is averaged together, there is a small decrease in ability beginning in the mid-fifties to early sixties. Beyond age sixty there is a steady decline in reasoning, spatial orientation, and word meaning, which becomes steeper at the very oldest ages. The result is the typical downward-sloping curve that was found in so many of the early studies of both mental and physical functioning.

But if the progress of individuals is measured, a very different picture emerges. In fact, only about 10 percent of the individual participants have a curve matching the group average. At age sixty, 75 percent of Schaie's participants maintained their level of functioning on four out of five abilities measured. At age eighty, roughly two-thirds of the group members had experienced no decline; in fact, they had actually improved their cognitive functioning on one or more abilities. (Perhaps this is a result of the increase in dendritic linkages found in Coleman's study between ages fifty and eighty.) Only about one-third of Schaie's sample experienced a moderate to large decline in overall mental abilities by the age of eighty, and usually this was associated with a specific illness.

Analyses from the Seattle study showed that people with cardiovascular disease tended to decline earlier in all mental abilities than those with no cardiovascular disease. Schaie then tried a fascinating intervention: he gave some of the cardiovascular disease victims training in inductive reasoning. Those who had received training had fewer episodes of illness and fewer clinic visits than those in the control group who had received no training.

Schaie's research is one of the most important bodies of work ever produced in the history of research on aging. Because of the size and constitution of the original group, and because the study was scrupulously well designed to begin with, there is no question about its meaning or its validity. Considering that two-thirds of the Seattle group experienced no decline in mental ability up to age eighty (and they were meticulously tested over and over again for more than thirty years), it is very clear that a decline in mental ability is not an inevitable, nor even a normal, part of aging. In a long-lived society, this understanding can free us from decades of misinterpretation, prejudice, and fear.

Equally clear are the messages about what we must do with this knowledge. On the collective level, the results of the Seattle study mean that we must exert more effort toward finding the causes of illnesses that affect mental functioning, and toward developing remedies for them. On an individual level, if you or someone you care about begins experiencing any kind of mental decline, consult a doctor. Symptoms of mental decline are not part of normal aging; they are indications of illness. If the first doctor you see is unwilling to look for the cause and dismisses the symptoms as "just old age," find a doctor who is more knowledgeable about the physiology of aging. Schaie's experiment in training cardiovascular patients suggests that many people who experience a decline can return to a higher level of functioning if they are given the right kind of support and instruction.

CREATIVITY AND HEALTH

There is one factor in human life that does seem to have a negative effect on creativity, poor health. For most of us, serious illness or severe physical pain can foreclose the question of creativity and accomplishment. There are, however, exceptions even to this general principle.

In her interviews for the Long Careers Study, noted artist Françoise Gilot spoke several times about how the great painter Henri Matisse, whom Gilot knew well during the 1950s, was relatively incapacitated following cancer surgery in his older years. In the most serious operation, many of his abdominal organs were removed, leaving him in almost constant pain and unable to stand or sit upright without support for more than a few minutes at a time. Since artists generally work standing or sitting before an easel, this was a serious handicap. Undaunted, Matisse turned from painting to making collages with cutouts of painted paper. He would have his companion, Lydia Delectorskaya, paint large sheets of stiff paper in brilliant primary hues. Then he would cut them into fanciful shapes and show Lydia how to position them on a canvas whose size he had already selected. He called this "carving in pure color." These collages, done when the ailing artist was in his mid-eighties, are among his finest works of art. Because of their vibrant graphic qualities, they are the most frequently reproduced and imitated of Matisse's work—one finds them on prints, T-shirts, towels, even ceramic tableware. It is useful to remember, whenever you see these joyous, brilliant, splashy shapes, that they are the work of an old man in his eighties, terminally ill, bedridden and in pain most of the time, who invented this form of collage so that he could continue to exercise his creative gifts and express his joy in life, despite the difficulty of his circumstances.

The message of Matisse's collages is that not even severe physical illness necessarily dries up the springs of creativity. Some people are able to continue creating and producing even when they are in ill health and physical pain. It is a purely individual matter.

In summary, here is what we now know about creativity in the older years:

• There is no set chronological point at which "old age" begins. This stage has been thought to begin at a variety of ages in different eras and different cultures; it is impossible to fix it at any particular chronological age.

• There is no inevitable biological decline either of the brain or of the mind. The available evidence seems to indicate that if you stop using your faculties—at any age—they may suffer, but as a result of disuse, not of chronological age. Some people do experience mental decline, but they are in the minority. When a loss of mental power or diminution of memory does occur, these are the result of specific illnesses, not of aging itself.

• Creativity is not just the privilege of youth. There are numerous examples of great achievements in every field—the arts, the sciences, literature, technology—by people in their sixties, seventies, and eighties. There are fewer examples by people in their nineties and beyond because, up until now, only a tiny percentage of human beings have lived to those ages. We can expect that the list of achievements by people in those decades probably will grow longer in the future, as the number of people living to those ages increases.

• The only element that seems to affect creativity to any marked degree is illness, at any age. People who are sick are less creative, whether they are seven or seventy. But this is not an invariable rule. There are people who remain creative even despite serious illness.

• In brief, staying creative is a highly individual affair. There is no intrinsic reason why you cannot remain creative throughout your life, regardless of how long you live. If you believe that your creativity will diminish, the psychological impact of that belief may indeed trigger a decrease, but it will be a product of attitudinal factors, not of biological inevitability. In other words, to a very large degree, it's up to you.

4

Patterns of Aging

DOES EVERYTHING GO DOWNHILL?

ONE MODEL OF AGING: CUMULATIVE DECLINE

The most widespread belief about the physical process of aging is that there is a particular age that is a biological watershed—a kind of chronological divide—at which your body begins an inevitable decline that cannot be slowed or reversed. We tend to believe that at a certain age, "everything begins to go downhill."

This is the popular reflection of the most widespread intellectual model of aging, the "cumulative decline" model. Dr. James Birren characterizes this idea as the "progressive dwindles": from a certain point in adult life the body starts to deteriorate, and that deterioration is inevitable and cumulative. This process has a snowball effect, carrying the body further and further downhill as it proceeds.

Usually this decline is thought to start in a preliminary manner in the late twenties or early thirties and become steeper at age fifty; it continues until age sixty-five, when it is thought to shift to a sharper downhill angle, bringing with it recurring episodes of increasingly damaging illness until it reaches a climax of institutionalization and eventual death. The cumulative decline model has been the most widely disseminated model of aging during this century: It does not offer us a cheerful view of old age.

A beautifully concise example of this model is the fictionalized account by Harvard geriatrician Dr. Jerry Avorn of the life and death of Oliver Shay. Shay is a composite of many characteristics drawn both from statistical tables and from Avorn's experience as a physician; Avorn himself believes that Shay's is the path most people follow. It is presented here not because this author shares that view but because it is an exceptionally good illustration of the scenario assumed in the cumulative decline theory.

Avorn's fictitious Oliver Shay was born around 1900 into a lower-middle-class household. He was well cared for as a child: fed amply, given enough liquids to drink, kept clean, and nurtured as well as were most other children of the time. The result of this was that he had a perfectly ordinary childhood and grew up to be an adult. Avorn gives us a one-sentence tour through Shay's adult life: he married and worked on an assembly line until he reached retirement age at age sixty-five, retiring in what appeared to be good health.

Shay's downhill slide began shortly after his retirement. He contracted a severe case of bacterial pneumonia and was hospitalized with acute respiratory failure. Treated with antibiotics, he recovered to apparently the same level of functioning that he had had before. But two years after his recovery—at age sixty-nine—he began to suffer from angina, and at seventy-three he had a bypass, followed by another apparent recovery. At age seventy-nine, degenerative arthritis led to a hip replacement and another recovery period. Shortly afterward, he had a stroke and had to be placed in a nursing home. Two years later he had a pacemaker installed. At eighty-four he began to suffer from Alzheimer's; at eighty-eight he experienced chronic kidney failure and was placed on dialysis for the remainder of his life. At ninety-one he died of an abdominal aneurysm, following ten days in intensive care. He had spent the last twenty-six years of his life struggling with a series of illnesses that led, one after the other, to increasingly poor health and a growing need for care from other people.[1]

For many years our vision of the older years of life has been based almost exclusively on an image like that of Oliver Shay. We believed that once an individual reached the traditional retirement age of sixty-five, the most important life events became medical events, with the prognosis being all downhill. Each episode would lead to an increasingly diminished level of functioning, ultimately ending in death. Although we have many ways of disguising our fear and dislike of this scenario, and many ways of distancing it from our everyday lives, most of us still accept it without question.

Where does this model come from? Partly, of course, from the experiences of real individuals. There are some people whose older years do follow this pattern, and most of us have known examples. The observation that old age is a period of physical decline has been around for a long time—it is a constant in literature, from the Greeks to the present day.

But in earlier times the decline of aging was presented more as a question of losing the physical strength and the dewy appearance of youth, rather than of tumbling headlong into an increasingly damaging series of illnesses. For one thing, in earlier times most people didn't live long enough to reach sixty-five, to grow old by modern standards, or to have a succession of cumulative illnesses—the first serious illness would probably have resulted in death. The downward slope as an avalanche of illness is a modern invention.

Osler's notion of the "uselessness" of people over sixty had been circulating generally in the national debate since 1905. But the concept of cumulative decline was popularized by the results of two different research projects on aging that date from the late 1950s and early 1960s, when research methods were still being developed, and when many unexamined biases still existed in the field of aging.

The results of these two projects were published fairly close together in time, so that even though they were not related to each other they appeared to validate each other. Because of this coincidental timing of their publication, each gained in credibility. And both appeared to confirm the accuracy of the downhill pattern.

THE KANSAS CITY STUDY

The first of the midcentury projects was a social-scientific study of 275 older adults between the ages of fifty and ninety living in Kansas City. It was conducted by Elaine Cumming and William Henry during the 1950s. This study found a pattern of gradual withdrawal from normal adult activity as the participants aged. The resulting book, *Growing Old: The Process of Disengage-*

ment, proposed an idea that became the first major theory in the social study of aging: disengagement theory.[2] It described an "inevitable mutual withdrawal or disengagement" between the older person and other members of the society. From a psychological perspective, this theory matched the analytic view then popular that the libido begins to wane in older people and as it does there is a simultaneous narrowing of their field of activity. The supposed purpose of this unconsciously motivated withdrawal was to provide a smooth transfer of responsibilities from one generation to the next.

From the beginning, disengagement theory was controversial because the authors saw disengagement as inevitable and inherent. It raised a furor among experts who did not regard disengagement as good or who believed that the disengagement process was socially generated rather than a biological phenomenon. In addition, a number of experts saw the conclusions of the study as indications of bias against older people.

Cumming and Henry did a fair amount of backtracking in the hubbub after the study was published, and each modified his or her position in some way. However, the study received tremendous attention at the time, made a very strong impression on researchers, and was infused into the mainstream of information communicated to the public.

EARLY REPORTS FROM THE BALTIMORE LONGITUDINAL STUDY

In the early 1960s Dr. Nathan Shock, one of the early pioneers of aging research, published a study showing a series of charts of many different kinds of physical functioning—breathing, heart function, kidney function, and so on—throughout the life course. In each chart there was a peak of functioning during the twenties and early thirties and then a long, gradual downhill slope. The apparent message of these charts, because of the way they were drawn, was that after the twenties, it's all downhill. The charts were much used in the medical community and were incorporated into medical school textbooks. For decades, every fledgling physician saw these charts as a factual depiction of continually deteriorating physical functions after the thirties.

There are four elements in these early charts that were unintentionally misleading. First, they were made from stress tests, not from ordinary functioning. Performance on stress tests falls much more sharply as you age than ordinary performance does. Older people in the 1950s and 1960s often didn't exercise regularly; lack of consistent exercise can also cause a steep decline on stress test performance, which does not show up in ordinary life. In other words, stress test performance is not necessarily an index of how well the person functions on an everyday basis. You can do poorly on a stress test and still get along quite well in everyday terms.

Second, as we discussed earlier, an average does not describe, and cannot predict, the experience of any given individual. The Shock charts were averages, and subject to the same weakness as Schaie later found in the results of the Seattle study.

Third, whatever decline may occur in physical functioning is in reality quite gradual. The charts from the Shock study had to compress a long period of time into a small amount of visual space. As a result, the lines appeared much steeper than the decline really was. If the chart had been, say, twelve inches long instead of three, the visual impression of the slope would have more accurately characterized the data, as it would have reflected a much more gradual decline.

Fourth, the assumptions drawn from the original Shock charts were somewhat premature—the results could not have been accurately judged so soon after the study began. Such perspective was gained, however, in the Baltimore Longitudinal Study's subsequent decades of research.

In fact, the results of the Baltimore study as they are assessed today, after thirty-four years of continuing research, are precisely the opposite of the impression given by Shock's early charts. "The study has shown that aging does not necessitate a general decline in all physical and psychological functions," write Drs. Nathan Shock, T. Franklin Williams, and James L. Fozard in the BLSA publication *Older and Wiser*. "Some abilities decline, but some remain stable. Others actually improve."[3]

The cumulative decline model is a medical model, and medical models are formed from the observation of illness, not health. Dr. Birren believes that this model has been heavily influenced by physicians themselves, who are in contact mostly with the sick and who often see a continuous decline in their patients. So any model that is predominantly medical is potentially biased in that it presents a picture of the experience of sick persons rather than those who are healthy. In a similar fashion, there are other professions that have built-in distortions of perspective—as, for example, social workers work with the indigent elderly.

Some illnesses do lead to a process of cumulative decline, even in young people. Multiple sclerosis, for example, can occur at any age and results in a cumulative deterioration of functions that results in death. But aging does not necessarily follow that pattern. As you can see from comparing the cumulative decline model with Svanborg's findings (chapter 2), there is a fairly substantial discrepancy between the two.

We also do not know to what extent lifestyle figures into these studies. Earlier generations of Americans, by and large, did not exercise frequently nor systematically once they were out of their twenties, and exercise is extremely important in maintaining good functioning. Recent research has yielded very interesting results about the relationship of exercise to strength and fitness in the older years (this will be discussed in chapter 15).

THE ATTEMPT TO CREATE ANOTHER MODEL OF AGING:

THE COMPRESSION OF MORBIDITY

At the end of the 1970s, a second model of aging was proposed by several scientists. It described a long period of sustained vitality lasting until very late in life, perhaps into the nineties or beyond, with only a short period of illness at the very end or, in some cases, no illness at all. The scientific term for this model is "compression of morbidity"—it is a model in which the period of sickness (morbidity) is shortened (compressed).

As is typical of medical models, this second attempt was also defined by reference to illness (a shortened period of illness at the end of life) instead of in terms of health (a longer period of healthy functioning before the end of life). I have chosen to describe this second model in terms of health, since that is its most important feature for those of us who are not medical professionals, and I thus use Dr. Birren's terminology for it: the "plateau of vitality." This model resembles the experiences of Svanborg's older people far more closely than does the model of steady decline.

The scientific basis for this model came from the work of a biologist named Leonard Hayflick, who in the 1970s discovered that human cells will multiply only a fixed number of times (approximately fifty doublings) in a laboratory culture.[4] This provided experimental evidence, for the first time, that there may be a fixed life span for human beings beyond which it is not possible to live: if cells have a built-in limit to how many times they will reproduce, the body itself may have a built-in limit to how long it can continue to replenish itself. Hayflick's studies triggered a great deal of interest and discussion among researchers in aging; the question of whether there is a biologically fixed limit to human life is one that holds endless fascination.

Another scientist, Dr. James Fries, picked up the implications of Hayflick's research and added a great deal of other data in an effort to decipher their meanings and to assemble the basis for a theory.[5] If there is a fixed life span, he reasoned, then within that fixed span it may be possible to increase the period of good health and shorten the period of illness at the end of life—so that the period of vitality is extended to the maximum and that illness is compressed into the shortest possible time. Perhaps we could avoid decline and maintain a normal quality of living right up to the very end of life. To the layman, this seems at the very least a harmless idea and at best a praiseworthy suggestion. But professional groups have their own dynamics, and Fries's first article, published in 1980 in the *New England Journal of Medicine,* raised a firestorm in the field of aging.

First of all, Fries's statement of his theory was somewhat more emphatic than scientific statements usually are; it was presented as if its elements had already been proven, when in scientific terms they had not been. To scientists, an idea is a hypothesis until enough evidence accumulates to substantiate it; then it can be considered a theory. As a hypothesis, Fries's concept might have gotten by. As a theory of how aging will develop in the future, it did not pass muster, because most scientists felt that there was not nearly enough evidence for it.

Scientists usually do not change basic theories easily. The cumulative decline model was already well established in the field of aging, and the compression of morbidity model is quite different from it. Since some people do experience a cumulative decline, there was a great deal of controversy about the relationship of the new model to the old one. Was it a replacement of the old model? If so, some experts rejected it out of hand because the old one matched observed experience in some ways. Or was it an addition? If this was the case, could the two models exist and be valid simultaneously? And where was the experimental evidence for the compression of morbidity model?

The second objection to Fries's idea was that it wasn't clear what implications the Hayflick experiments would have for live human beings. As you can imagine, what happens to cells growing in a laboratory dish can be very different from the behavior of cells in a living human body. Do cells in a living body follow the same pattern of replication as those in a petri dish? And what about the enormous variety in cell type? Conceivably, some cells might divide faster or slower, more times or fewer times. The Hayflick experiments are a fascinating and provocative first step—nothing further can be proved without a great deal more research. So the scientific basis of Fries's hypothesis seemed weak or nonexistent to some scientists.

At a deeper level, however, a large part of the controversy was about the image of aging that the model portrayed. Many practitioners in the field of aging work with people who are in desperate need: poor, frail, ill, and unable to care for themselves in any one of a variety of ways. The physical reality of these ill older people is far more powerful than any written description can convey. When these are the people you work with, day after day, their image becomes the image of all older people, and it can be tremendously compelling.

Moreover, this image is a key part of the process of obtaining the monetary resources necessary to care for the needs of frail and ill older people. The only avenue available for receiving funding for programs that serve the ill elderly is an appeal to public compassion. Without the money provided by charitable giving and by tax dollars, the situation of the frail elderly would be far worse than it is now.

To broadcast a theory proposing that older people can stay healthy and vigorous very late in life, with little or no period of illness and frailty and without an iron-clad scientific underpinning, seemed both irrational and cruelly dangerous to many professionals in the field of aging. Many of the improvements brought about over the past sixty years in the circumstances of people over sixty-five have emerged from public compassion for the truly unfortunate living conditions of the needy elderly. If the public were mistakenly led to believe by Fries's theory that all the problems had been solved, that we had no more need for concern about the future, then years of painful effort and hard-won support for the genuinely disadvantaged might be swept away.

For two or three years a debate raged across the field of aging about the Fries theory. Finally, in 1983, Fries published an article in the *Gerontologist* summarizing and responding to the various arguments. He pointed out that, first of all, the period of illness at the end of life *is* being postponed to older ages, and that this is a matter of historical fact. During the following ten years, according to Fries, the patterns of health and illness among older people would themselves demonstrate whether he was right or wrong. And he noted that there was already an indication that some older people die simply of "old age," not of any specific illness; according to research by R. R. Kohn published in a 1982 volume of the *Journal of the American Medical Association*, "30% of elderly individuals do not have post-mortem evidence of disease sufficient to have caused death in a more vital individual." Finally, Fries urged again that more attention be placed on learning how to prevent illness in the older years of life, instead of on treating it once it has developed.

The controversy rested there, and it has gradually receded. As this book is being written, almost ten years have passed since Fries's article appeared in the *Gerontologist*. What has happened has been unexpected, a kind of combination of both views. The period of good health has, in fact, lengthened. But the period of illness at the end of life has stayed the same. Still, some professionals did believe that Fries had acted irresponsibly in proposing a theory that was not adequately grounded and could have destroyed many of the programs for needy older people that had taken years to establish and build up. On the other hand, the debate planted a tiny seed of doubt in the minds of the aging community that perhaps other models might be possible—although certainly none has been proven, according to scientific criteria, so far.

THE PLATEAU OF VITALITY MODEL

Setting aside the Fries controversy, it is important to observe that in terms of human experience, the cumulative decline model does not describe, and has never described, everyone. In each generation, there have always been some older people who remained healthy and active consistently until very old ages and who died with virtually no period of illness or only an extremely brief one.

This observation was made by Dr. James Birren some years before the Fries controversy erupted. Birren himself had become aware of it when he received an unexpected visit one day at the Andrus Center from a woman who told his receptionist that she was 102 and she had just dropped in because she was curious to see what a gerontology center did. Birren hurried out to the reception area, eager to see what a 102-year-old drop-in visitor would look like. He found a woman who appeared to be about 70. "You couldn't tell how old she was," he said. "She didn't use a cane; she wasn't enfeebled in her walking or in her manner; and you reacted to her as if she were Mrs. Everyday or Mrs. Everyperson, not as if she were a fragile hundred-and-two-year-old woman." He was even more astonished when she told him that to reach the Andrus Center she had taken the bus—a heroic feat in Los Angeles at any age. Just as interesting was the reason for her visit: she was curious to see what a university gerontology center did, whereas, according to the ideas predominant in the late 1970s, when this incident occurred, older people were widely believed not to be curious about new ideas nor interested in the external world.

The woman returned several more times over the next few years, developing a very cordial and interested relationship with Birren and his staff. Then Birren received a letter from one of the woman's friends telling him that she had died in her 104th year, without any trauma or apparent illness. She just simply "faded out" over a period of a few months.

The incident piqued Birren's interest, and he began to collect anecdotes of lives similar to this woman's. He has accumulated a number of them, about equally divided between women and men. In many of the examples he has found so far, the lifetime extended past 100, often to 104 or 105, without any significant change in the person's abilities right up to the end of life.

Birren observes that some people seem to reach a "plateau of healthy aging" at a point in their late sixties or early seventies. They maintain the same level of functioning until the very end of their lives—sometimes for thirty years or more. For them, there is no slow decline, no long period of ill health, and no real impairment in functioning.

The difference in this formulation and Fries's is that Birren's thinking is based on observation (rather than being an assumption made about the future). And Birren makes no speculation about the limits of human life expectancy.

Several of the Long Careers Study participants had relatives whose lives followed this pattern. Interviewee Ollie Thompson told about his grandmother, who at 103 could thread a needle without glasses and did all her own housework. One day, for no particular reason, she called Thompson's mother and told her to bring all the grandchildren over for dinner, because she felt a bit weak. She took everyone out to a movie and then for ice cream afterward; then the group caught a bus back to her house and had dinner. After dinner she told Thompson's mother, Martha, that she was tired and thought she would turn in. Martha went upstairs to her bedroom with her, tucked her into bed, and returned to the living room. An hour later, Martha went up to check on her and found she was dead. "She wasn't sick at all," Thompson remembers. "She just slept away."

Dr. Irving Wright told a similar story about his father, who lived to be eighty-eight. An inventor and a machinery pattern-maker, Perry Wright at the age of seventy-two helped to design the B-29 bomber, which carried the atom bomb during World War II. After the war he continued to be active and kept up his pace of invention. Then, in 1950, Dr. Wright said, "my father was presiding at our annual Thanksgiving dinner, when suddenly he said, 'I think I'll take a nap.' Nobody had ever heard of Perry Wright taking a nap in the afternoon. They all commented on it. He went up and went to sleep and was dead three days later. It was as simple as that."

Regardless of the scientific controversy, it is clear from these examples that there are some people who have a long, healthy older adulthood, without a cumulative decline and with little or no illness at the end of life. It is a life pattern very much like that found in many of Svanborg's participants.

The Long Careers Study provided another form of confirmation of this model. During the five years of the study, fourteen participants died; seven of those fourteen people followed the plateau of vitality model, having only short periods of illness or none at all prior to their deaths. Although the Long Careers group is not a scientific sample, it is nevertheless very interesting that such a high percentage to date followed the plateau of vitality model.

Because of the dominance of the cumulative decline model for almost fifty years, we currently know very little about the plateau model. We don't know, for example, how prevalent it is in comparison with cumulative decline. How large or small a percentage of older people are healthy and functioning until a short time before death, compared with those who experience cumulative declines? Is it just a few, or almost half, as with the Long Careers Study group to date? We don't know. Because people who stayed healthy throughout their old age have been regarded as exceptions, the question hasn't been pursued.

Perhaps when we know more about it, we may find that, without the intervention of specific disease, the plateau model represents the normal progression of late life. Or it may be a model that represents only a small percentage of people but with the assistance of modern medicine is being extended to much larger numbers of people. Certainly it is a question that calls for a great deal more attention in future research.

A THIRD MODEL OF AGING: THE EPISODIC MODEL

A third model of the physical aging process is a kind of halfway point between the first two. It is suggested by the experience of several participants in the Long Careers Study, most strikingly by the life of the late Norman Cousins. In it, the person does experience bouts with illness but recovers completely from each one and regains the same level of functioning as before the illness. The person's health does not go gradually downhill; and there is no long period of illness at the end of life. Instead, there is a zigzag pattern of periods of good health interspersed with periods of illness.

Cousins experienced and recovered from two bouts with potentially fatal illness after the age of fifty. The first was a degenerative disease of the connective tissue called ankylosing spondylitis, which he contracted in the early 1970s. He recovered completely. An article he wrote about the experience for the *New England Journal of Medicine* received such favorable comment that he expanded it into a book, *Anatomy of an Illness*. Published in 1974, it revolutionized the attitude of Americans toward participating in their own health care and, moreover, did so without alienating the medical profession.

About ten years later, Cousins suffered a heart attack. Again, he recovered from this so completely that he returned to all his regular activities including playing tennis and golf. He and his wife, Ellen, had just moved to southern California, where he was an adjunct professor at the UCLA medical school, designing and taking part in research that documented the effect that the mind has on physical health via brain hormones. This project lasted for almost a decade and yielded major advances in our understanding of the role of the mind in physical illness.

After ten years of vigorous health, with no preliminary warning signs and no indication that anything was wrong, Cousins died suddenly at around 4:30 P.M. on Friday afternoon, November 30, 1990, at the age of seventy-five. The physician's diagnosis was full cardiac arrest. One day earlier, Cousins had played sixteen holes of golf.

Another study participant, Max Lerner, also exhibited this pattern. He went through two bouts with cancer and a heart attack and recovered from all. At eighty-eight, he continued to keep his regular travel schedule, write his syndicated column for the *New York Post*, and publish books. His last book, *Wrestling with the Angel*, the story of how he confronted and triumphed over his illnesses, was published in 1990 to universally favorable reviews. In 1991, his cancer recurred; in the process of battling it to a standstill once again, Lerner had a stroke and died.

The episodic model may be a product in part of modern medicine: the people in this category might have died if they had existed in previous eras. They now are able to recover completely because of our advances in medical technology.

In conclusion, there is not just one model of physical functioning in old age. At present, there are at least three—and there may be more that have not yet occurred to us. There is no set chronological age at which everything—or even anything in particular—begins to "go downhill" for everybody. There is an undetermined number of older people for whom, past the sixties and early seventies, nothing much really goes downhill at all. And there are some who have episodes of illness, with periods of recovery and undiminished functioning in between. There are many possible patterns or types of aging. We need to acknowledge their diversity and begin to examine them more objectively.

We need a more complex view of older people and the physical aging process. Older people are not a monolithic group. They are just the opposite: people seem to become more individual and more different from each other, the older they get. It isn't true. Older people are not universally poor, sick, and frail, just as they are not all glowingly healthy and out playing tennis. There are people in each category, and others in between.

We don't need to replace the image of the frail sick older person with the image of what Mary Catherine Bateson terms a super-elder, who leaps tall buildings at a single bound.[6] To do that would be a terrible disservice to all older people, the healthy and the ill alike. It is as oppressive to expect all older people to be super-achievers as it is to expect them to be helpless and incompetent. Neither image is truthfully representative of all older people as a group. Our objective should be more diversity of image, not less.

Just as we must begin to identify a variety of patterns, we must also try to find out what factors contribute to their development. This is a formidable task because there are so many different variables involved. But it is vitally important, because the real answer to the physical ills of aging in the long term—for those Americans who are now in their thirties, forties, and fifties—is in preventing those illnesses from the development of those illnesses in the first place. Perhaps in the decades ahead, medicine will move increasingly in that direction, building on some of the steps it has already taken.

5

The Long Careers Study

In 1987, when I first began studying people who continued to work beyond age sixty-five, I believed that there were not very many of them. Though I knew several people who were still working in their seventies and eighties, I assumed, as most of us probably would, that the majority retired at some point in their sixties, and then spent their time in family and recreational activities, with perhaps some volunteer work on the side.

But the more I looked, the more older people I found who were still at work in one capacity or another—and who were working because they enjoyed what they were doing. I decided to find out what a very long life was like, and what people did with the added time.

Examinations of the research literature and of population statistics convinced me that this was a new phenomenon, one that had not yet been identified or described. There were simply too many people who were labeled "retired but working" or "never retired" to fit the old definitions.

Government population statistics tell us that there has been a sharp decline during the past thirty years in the number of people over fifty-five who remain in the work force. In themselves, the figures are convincing: in 1950, 65 percent of all men fifty-five and older were still employed; by 1990, there were only 38 percent in this category. The women's work-force participation curve has been somewhat different from that of men because more women joined the work force during those forty years: in 1950, 18 percent of women over fifty-five were employed; by 1990, the figure had risen to 22 percent. But with women and men combined, the percentage of employed people over fifty-five fell from 41 percent in 1950 to 29 percent in 1990.

Looking at work-force figures for those fifty-five and older does not give us a complete picture, however; we must also look at figures for those between the ages of forty-five and fifty-four. The traditional boundaries of retirement began to expand in the 1970s and 1980s, when a trend toward early retirement appeared in corporations and businesses—the practice of allowing or encouraging employees to retire before they reached age sixty-five. Early-retirement offers have been extended to people as young as fifty; in a few well-publicized instances, companies like Atlantic Richfield and CBS offered age-fifty early-retirement packages to thousands of employees at one time. The percentage of employed men aged forty-five to fifty-four has also been falling—from 91.9 percent in 1950 to 87.4 percent in 1990.

These figures seem to show that now, when almost twice as many adults are over fifty-five as under this age, participation in work is steadily declining in both of these age categories. In such a situation the older people who are still in the work force might be there because they need the money—in other words, financially, they can't afford to retire.

To some degree, our social environment should reflect this statistical profile. There should be relatively few older people around who are still working. The individual level of experience—what scientists call the "anecdotal"—isn't necessarily a reflection of what is happening on a large scale; nevertheless, large-scale trends are frequently apparent in everyday life. But here the environment showed something that was the opposite of the statistical picture. Wherever I went, I found active older people, working at an enormous variety of pursuits in many different circumstances, apparently enjoying what they were doing.

That there were so many people who continued to work—by choice, not just because they needed the income—raised a host of fascinating questions. Why were they still working, if they didn't need the money? Was there something different about them that kept them engaged, while others were enjoying their well-earned leisure? Was it a positive difference or a negative one? Were they just workaholics who couldn't give up their way of life? Were they afraid of retirement, classic cases of people who couldn't "adjust"? Or were they all exceptionally creative people, like Picasso, capable of practicing their craft indefinitely, whereas the rest of us at some point give out and give up?

Researchers in the field of aging have speculated about the effect of having so many increasingly vigorous older people and so few ways for them to participate in the society as a whole. Traditional retirement has been called a "roleless role": although it is treated as if it gives the retiree a role, it offers few models and no real way of staying involved in the life of society. Many retirees do find a creative outlet for their energies in individual pursuits or in organizations geared to "seniors." But not all retirees have creative outlets, and as the number of older people increases, the need for more alternatives is becoming greater. Drs. John and Matilda White Riley point out in their article "Longevity and Social Structure" that in our society there is a serious lag in finding new roles for healthy older people. "As members of successive cohorts retire at young ages and are better educated and perhaps healthier than their predecessors," the Rileys observed, "it seems predictable that pressures from old people and from the public at large will modify the existing work and retirement roles.... Study after study suggests that the need for involvement and participation in the larger society does not end with formal retirement. Yet the needs still outstrip the incipient opportunities."[1]

In other words, older people might choose, as one of their options, to continue to work, and this impulse would be generated by individuals, since institutions and organizations are doing very little to deal with the lack of roles. "One inference seems inescapable," noted the Rileys. "The presence of increasing numbers of capable people living in a society that offers them few meaningful roles is bound to bring about changes.... Capable people and empty role structures cannot co-exist for long."

It is worth noting that the Rileys are justifiably experts on this phenomenon, not solely on the basis of their academic credentials. Born in 1908 (John Riley) and 1911 (Matilda White Riley), they have been active in the field of aging since it was inaugurated in 1947. And both are still working: he as a consultant for the Equitable Life Insurance Society and the International Association of Aging, and she with the Behavioral and Social Science Research

Section of the National Institute on Aging, first as its director and since 1992 as a senior scholar.

It seemed reasonable to conclude that working older people might be doing just what the Rileys predicted and had done themselves: creating new roles where no other satisfactory roles existed. I decided to organize a research project, which I called the Long Careers Study, that would allow me to explore this phenomenon. The study's goals were qualitative: to begin learning about how people are using the time that has been added to adulthood by longevity; to gain some insights into how a long career differs from a career of conventional length; and to begin the process of rethinking the individual life course, so that people can form a less negative and more realistic sense of their options in the decades of life after sixty. The next step was to find active older people who would be willing to take part.

FINDING THE LONG CAREERS STUDY PARTICIPANTS

Other studies of adult life have generally been done with a controlled population of some kind. The researcher would enlist members of a particular college class or employees from a specific corporation or cluster of corporations; members of an organization; or a scientifically random sample drawn from a limited geographic area. In order to do this, the researcher would have to have available some central source for potential participants. But no such source of names exists for people over sixty-five who are still working. Nor was there a single institution or organization in which a number of these individuals was likely to be gathered. Corporations and universities were not sources of participants, because mandatory retirement had pushed most people above a certain age out of the workplace. Another obvious source was the American Association of Retired Persons. Despite its traditional emphasis on retirement, it has many members who are not retired in the usual sense of the word; it is rapidly changing into an organization of people over the age of fifty, regardless of their employment status. However, the AARP does not maintain detailed information on its thirty-six million members—perhaps the sheer size of the membership makes this prohibitive—and I was told that the organization does not have a mechanism to provide information of the kind I needed.[2]

Similarly, there were no available government sources for such information. The Social Security Administration has on record the work and income status of everyone in the United States, but its files are confidential and legally sealed to outside inquiry. The Bureau of Labor Statistics maintains collective data on the work force, and it also has data on retirement ages of both men and women, but it does not have individualized information either on those who retire or on those who continue to work.

Essentially, I found that if I wanted to locate people with long work lives, I was on my own. I had expected to be able to find a way of obtaining a scientifically random group. Instead, what I had to settle for was genuine randomness: finding each interviewee by chance, or in whatever way I could devise.

The task turned out to be easier than expected. I wrote letters, buttonholed professional friends at meetings and lectures, telephoned people I knew, combed newspapers and magazines. Everyone I approached knew several people who fit into this category. One dinner with three professional friends yielded a total of thirty-three names. The lists grew steadily. The names most people contributed initially were those of public figures. If I questioned them further, they would begin to think of people who were not particularly well known, so it became clear that the trend was not restricted to celebrities.

The list continued to expand after I began interviewing. All the participants had names of others to suggest. Bostonian Thomas D. Cabot reeled off a list of twenty-five names of personal acquaintances in their eighties and nineties who were still active, and then he told me how sorry he was that I had missed meeting a friend of his, Herman "Jackrabbit" Smith, who lived to be 111½ and went skiing with Cabot three months before he died. Needless to say, I, too, was sorry I had missed him. But I was happy to talk with Cabot, who at ninety-five still went to his office every day and had just come back from a three-week trip to Antarctica with his ninety-three-year-old wife.

This first list of potential interviewees soon contained several hundred names, mostly of men. There were few women and very few minority group members of either sex. This lopsidedness made sense because in the decades when the participants were growing up, most career tracks were closed to women and just as tightly barred to blacks and other minorities. There were many more white males over sixty-five whose work history would make it easy for them to stay active.

It took a lot of time and conscious effort to expand the list of possible interviewees so that it included more women and minority group members. Ultimately, a reasonable balance between men (57 percent) and women (43 percent) was achieved. Although the percentage of women does not match the figures for the population as a whole nor the percentages for women in the over-sixty-five age group—where women outnumber men two to one—it is still better than that in most prior research.

Locating minority group participants was much harder than finding women, even though I was both experienced and motivated. The final group included eight blacks (four men and four women) and two Hispanics (one woman and one man). Several minority group members whom I approached declined to participate, and the constraints of time and money limited my efforts to locate a representative minority percentage.

THE INTERVIEWS

The type of interview I employed is known as a focused life history. Every interviewee was asked to give a concise history of his or her life beginning with birth, emphasizing the area of particular interest to the study—in this case, the person's career pattern. From these accumulated narratives, I could draw larger conclusions about overall patterns.

Most interviews required two sessions of an hour and a half each; some were broken up into shorter and more numerous sessions because of the interviewee's schedule, and a few took up one longer session instead. Style differed enormously: one energetic and strong-minded man in his seventies condensed his entire life history into approximately fifteen minutes and then told me he couldn't think of anything else to say. (I was able to draw him out beyond that point, but not without effort.) Another interviewee, a woman in her late eighties, was reportedly frail and had a heart condition. I arrived fearful that even half an hour would overtax her. To my delight and amazement, she talked for more than five hours at the first (and only) session, telling story after story, delving repeatedly into the intricacies of how certain life experiences and events really took place and what they meant, and pointedly asking me if I were tired whenever she saw my attention lag for even a few seconds. I interpreted this in part as the desire to demonstrate to someone roughly half her age that determination and stamina count more than simple chronological youth. The point was well taken.

Generally I met the participants on their own territory, partly as a matter of courtesy and also to gain a clearer understanding of their life and personality through their environment. I also learned not to be directive in the early part of the interview, saving my list of standardized questions for the end of the conversation. If allowed simply to speak freely, the participants gave me information and made observations I would not have known to ask about.

In addition to the interviews, I also asked for copies of the interviewee's résumé or other biographical material. In some cases, in which the interviewee had written books or articles or there was published information about the person, I acquired and read as many of these items as possible before the interview.

Ultimately, 150 people—86 men and 64 women—were interviewed for the Long Careers Study over a period of roughly five years, from December 1987 to November 1992. Collectively, they had lived a total of almost eleven thousand years. They ranged in age from a few months short of their 65th birthday at the time of the first interview to 101. The interviews produced over nine thousand pages of raw transcripts, which were edited down to around six thousand pages of monologue transcripts containing the participants' narratives alone.

THE PARTICIPANTS: LOCATION, AGE, AND OCCUPATION

In putting together the group, I looked for variety in age, geographic location, background, social class, type of career, even personality.

GEOGRAPHIC DISTRIBUTION

Most of the study participants were born in the United States. Although I wanted to obtain an even geographic spread from across the country, during the course of the interviews it was made clear that any attempt at simple geographic score-keeping would be a lost cause. During the participants' long lifetimes, only a very small percentage of them had remained in the town (or even the region) where they were born and grew up. In the final group, there were only ten people who had stayed in the city where they started out: eight in New York; one in Memphis, Tennessee; and one in Houston, Texas. All the rest had moved several times at least, as children or adults or both. Most of the participants had moved so many times that it was impossible to assign to them a geographic label of any kind. They lived in a century of extraordinary mobility, and almost all of them had been swept along by it.

AGE DISTRIBUTION

The average age of the study participants was seventy-nine. There were relatively few people in their sixties, because those were the youngsters of the age group and I wanted the majority of interviewees to come from the older decades. At the end of the study, in 1992, there were twelve participants in their sixties; sixty-seven in their seventies; fifty-three in their eighties; fifteen in their nineties; and three centenarians.

It was easy to find people in their sixties and seventies who were still active, because there were a great many of them. People in their eighties were not hard to find either, although they were not quite as plentiful. People in their nineties were much scarcer—but, if anything, they were harder to make contact with than the younger people because they were generally so busy that it was difficult to get a foot in the door! By and large, they were very conscious of the preciousness of their time and were working intensely on the things that were most important to them.

Dr. Linus Pauling, for example, who was almost ninety when the study began, agreed to be interviewed but asked that I come to his ranch on the Big Sur coast of California. His weekly two-day visits to the Linus Pauling Institute of Medicine in Palo Alto were so packed that he did not have time for an outside interviewer. When I arrived at his home, he was analyzing the nuclear structure of rare earths, his large worktable strewn with charts of various elements. Although he was gracious, clearly it was a sacrifice for him to tear himself away from his project to talk to an unknown interviewer.

The three centenarians were Edward Bernays, Dr. Michael

Heidelberger, and Theresa Bernstein Meyerowitz. All three were quite functional at the time of their interviews. Dr. Heidelberger, a research chemist, still went to his office at New York Hospital three days a week until shortly before he died at the age of 103. Although he no longer did active chemical experiments at that point, he continued to write articles, and he edited the writing of all the other chemists in his department—enough, I imagine, to keep anyone busy at least three days a week.

Edward Bernays, the founder of the field of public relations, is still active as a public relations consultant and charges his standard fee of $1,000 an hour. During the period when I interviewed him, he was helping Hill and Knowlton plan his hundredth birthday celebration for November 1991, a two-day conference at Northeastern University to celebrate the birth of the field of public relations. He was amazed at the growth of this field, which at its inception consisted of just one man, himself, but now employs hundreds of thousands of people all over the world.

Theresa Bernstein Meyerowitz, a painter contemporaneous with the Ashcan school of art, had just had a retrospective show at the Museum of the City of New York. At the time of her interviews she was still drawing and painting avidly, getting ready for another show despite a broken hip.

There is roughly a forty-year age spread between the oldest participant, Dr. Michael Heidelberger, who would have been 104 in 1992, and the youngest participants, the 65-year-olds, who are the teenagers of the group. It is important to remember that this is a difference of two full generations. We tend to place everyone over 65 in one category, as if people magically become the same age once they pass their 65th birthday. But these people belong to very different age cohorts, separated by as much time as, in the case of Dr. Heidelberger and someone who turned 65 in 1992, the amount of time separating a 41-year-old from a newborn. The 103-year-old could be the parent, or even the grandparent, of the 65-year-old.

OCCUPATION, ACHIEVEMENT, AND STATUS

About half the group was made up of people with distinguished reputations. There were two reasons for this. First, relatively well-known people were easier to find than those with more ordinary occupations. When I did find people who were secretaries or factory workers, for example, I signed them up immediately if they were willing. The trouble was that most of them were not willing; they did not want their age to be generally known and were afraid that being interviewed would have a negative impact on their work. Several people in this category turned me down flatly, including a department store saleswoman in her seventies who was panic-stricken that she would lose her job and fled to the stockroom to escape me, begging me not to tell to anyone her age.

The second reason, however, was more important. The publicly known participants have great value as role models. Older people have been the object of considerable prejudice in our society in the past. In every group that is the object of prejudice, there are a few members who are able to make outstanding contributions because of unusual circumstances. They have a talent so exceptional that it is recognized regardless of their status as part of a discriminated group. Or they have sponsors or powerful friends who enable them to overcome external obstacles and gain the recognition they deserve. Or they are just simply lucky; everything falls into the right place at the right time.

Whatever the reasons that they have been able to thrive and to produce in a generally unfriendly climate, these people are the exceptions that disprove the rule. If one member of the group has been capable of achieving at that level, then there are other members of the same group who had the native ability for similar accomplishment but did not have the circumstances necessary to overcome the barriers to achievement raised by prejudice.

The aftereffects of the civil rights and women's movements have amply demonstrated the truth of this principle. When both minorities and women were the object of overwhelming prejudice in the society at large, there were a handful of blacks and a few women who because of exceptional circumstances were able to succeed far beyond the levels accessible to blacks and women in general. Those individuals are clear testimony to the fact that without the existing prejudice, many more people belonging to those groups would have been able to excel.

The people I have interviewed for the Long Careers Study are but a tiny percentage of the millions of Americans over sixty-five who are creative, productive, and engaged in worthwhile and fascinating pursuits. The Long Careers Study participants are one row of waves in a large and lively ocean.

LOOKING FOR CLUES

Once the interviews began to accumulate, I began to look for similarities in background and patterns of career development that would help explain this group's commitment to working and staying active. Some patterns that I had anticipated never appeared, whereas there was an emergence of other surprising trends.

FAMILY BACKGROUND

FINANCIAL STATUS

Regardless of their accomplishments or their relative financial security by the time of their interview, the great majority of the study participants began life in households with modest incomes. Ninety percent were born into either middle-class or poor families. A majority of them came from families in which only the father worked outside the home (no surprise, given the time period in which they grew up), his efforts providing a livelihood that was just enough for the family to get along on. Their fathers were teachers, businessmen, ministers, merchants, tailors, and small-town lawyers and doctors in times when such professions were neither well paid nor prestigious.

Businessman and philanthropist Milton Petrie, for example, recalled growing up in Detroit in a family that tried to live on a policeman's small salary, and he remembered his mother's constant struggle to make ends meet. He determined that when he was grown up he wanted to make money so that he would never have to be poor again. Later in life, after his decades of effort in building Petrie Stores had made him wealthy, he became famous for his spontaneous charitable gifts to victims of crime and to policemen injured in the line of duty.

Only six of the participants came from families that consistently had a good deal of money during the person's childhood. However, being born into a well-to-do family did not necessarily mean either that the person's childhood was idyllic or that adult life would be carefree. For one, this childhood environment affected her life in a very unexpected way. Mrs. Henry Parish II grew up in a family that had not only money but exquisite taste; she was constantly surrounded by beauty. Furniture, paintings, rugs, objects d'art—were all chosen by her mother with great care and exquisite taste. Parish had no career aspirations as a child and never expected to have any, because she believed that her highest role would be to marry, have a family, and create a home.

When the depression badly affected the finances of her young family in the early thirties and she was forced to try to find an additional source of income, as were many depression-era women, Parish hit upon the idea of being an interior designer. With a friend, Albert Hadley, she later founded one of the greatest American design firms, Parish-Hadley Associates. Her eightieth birthday was recently celebrated with great festivity at the Cooper-Hewitt Museum of design. Parish is still active in Parish-Hadley as a consultant and continues to serve a large number of devoted clients.

HOME LIFE

Another question that arose was whether the participants owed their success to a happy and trouble-free childhood. The interview material showed that most of the participants grew up in a traditional nuclear family. The majority seemed to come from relatively happy families, but there were some whose families were not at all happy. Many more than I expected (25 percent) were raised by only one parent, usually the mother. In most cases this was because the father died relatively young, but in a few it was because the father was working in a different city.

A number of the participants suffered early traumas or deprivations that they had to overcome. In some cases the trauma was the loss of a loved one, most frequently a parent, as mentioned above. Some found their lives dramatically changed because of this; their families were plunged almost instantly into poverty because of the father's death. In every case, the child gained a very different view of life as a result of this early tragedy.

SIBLING ORDER

One's place in the sibling lineup has been said to contribute to the development of certain character traits; for example, oldest children are assumed to be hard workers, leadership-oriented, and more responsible than the younger siblings, whereas younger ones are considered extroverted and free-spirited.

Even though in general the participants were responsible and achievement-oriented, they were not all oldest children. In fact, the participants' places in the sibling lineup and the overall sizes of their families of origin varied enormously. Some came from very large families—two were the youngest from families of eleven and twelve children. Of the group, 3.6 percent were the only child in the family, whereas most had two or three siblings: 41.7 percent were the first child in the family, and 29.7 percent were in the middle of the family lineup. The remaining 25 percent were the youngest child in their respective families.

CHILDHOOD ILLNESS

Combating illness successfully at any age, but particularly in childhood, contributed to participants' sense of purpose and vitality. Several participants who were ill during childhood found that their lives were shaped by this experience—though not always in predictable ways. Norman Cousins was a sickly child, and his early childhood was a dreary round of being taken to one doctor after another. When he was seven, he was placed in a tuberculosis sanitarium for a year, to his great distress. "It was a very wistful experience when the parents came to visit their kids on Saturday mornings," he said. "I would sit on the wall near the entrance and get a whiff of the healthy outside world: healthy parents and healthy youngsters coming to visit the sick kids and then going back to this larger world. I began to value life."

The experience gave Cousins a lifelong interest in health. "I learned that you had to make your choices very early," he said. "I observed what it was about these kids who didn't make it and what it was about the kids who did. The kids who didn't make it regarded their illness as a verdict. Kids who did make it regarded the illness as a challenge. There weren't very many of the latter. That puzzled me at the time. There was no doubt in my mind that I would walk out of that place."

But apparently similar events can affect people very differently. Actress Jessica Tandy was also sent to a tuberculosis sanitarium when she was a child. When she related this during her interview, my first response—primed by the stories of Norman Cousins—was to assume that it was a wrenching experience and to feel great sympathy. But when I asked her what the experience was like, to my utter astonishment she replied, "Just *marvelous!*"

Tandy went on to tell me that she came from a tense and stressful family, and that the institution where she was sent was more like a convalescent home than a real hospital. Being away from home was like a wonderful vacation for her. It was the one time when she got some freedom from the constant tension of her parents' marriage and could do things that she enjoyed.

CAREERS: ASPIRATIONS AND PATTERNS

It is popularly assumed that successful people know early in life what they want to do and move directly toward their goal. But, surprisingly, only a very small number (15 out of 150) of the Long Careers Study participants knew what they wanted to do early in life and followed through on that knowledge. The rest of the participants figured out their career choices in high school, in college, or later, largely by trial and error, as most of the rest of us do.

Sometimes the search was easy; sometimes it was difficult and discouraging. There did not seem to be any correlation between the length and type of career search and the subsequent degree of success.

Career development among the study participants did not fall into any neat and consistent pattern. The timing and circumstances of their decisions varied greatly. However, a few specific types of patterns did emerge upon further examination. A few examples of the evolution of career decisions are included next to give you an idea of some of the patterns that emerged from the group of study participants. These patterns will be described fully in chapters 6–12.

FIRST VERSUS SECOND CHOICES

Many of the people who were not able to pursue their first choice in careers became not just successful but very distinguished in their field. The most startling example among the participants was Dr. Jonas Salk, creator of the influenza and polio vaccines. In his childhood, Salk wanted to be a lawyer—a choice that was emphatically vetoed by his mother, who was determined that her cherished eldest son would become a schoolteacher. Salk, however, had no interest in being a schoolteacher; he simply was not drawn to it. Deprived of his first choice, he then decided to become a medical research scientist and insisted on his second choice. He enrolled in medical school and went on to become one of the century's greatest medical research scientists.

CAREERS FOUND BY TRIAL AND ERROR

A correlation was found between the degree of public familiarity with the career and the ease with which the candidate found it. Several people clearly had their search lengthened because the work that turned out to be ideal for them was something they had never encountered in any form. As a result, they had to find it by wandering through a maze of other possibilities, sometimes for several years.

Oscar Dystel, for twenty-six years the president of Bantam Books, is perhaps one of the most striking examples of a person whose exceptional gifts lay in a field he didn't even know existed when he began his career. When Dystel was a child, his mother thought he had talent as a musician, and he spent years studying the violin before he realized that he did not have outstanding concert ability. Next he took up running and won a track scholarship to New York University. But there Dystel, who had planned to major in accounting, discovered that he was good but not great at running and that he had no real affinity for accounting. He gave up his athletic scholarship, got several part-time jobs, and switched to a major in marketing and advertising.

In Dystel's senior year, one of his finance teachers suggested he apply for a scholarship to Harvard Business School, and he did. At Harvard, one professor asked him to write an original analysis on magazine circulation. The article was published and attracted a great deal of attention, leading to a number of job offers after graduation. At first he worked in magazine publishing; later he moved into book publishing, where he found his real vocation and became the architect of the paperback book revolution. The paperback industry had been, until then, limited to college texts and classic fiction. Dystel aggressively and innovatively developed paperbacks and by so doing forever changed the book buying and reading habits of the world.

Although his name is not well known publicly, Oscar Dystel's broad recasting of paperback publishing has touched the lives of every American in the last half of the twentieth century. Yet, remarkably, he did not have a clear sense of his real career until he was a mature adult, and had spent many years working his way diligently through other occupational possibilities, discarding each inappropriate goal and finding another one.

CAREERS FOUND THROUGH PURE COINCIDENCE

Some careers are launched by an entirely unexpected and fortuitous coincidence. Record store owner Sam Goody experienced just such a coincidence early in his own career. After his first company, a wholesale millinery supplies firm, went bankrupt in the depression, Goody started a small-goods shop that carried toys, books, and various random items. One night, he went down to see the superintendent of his apartment building for some reason and during the conversation noticed a box of old phonograph records. They had been discarded by a tenant, and the superintendent intended to throw them out. The following morning, a man came into Goody's store and asked him if he had any old-fashioned Victrola records. Goody said he might have and, with the man's promise that he would return the next day, that night Goody bought the records from the superintendent for a quarter. But the man didn't come back for several weeks and Goody became angry; a quarter in those days was a lot of money, Goody said, and he felt he had spent it for nothing.

When the man finally returned to the shop, he looked through the large stack of records and chose only one record to buy. Goody was put off that the man was buying only one, after he had prepared dozens for him. Then the man said: "I'll give you five dollars for it."

Goody exclaimed, "Five dollars?!" It was an enormous sum.

The man, thinking his bid too low, said, "Eight dollars, but that's my best price."

"And that," Sam Goody told me, "is how I got into the record business!"

MENTORING

Two-thirds (67 percent) of the participants said that mentors had given them substantial support and guidance in finding, maintaining, and changing careers, particularly early on. These mentors—

parents, teachers, older colleagues, even friends—often played key roles in helping the participants make their choices.

Dr. James Dumpson, raised in a low-income area of Philadelphia and currently vice president of the New York Community Trust, owes the evolution of his career in large part to a series of important mentors who guided and encouraged him. His early mentors were his mother, who had been a teacher before her marriage, and a high school teacher who had him write a paper on the first black Rhodes scholar, Alain Locke.

After high school, Dumpson was mentored by a series of employers. One employer, for whom he worked as a butler and cook, suggested he attend the state university and work only part-time for her. Later he worked as a waiter for Richard Beamish, who became Pennsylvania's secretary of state and hired Dumpson to work in his office for a year after his college graduation. A few years later, Dumpson's supervisor at another job in the Department of Public Assistance encouraged him to get a degree in social work. Once in school again, he met Dorothy Kahn, a faculty member and head of his department, whom he credits as one of the people most responsible for his going to New York and working for the United Nations. From that point forward, Dumpson has had a brilliant career as executive director to several federal and state agencies; commissioner of welfare for New York State; and dean of the schools of social work at Hunter and Fordham colleges. He is currently chairman of the Health and Human Resources Department of New York City.

As testimony to their understanding of the importance of mentoring, nearly all the Long Careers Study participants have in their turn mentored younger people. Ninety-two percent say that they have mentored others.

THE PARTICIPANTS AND POSITIVE AGING

In professional groups where I periodically discussed the Long Careers Study, negative images of older people continually surfaced. This suggests that negative stereotypes of older people are still very widespread in our society, even in groups that one thinks should be more knowledgeable. As we grow more long-lived (assuming that the trend toward longer lifetimes continues), one of the most important tasks we face is that of dismantling our negative assumptions about old age.

THE LOUIS HARRIS STUDIES

Two famous polls conducted in 1974 and 1981 by participant Louis Harris for the National Council on Aging illustrated the presence of negative stereotypes. They showed major discrepancies between the way that people aged eighteen to sixty-four imagined the lives of older people, and how those over sixty-five experienced life themselves. The results of the studies were similar, so I shall use only the 1981 figures here.[3]

The Harris studies showed that the public in general believed that older people did not have enough money to live on (68 percent); were in poor health (47 percent); were lonely (65 percent); were afraid of crime (74 percent); and did not have enough job opportunities (51 percent), medical care (45 percent), nor education (21 percent). In the public mind, the typical older person is poor and lonely, desperately afraid of crime, most likely in poor health, and lacking in medical care. Nor does he or she have enough job opportunities.

The responses of those who were actually over sixty-five gave a very different picture. What was most telling about this survey, however, was that *older people themselves* believed that these problems were of much greater magnitude to the old in general than they had been to themselves personally. Only one-sixth (17 percent) had experienced not having enough money to live on as a serious problem, yet half of the respondents believed that not having enough money was a problem for older people in general. Only one-fifth (21 percent) had been troubled by poor health, yet 40 percent believed that it was a problem in general for old people. Only 13 percent felt that loneliness was a problem for themselves, whereas 45 percent said that they believed most older people suffered from loneliness. And only 25 percent were concerned about crime, though 58 percent felt it was a general problem for the elderly. The respondents' concern about not having enough education (6 percent), job opportunities (6 percent), and medical care (9 percent) fell far below the public's beliefs, while 17 percent, 24 percent, and 34 percent, respectively, said that these were problems for the elderly in general.

In short, the negative image of aging is shared by young and old alike, and it persists among older people despite their own experience to the contrary.

The participants in the Long Careers Study affirm the results of the Harris studies; if anything, the study group conforms even less to the stereotyped images. All of them, at the time of their interviews, were actively engaged with life and were not pessimistic about being older; three-quarters of them felt that growing older was a positive experience. Their time was filled with activities—work, relationships, family, hobbies—just as are the lives of younger adults.

By and large the Long Careers Study participants did not fit any of the negative stereotypes of aging. They were not self-centered, moody or irritable, rigid, abrasive, or consumed with fears. They behaved and operated like normal adults, with little intrusion of any effects of their chronological age into their activities or their relationships.

All of the participants were financially stable, though within a very broad range. Their incomes ranged from Social Security benefits supplemented by money earned from their work; through middle- and upper-middle-class incomes; to substantial wealth, whether earned or inherited.

The widespread negative stereotypes of aging were well known to the interviewees, and some were consequently wary about participating in the study. Two women who were invited refused to take part in the study specifically because doing so would identify them as being over sixty-five—even though they were both publicly known to be past that age anyway. Three of the women who did agree to take part in the study refused, politely but firmly, to tell me their ages because they felt it would hurt them professionally—even if the information was already available in published sources.

Despite this wide awareness of our negative image of "old age," only one-fifth of the study participants said that they had had personal experience with age discrimination. However, well over a third said they had experienced other kinds of discrimination (gender, racial, or religious). And eight out of ten firmly believed that mandatory retirement is a form of age discrimination.

In general, the study participants did not seem to be concerned about being alone or lonely. They had accumulated a lifetime of well-used friendship networks. Although they had lost or grown out of touch with some friends along the way, they had also acquired new ones, so that their address books generally had gotten fuller as the years passed.

Their families also had grown. Most participants had children and grandchildren, and some had great-grandchildren as well. Those who didn't have children themselves had networks of other family members and friends. Samuel Allen Williams, the ninety-two-year-old Chicago stockbroker, has no children but does have large numbers of nieces, nephews, grandnieces, and grandnephews. Judge Lucy Somerville Howorth, a ninety-five-year-old lawyer in Cleveland, Mississippi, likewise has no children but has maintained a huge friendship network that stretches throughout the country.

Although they were not lonely, a number of the interviewees did mention that they had found it difficult to lose friends and family members through death. It was an experience that all found painful, and it is very common in long-lived populations. Losing a spouse, parent, relative, or friend of many years' standing late in life can be profoundly disturbing. Many years of shared experiences and affections are lost, and the person left behind feels cut off from a large segment of his or her personal past.

AN ORIENTATION TOWARD THE
PRESENT AND THE FUTURE

The people in the study were not absorbed with the past but with the present and the future. For example, despite their age, many of the participants did not view their careers as complete: only 63.3 percent said they felt they had accomplished to a great extent what they intended to do. Some of them, in fact, thought about the past so infrequently that it was hard to direct their attention to it long enough to interview them.

Mrs. Sayra Lebenthal—who at the time of our interview was ninety and still chairman of the bond firm, Lebenthal and Company, that she and her husband founded in 1926—was so little focused on the past that she became impatient with the standard interview questions I asked about her childhood. "I'm thinking about bonds that will come due in 2026," she reminded me. "That's what's important to me—the future! I don't have time to think about the past!"

The negative images we harbor of the older years of life are a tremendously destructive influence. Even so, this wide disparity between the stereotypes of old age and the reality became one of the most important, and one of the most hopeful, features of the Long Careers Study. The stereotypes present us with an extremely narrow and constrained view of human possibilities. But the experiences of the study participants should reassure us that these standards are certainly not iron-clad models, and that even in an atmosphere where they are widely accepted they do not dictate what we can accomplish.

PART II

THE PATTERNS OF LONG CAREERS

A typology is a kind of metaphor; it is the analysis of the different patterns in a group and the naming of those patterns. We use a typology to understand an unfamiliar phenomenon by comparing it with a familiar one. To a degree, all typologies are suits of secondhand clothing: they communicate meaning by draping new ideas on a familiar frame, and they always fit well in some respects and poorly in others. The jacket may hang perfectly, but the trousers may be too short.

This useful but imperfect fit is true of the typologies I have chosen to describe the career patterns of the long-lived adults from the Long Careers Study. The image of the frontier is characteristically American, and I have drawn on it freely. But in our age, the frontier is not a real place; it is a part of history, a well-loved cliché. The original frontier vanished long before our time; now its mythical prairies and forests have become the assets of agribusiness companies, the sites of populous suburbs, and the seedbeds for edge cities that spring from the soil like settlements from outer space, miles from any other habitation.

What confronts us now instead is a frontier in time and personal experience. In surpassing the fifty-year life span we have entered unknown territory. We do not know what it will be like to inhabit a society in which large numbers of people have accumulated three-quarters of a century or more of life experience. The Long Careers Study participants and their agemates throughout our society are the vanguard, the settlers of this unfamiliar and unexpected new stage of life.

6

The Homesteaders

Forty-eight (roughly one-third) of the Long Careers Study participants had a career pattern in which they remained in the same job or profession, and in some cases in the same organization or company, for their entire working lives. Like the homesteaders in the American West, who chose a piece of land, tilled it, and made it produce, these people selected what they wanted to do early in life and stayed with it.

LIVING THE AMERICAN IDEAL

The Homesteaders are interesting because they have lived out a pattern that until the 1960s was the American ideal. During the first two-thirds of this century, it was assumed that a young person, whether a professional or a factory worker, would start work in a particular company or field around the age of twenty-one and remain there for the rest of his or her life. Work was expected to be a single track down which the individual traveled.

"When I was growing up, stability in a job was a great virtue," said Horace Deets, executive director of the American Association of Retired Persons. "My father spent forty-one years in the same workplace. He wasn't doing the same thing; he went in as an apprentice in the Charleston Naval Shipyard in the electric shop and he retired as the director of the electronics shop. He was the top manager. He had five or six hundred people working for him and he was in charge of all the electronic installations and repairs for the Sixth Naval District."

"He never missed a day because of sickness," Deets continued. "He had all of his sick leave accumulated. Just an amazing thing. It wasn't that he never had an illness or a legitimate reason for staying home, it was just that he didn't do it."

This mystique was particularly compelling for those who went into the business or corporate world, assuming a role of service to a larger, paternalistic organization. The young man who began his working life in the mail room and rose to be company president was part of the banquet of legends on which generations of Americans nourished their dreams.

Behind the myth lay a number of key assumptions about the relationship of employee to employer and about the basic values ruling the workplace. Loyalty was a primary consideration, and it meant sticking with something once you had started it, staying with the company once you had signed on, seeing things through. The myth whispered seductively that the company would take care of its own. Good work and devotion would be rewarded; talent would inevitably rise to the top, like the thick layer of cream in an old-fashioned glass milk bottle.

These beliefs were so strong that looking for another job when you already had one was often regarded as disloyal; if your job search became known to your boss, it could be grounds for being dismissed. At the very least it might bring criticism both from co-workers and friends. The practice of staying with one job may have foreclosed other opportunities. But in the aftermath of the Great Depression when so many men lost their jobs and so many family fortunes crumbled, this mutual contract of loyalty was valuable to employee and employer alike for the security it provided.

The reality was that many working men in the early part of this century did stay with the same company pretty much for the duration of their careers. And some people did rise to the top of their divisions or organizations, although not all those who worked hard and were loyal succeeded to the degree that they hoped.

Contemporary patterns of work have evolved quite differently. Beginning in the 1960s, expansion and shifts in the economy began to exert pressure on workers, moving them toward a change in career patterns. An expanding economy meant that growing companies needed more employees. The logical place to get these people was from other companies, by offering incentives tempting enough so that people could be lured into turning away from their loyalty to their current employer.

It was a break made, however, for an ostensibly good motive, one consistent with the most compelling American value: the drive for growth and progress. Moreover, Americans in the 1960s felt that they were engaged in a war, albeit a cold one. The launching of the first satellite by the Russians in 1957 pushed the U.S. into a race for technological achievement. The competition was vital: the future of the nation seemed to depend upon the outcome of industry's efforts. Securing the best workers, even if you had to get them from other companies, was in the national interest.

In the aftermath of the 1960s, we moved so far from those earlier ideas of job stability and employee loyalty that many of our subsequent values became their direct opposites. Frequent moves became synonymous with advancement and upward mobility. The notion became widespread that everyone should change jobs periodically—every five years and every ten years are the two intervals most frequently cited. Staying in one place too long was believed to invite "burnout," a failure of creativity that resulted in the carrier's becoming "deadwood" before his or her time. Remaining in one job or career for an entire lifetime came to be regarded as outmoded, dull, even dangerous.

This trend, in turn, has begun to disintegrate in the economic recession of the 1990s. As companies relocate or close, as more and more jobs are eliminated each year, employees whose lives were once secure find themselves out of work and unable to find a job equal to the one they lost. We have come full circle—from the ideal of one job or career; to the ideal of the upwardly mobile corporate nomad; and back once again to the longing for stability.

DEEPLY ENGAGED AND CREATIVE

Two things are especially intriguing about the Homesteaders in the Long Careers Study. The first is that although they stayed in the same field all their lives, contrary to the mythology of the 1970s and 1980s they are resolutely and vigorously not dull, outmoded, or burned out. They are still deeply engaged by what they do. The Homesteaders have remained in the same field all their lives precisely because they were not bored. They loved and were endlessly fascinated by the work they had chosen. None of the people in this category felt that they had exhausted their possibilities for growth in what they were doing, despite the length of time they had spent in it. In fact, many of them told me that they felt they had not had enough time in their field, although they had already spent a lifetime engaged in it.

This satisfaction with their work did not appear to be unrealistic nor smug. When the Homesteaders talked at some length about their work, they also discussed the difficulties they had confronted. They are realists; no fairy godmother hit them on the head with her wand to make their work easy in every respect all of the time.

The second characteristic of the Homesteaders is that the majority of those in the Long Careers Study did not build their careers in corporations or institutions. More than half (twenty-nine out of forty-eight) of the Homesteaders were creative artists or scientists; twelve were institution builders—businessmen, entrepreneurs, publishers; and the remaining seven were highly oriented toward interaction with other people as part of their work (to use a colloquial phrase, they were "people people"). Many of the Homesteaders in the first two clusters also had an affinity for human contact and found this a professional as well as a personal asset.

Because mandatory retirement rules have forced retirement on most corporate and industrial employees by the age of sixty-five, and because the study focused on people over sixty-five who were still working, it is not surprising that most of the people I located did not have careers in such settings. Some of the participants who worked in corporations did get caught by mandatory retirement rules. As a result, they were compelled to change jobs or careers. They went out and found new careers for themselves in other organizations, often nonprofit, and in volunteer work. For most, the change was substantial enough to place them in another category of career pattern.

EARLY CAREER CHOICES

About one-quarter (twelve) of the Homesteaders group had powerful childhood experiences of being deeply fascinated by a particular occupation, or of feeling "called" to one type of work. These Homesteaders went on to develop careers based on their early aspirations. This was not true for the other career patterns.

The earliest career recognition in the study was that of Celeste Holm, who decided what she wanted to do at the age of two and a half, when her grandmother took her to the theater for the first time. She had not been told where they would be going that day, and when they entered the theater, she was surprised by the sight of the audience—more people than she had ever before seen in one huge space, all sitting quietly in rows, with very formal, closed faces. When the curtain rose, it was on a performance by Anna Pavlova, the most famous ballerina of her time.

It was, Holm recalls, sheer magic. She loved every second. But even more astonishing than the beauty of the dance itself was that when the performance was finished, Holm saw that the appearance and behavior of the audience had completely changed; their faces were alive with feeling, and they were laughing and talking among themselves with great animation. Their cold formality had vanished; it was as if everyone had been transformed. Holm decided on the spot that she wanted to be able to do that for people, and announced to her mother that she would like to take ballet. Her dance training later opened a door for her into the theater, where she became enormously successful, playing Ado Annie in the first production of *Oklahoma!* and then going on to numerous movie, stage, and television roles.

Another creative Homesteader, artist Françoise Gilot, realized at the age of five that she wanted to be a painter. Gilot's maternal grandmother was a very cultivated woman who knew a number of artists and had Françoise's portrait painted when the child was quite young. This gave Gilot a chance early in life to see firsthand what artists did; she was curious, fascinated, and excited by the experience and thought about it a great deal. On New Year's Day following her fifth birthday, Gilot woke up with a powerful sense of resolution: she knew that she wanted to be a painter. She told her grandmother about it and was immediately enrolled for her first drawing lesson.

Several of the Homesteader physicians who recognized their vocations early in life had family losses in childhood. For example, Dr. William Cahan, a well-known New York chest surgeon, was about fourteen when his beloved grandmother died in his arms of a heart attack on the front porch of their summer home. She had driven down to the New Jersey shore on an extremely hot day to visit her son and his family, and she collapsed upon arrival as she was getting out of the carriage. Cahan felt that if a doctor had been present at the time, she could have been saved, and he made up his mind that he would become a doctor so he could save the lives of other people.

Eda LeShan, the well-known child psychologist, grew up in a family where enlightened childcare was considered extremely important. LeShan's mother worked in one of the nation's first parent education programs; her father was originally a grade-school teacher. An involvement in psychology and in child development came naturally to her, because it surrounded her at home. She never thought of doing anything else. "Basically it was a very happy childhood," she said. It enabled her later to explore childhood issues very deeply and develop a tremendous resonance with children, a great gift as a therapist.

A few of the Homesteaders had childhood aspirations that were different from their subsequent careers. Retail magnate Milton Petrie wanted to be a baseball player (as did J. Peter Grace, discussed in the following section). Petrie, whose company is one of the most successful in the United States, was born into a family that always had to struggle to make ends meet. He was fascinated by baseball, but he also had a determination to make enough money so that he would never have to struggle again. When he was in high school his older sister got a job in the advertising department of a local department store. Petrie followed suit, and a few years later, during the Depression, he was able to open a store of his own. Now one of the wealthiest men in the United States, he owns a chain of more than sixteen hundred Petrie Stores nationwide and has become famous for his philanthropy.

FOUR CLUSTERS OF HOMESTEADERS

The Homesteaders further divided into four distinct clusters: artists, physicians and scientists, institution builders, and people-oriented Homesteaders. The largest of these clusters is the creative artists and scientists—people who are dominated by a strong inner drive that is the central motivation of their work life. Painters, writers, actors, dancers, musicians, and scientists are all engaged in the difficult task of creating things that did not exist before, using their own mental and physical resources. Although the fields in which they work are different, the process itself has many similarities. It has been widely recognized that people in a few career areas—particularly physicians and creative artists—have a tendency to stay in the same area of work for a lifetime, often a very long lifetime. Orchestra conductors, concert musicians, painters, and sculptors are particularly famous for their longevity in their professions. The great Renaissance artist Michelangelo, for example, lived to be eighty-eight and continued working to the very end of his life, producing some of his greatest work in his last years.

There are a couple of factors that distinguish the second group of Homesteaders, the institution builders, from the third group. One factor concerns interaction. The third cluster of seven Homesteaders, all women, were "people people," oriented essentially toward interaction with others rather than toward ideas, theories, or systems. They enjoyed working in fields that involved a great variety of individual human contact. Some of these people-oriented Homesteaders started organizations through which they developed their work; but the emphasis of their careers was always on people, not on institutions. Another factor that distinguishes them from the institution-building Homesteaders is the size and scope of the organizations founded. The organizations begun by the people-oriented Homesteaders tended to remain small and to be essentially an extension of the founder's identity; whereas the institution builders created organizations that grew exponentially and acquired an identity larger than, and separate from, the identity of the founder.

The similarities of patterns among the Homesteaders can be seen from comparing their life histories. I will include here examples of the different types of Homesteaders: artists, physicians and scientists, institution builders, and people people. The activities they engage in are vastly different from each other, but as you will see, there are underlying similarities in the development of each career.

ARTISTS

ISAAC ASIMOV

The great science fiction writer Isaac Asimov was a Homesteader who found his major interest very early in his life. It took the form of a strong, continuous drive: he passionately loved books and reading. Beginning when Asimov was about six, his father would take him to the public library once a week. On each visit Isaac was allowed to take out three books—two nonfiction and only one fiction. It was, of course, the fiction book that Asimov wanted most, and which he would read immediately in one great gulp. Then he was left with no other fiction book for the rest of the week.

Asimov's account of how he tried to resolve this problem was delightfully funny. Although it did not come through often in his fiction, Asimov had a gift for humor equal to any of the world's best stand-up comedians.

First, he said, he decided he would copy the week's fiction book. That way, he could keep it, and eventually he'd have a lot of them. But he soon had a further insight; as he put it, "My hand might fall off before I could finish the copy." He pondered this and came up with another solution: he could write a story himself. Enthusiastic, he plunged into the project. But he was too impatient to finish the stories he started, so for years he would begin stories and leave them unfinished in his eagerness to get on to the next story.

In the meantime he discovered a second solution for his reading problem: a monthly called *Science Wonder Stories*, which he found on the magazine rack in his father's candy store. The senior Asimov thought fiction was a waste of time, but Isaac was able to persuade his father that *Science Wonder Stories* was really about science. "My father thought awhile," Asimov said, "and he knew that science was nutritious." From that point, at about the age of nine, he read every science fiction magazine that came through the store.

At seventeen, Asimov decided to actually finish one of his short stories. At his father's urging he took it to a magazine to see whether they would buy it. The editor of *Astounding Science Fiction,* John Campbell, liked Asimov, and although he did not buy that story, he eventually bought another one. Asimov's career was launched.

It was not immediately clear, however, that Asimov would be successful as a science fiction writer or would be able to build his entire career in the field. Between the ages of twenty-one and thirty, he earned a Ph.D. in physics from Columbia University. He delayed the publication of his first science fiction book until after his dissertation was accepted because he was afraid that if his professors knew, they would consider him flakey.

Once Asimov had achieved enough fame and financial security to choose his own lifestyle, he simply stayed in Manhattan and wrote all the time. Paradoxically, for a man who roamed the entire universe in his imagination, Asimov hated to travel and couldn't stand flying. In his mind he could soar through distant galaxies and other universes; in his body, however, just the idea of a plane ride evoked discomfort, which he inflated into funny stories for his friends.

The diligence with which Asimov had invested himself as a writer marked his earlier career. By the time he died at the age of seventy-two in April 1992, Asimov had published 520 books and an immense number of short stories. He had branched out from science fiction to numerous other subjects, such as in *Asimov's Guide to the Bible* and *Asimov's Guide to Shakespeare.* "You know," he had said in his interview, "these later years, what am I going to talk about? It's just: and then I wrote; and then I wrote; and then I wrote."

JESSICA TANDY

Actress Jessica Tandy is known around the world for her remarkable portrayals of older women: from her Oscar-winning Daisy Werthan in *Driving Miss Daisy* to her Oscar-nominated Ninny Threadegoode, who taught Kathy Bates to find joy in life in *Fried Green Tomatoes.* Although Tandy's talent may have received worldwide recognition only in the last decade, she has been a successful working actress since age eighteen.

Born in London in 1909, Jessica Tandy always wanted to be an actress; her first performance was at age five, in an operetta directed by her older brother and staged in the family living room. Her mother encouraged her interest in acting and took a second job at a night school to pay for Tandy's training at an acting academy. Tandy got her first professional role at the Birmingham Repertory in 1928, playing Gladys in *The Comedy of Good and Evil.* Since then, she has appeared in a staggering number of plays, movies, and television programs and has repeatedly been honored by awards, including the Kennedy Center's Lifetime Achievement Award.

One of the great talents of the theatrical world for many

years, Tandy has found most success in portraying older women who are dealing with aging. Onstage in *The Gin Game* and *Foxfire* (her costar in both plays was her husband, Hume Cronyn) Tandy played women facing not only their own aging but their spouses' as well. In the film *Cocoon,* Tandy and Cronyn teamed up again to play an aging couple given the gift of renewed youth.

If Cronyn and Tandy have found the fountain of youth, both agree that for them it is their work. "There was never any question of [retirement]," says Tandy. "I was working full-tilt. It never crossed my mind, and still doesn't. Except that I hope that I will stop before somebody tells me I should because I am not giving full measure. I think you get back what you put into life."

In her recent film roles, Tandy has played older women who are alone and coping as best they can with their loneliness. She endows these characters with a magical combination of strength and vulnerability, which gives them tremendous dignity and poignancy. And she always brings her trademark twinkle to the eyes of all her characters. Those who have seen her in these films have had a rare opportunity to witness the experience of aging on a personal level.

WILL BARNET

Like Asimov, painter Will Barnet loved to read and remembers from early childhood going to the library in his hometown of Beverly, Massachusetts. But for Barnet it was not the text but the illustrations that particularly enthralled him. At the age of six, Barnet happened to pick up a book with fantastic, wonderfully colored drawings. He was enchanted by these illustrations and said to himself, "That's what I want to do."

With unusual determination for someone so young, he set about shaping his education so that he could become an artist. His parents had very little money and knew nothing about art, although they gave him unquestioning emotional support. At fifteen he applied for and received a fellowship to the School of Fine Arts at the Boston Museum, where he began his formal artistic training and completed his high school degree.

Three years later, feeling that he had learned everything he could in Boston, he applied for and received a fellowship to the Art Students League in New York City. He earned money in a variety of ways to supplement his fellowship: he drew cartoons for *The New Yorker,* worked as a librarian, and did lithograph printing, in which he decided to build a career. He was hired by the league as the school's printer and within two years became the youngest instructor in the league's history.

Most of his work consisted of oil paintings. But in 1939, he did a woodcut called "Early Morning" which was one of his most important prints of the period. "That was the beginning of the development of my work towards a more abstract concept," explains Barnet. "I was always seeking to break away, to become more contemporary on the way I handled my language and form. So 'Early Morning' became a symbol."

During World War II, Barnet was not drafted because he had three young children, but he was recruited to work at a lithograph company, printing secret war documents at night while continuing to teach during the day. When the war ended, veterans flooded his classroom, and Barnet began to shape a new generation of artists. Throughout his career Barnet has served as an important mentor to younger artists, encouraging their experimentations and the development of their personal styles. Many of his students have gone on to achieve world fame.

Barnet continued to work both in oils and in printing, combining abstract concepts and symbols with figurative forms. He called his own unique style "figurative abstraction." By the 1960s, he had achieved recognition within the art world as one of the most accomplished contemporary painters. In the 1970s he became more widely known, through a renaissance in prints that highlighted his striking and beautiful style. Since then, he has had major exhibitions in museums across the country. In his early eighties, Barnet has been at the peak of his powers for many years. His work has grown simpler and more richly evocative as he has matured. It conveys a sense of profound mystery. For painters, Barnet says, "maturity is more important than being young. . . . If you study the history of art, you will find the greatest painters were those who were trying to understand their language and develop it as they grew older. That's what it's all about. Maturing and then letting it flourish into a wonderful painting."

FRANCES WHITNEY

A year younger than Will Barnet, Frances Whitney followed a very different route to becoming an artist. Brought up in a well-to-do family, she was educated to be a wife and mother, although her drive toward creative expression was clearly unusual even in childhood. In her teens she began making hats that were really art forms, including, in 1946, a group of Millinery Mobiles—circles of fabric cut into spiral curls and suspended delicately over the wearer's head. In an interesting synchronicity, the shapes that she devised were similar to those later adopted by Alexander Calder; eventually she met Calder and they became friends.

For the next ten years Whitney worked in the fashion industry adapting her patented designs to the mass market, and exhibiting in many prestigious institutions, including the Metropolitan Museum.

Her career was interrupted for several years by a bout with tuberculosis, which also helped break up her marriage. When she recovered, she gradually abandoned the pretense of fashion design. "I went from hats to sculpture," she said, "because the millinery people didn't want to buy the hats. So I thought, okay, if they don't want to buy the hats, I'll make them out of silver and gold and put them on the dining room table." She expanded to larger forms, then invented a series of jewelry shapes which she called "body sculpture," and eventually began combining large pieces of sculpture with the effects of varying types of light.

In her Soho loft, she has devised an innovative technique for creating an art work using sculpture, a laser, and computerized video equipment. Taking one of her pieces of sculpture as a model, she draws with the laser beam onto a digitizer tablet. The drawing is taken by the computers, scanners, and synthesizers, and electronically changed from a light wave into a sound wave. Then the drawing is projected by the laser back onto the sculpture, accompanied by the sound. At that point Whitney adds video feedback, which superimposes a whole performance onto the original sculpture. The result is a pulsing, swirling ballet of red light, alternately caressing and assaulting the monumental bronze shape whose form helped create it. It is a stunning combination of a conventional art form with the most up-to-date space-age technology. She has had shows in several major galleries recently, including one in New Haven, and more are planned for the future.

Whitney is a Homesteader who did not know what her real career was and had to find it, slowly and painfully, in her thirties and forties. Because sculpture was not a conventional career choice for a woman, and there was little contact with art in her family, her search was probably made longer and more intricate. Now a fully developed artist in her early eighties, she has made up for lost time by choosing a medium so technologically advanced that she has moved beyond many artists young enough to be her grandchildren.

PHYSICIANS AND SCIENTISTS

DR. IRVING WRIGHT

Even as a Boy Scout, Irving Wright was most interested in first aid. He always wanted to be a doctor; "I can't remember ever wanting to be anything else," he recalled. For sixty-six years, Dr. Wright has been active in his cherished profession. Although he has shifted his role as he grew older, at ninety-two he is still professionally active.

Born in New York City in 1901, Wright graduated from Cornell University Medical School in 1926. He became a professor of clinical medicine and later director of the Department of Medicine at Columbia University. In 1946, he was appointed to New York Hospital–Cornell Medical Center as clinical professor of medicine and attending physician. He has remained in that position up to the present, becoming emeritus in 1968.

Wright established a private practice as an internist and cardiologist, maintaining it for many years. But he also made outstanding contributions in medical research and geriatrics and in the organization of several important medical associations, among them the American Heart Association.

Although it has not been widely recognized, Wright's most outstanding innovation was one that has been instrumental in saving literally millions of lives, especially those of older people: he was the first physician to use anticoagulants in a human patient, in 1938. This work formed a base for all subsequent use of anticoagulants to dissolve blood clots and thromboses, as well as to minimize damage from heart attacks. And it made possible the later development of fine surgical technologies that depend upon the blood's remaining liquid when exposed to air: open-heart surgery, arterial bypasses, organ transplants, kidney dialysis, and knee and hip replacements. The implications of this one discovery are staggering, for these surgical procedures have been responsible for either saving or improving the lives of countless numbers of people throughout the world.

Wright had learned about the anticoagulant heparin from Dr. Charles Best, the Canadian physician who purified it; at that point he had tested it in animals but not in humans. Heparin was originally derived from a type of rat poison, but Best immediately saw its capacity to prevent blood clotting as an extremely important medical tool.

One day in 1938 Wright was consulted by a patient named Arthur Schulte who had severe thrombitis; his circulatory system was filled with clots and he was failing rapidly. In desperation, Wright called Dr. Best, who flew down to New York with the world's supply of heparin in his jacket pocket. Wright administered the drug by injection, guessing at the amount because it had never been used before. Then he stayed at Schulte's bedside for sixteen days to monitor his progress. Schulte recovered; he is still alive, in his eighties, as this book is being written, and he has been on anticoagulants ever since that period in 1938. He has been the beneficiary of more than fifty extra years of life because of Wright's passion for saving lives.

Dr. Wright continued to see patients until age seventy-eight. "I didn't want to retire altogether. Life would have been too boring and it would have been a waste of my life's experience," he explains. He began to spend more time on a hobby, archaeology, which has taken him to sites around the world to investigate ancient cultures. At ninety-two, his eyesight is problematic, but he still lectures to students at Cornell, conducts grand rounds, and is tape recording his recollections of twentieth-century medical history for Cornell's archives.

About his future Wright says: "I would like to have a very comfortable chair facing a very large screen where I could see all of the things that the human race will do in the next twenty-five years. And just think about the direction the world is going. My curiosity is so great that I do not want to die without being able to follow the future."

Wright is extremely aware of what the longevity factor has meant for his career and his life. "Looking back, I wonder how I was able to accomplish so many interesting aspects of life," he said. "I suppose in part it is because I have been granted so many extra years. When I started to practice medicine, the average life expectancy was forty-seven years. Now it's seventy-four years—and I've gone beyond that by almost two decades!"

DR. ALAN COTT

Dr. Alan Cott, one of the first medical doctors to become involved in nutritional (orthomolecular) medicine in the 1950s, similarly became interested in his field when he was quite young. The youngest of a family of twelve children, he was born in 1912. He learned very early on that several of his brothers and sisters were "missing"—apparently they had died. He felt intense grief over their absence, and great curiosity about what had happened to them. As was characteristic of many families in the early 1900s, death, illness, and birth were never discussed. Cott never found out the fate of his missing siblings, and his frustration pushed him toward an interest in medicine.

Cott began practicing medicine in 1936, after graduating from Case Western Reserve Medical School, at that time one of the last medical schools to train physicians in both allopathic and homeopathic medicine. He was licensed in both. An internship at Jersey City Medical Center convinced him that he didn't like surgery; he decided to become a psychiatrist instead.

Four years later, with the beginning of World War II, he served in Iran as a consulting psychiatrist to the Persian Gulf command.

On returning home in 1945 Cott became interested in psychoanalysis. He opened an office and spent seven years studying with the pioneering psychoanalyst Wilhelm Reich. Cott worked as a psychoanalyst himself for the next twenty-two years, during which time he became increasingly interested in orthomolecular medicine. "I remember that what I learned in medical school in a course called physiology was actually nutrition. That's what led me into thinking about checking up on these sick people, to see what they were eating," he recalled.

Cott's first breakthrough was his work with megavitamins in treatment of childhood schizophrenia and autism in 1965. At first, this new treatment met with resistance, even ridicule, among many other doctors. "When I began at the hospital treating patients with vitamins," Cott explained, "at first [the doctors] laughed. Then they began to see how many more nutritionally treated patients improved than the patients they were treating, and some of them came around."

Over the next twenty years Cott concentrated on orthomolecular psychiatry, the most substantial part of his practice being with autistic and schizophrenic children. During the early 1970s, after visiting the Moscow Psychiatric Institute as a lecturer and an observer, Cott heard of a fasting treatment for schizophrenia and soon adopted the treatment, with much success. Two years later, in 1974, he authored the widely successful *Fasting: The Ultimate Diet*.

Now retired and living in Miami, Cott looks back on his career feeling most proud of his ability to help others and make a positive difference in their lives. And he admits that, in his attempts to promote orthomolecular treatments, he needed the resolve to "handle the things they said about me."

DR. BARBARA MCCLINTOCK

It was over the radio that Dr. Barbara McClintock learned about winning the 1983 Nobel Prize for medicine. She had refused to have a telephone in her house because she wanted "to be free."

Born in Connecticut in 1902, McClintock insisted on playing with a real tool set as a child. She became fascinated with physics in high school and decided that she wanted to go to Cornell University, although they accepted few women in those days. In order to pursue her interest in chemistry and biology, McClintock, like Dr. Linus Pauling, had to apply to the agricultural college rather than the regular liberal arts school. Because of the practical need for biology and chemistry in agriculture, only these institutions early in the century had developed advanced programs for their study. McClintock was the only woman in the program, and a real maverick, cutting classes regularly to go ice skating, then passing exams with exceptional marks. She scandalized her classmates by bobbing her hair and having long trousers made for her fieldwork, and she got great satisfaction when the other Cornell women followed suit within a few days.

After receiving her Ph.D. in 1927, McClintock taught at several universities and won a series of fellowships to study abroad and participate in research projects. In 1941, she joined the staff of the Carnegie Institution, where she subsequently conducted all her prize-winning research. She remained affiliated with the institution until her death in 1992.

At Carnegie, McClintock began to explore and analyze the genetic structure of plants (cytogenetics) and soon became known as the foremost investigator in the field. She chose the maize plant as her study material, which later earned her the title of "Corn

Lady" in *Time* magazine. Her work yielded radical new information about the structure and activity of chromosomes and genes. Previously it had been held that chromosomes could not move around on the DNA strands; McClintock, however, proved that they not only could but that they do. She had a profound influence on a whole generation of geneticists and an enduring impact on the study of the evolution of species. Her discoveries remain at the very root of much of today's research in genetic engineering. She won dozens of awards and honorary degrees over the years, including the National Medal of Science. When she was eighty-one, McClintock finally received the international acclaim she long deserved, receiving within a short time both a MacArthur Prize Fellowship and the Nobel Prize.

An important aspect of McClintock's career is the degree to which her ideas and observations were ignored by the scientific community until her findings were ultimately proved correct. Her ability to disregard naysayers and persevere is a quality shared by many of the study participants. "I knew when I was working that what I was doing was not acceptable, that people's tacit assumptions would not allow what I was doing to be understood," McClintock remarked. "But you cannot work with something and have it tell you some very striking things about what was going on without knowing that sooner or later it would be found in other organisms. You have to know that sooner or later it will come out in the wash, but you may have to wait some time."

When asked if she had ever planned to retire, McClintock said, "I just had been so interested in what I was doing, and it's been such a deep pleasure, that I never thought of stopping and I never had a time when I didn't know what I wanted to do next. I can't wait to get to the laboratory in the morning and I just hate sleeping." Like so many of the participants, McClintock's work kept her energized and happy; she continued to work seven-day weeks, sometimes sixteen-hour days, up until four months before she died of natural causes on September 2, 1992.

DR. ROSALYN YALOW

Another Homesteader woman scientist, Dr. Rosalyn Yalow arrived at the same peak of distinction as Dr. McClintock—the award of a Nobel Prize—by a route that was virtually different in every respect. McClintock's father was a relatively prosperous attorney; Yalow grew up on the Lower East Side in a hard-working immigrant family. Her father had a paper and tiling business; Yalow remembers as a child helping her mother make collars for her uncle's neckwear firm to earn extra money.

McClintock knew early in life that she was interested in science. Yalow's earliest aspiration at age six was to be a school teacher, "like all Jewish girls. That's what I was told to be." Her interests shifted to science in high school, because she had a terrific math teacher who thought she was special. In college, she was drawn to physics; she worked her way through Hunter with a part-time job as a secretary. She couldn't afford to go to graduate school unaided, and her teachers doubted she could get a graduate assistantship in physics because she was a woman. But through a combination of talent and good luck she got one anyway. "When I got my graduate assistantship, I tore up my steno books," she said, obviously still relishing the victory.

After receiving her M.A. and Ph.D. in nuclear physics from the University of Illlinois in 1945, she took a job as an electrical engineer at ITT. She did not like working in industry, however, and returned to Hunter to teach physcis. In 1947 she joined the Bronx Veterans' Administration Medical Center to explore the use of radiation in biomedical research, and developed the process or radioimmunoassay, a diagnostic technique now used in thousands of laboratories around the world to measure biological substances in blood and other body fluids. In addition to the Nobel Prize, in 1988 she won the National Medal of Science.

McClintock never married, feeling that she could not maintain her intellectual independence and her career if she did so. Yalow married very happily, had a family, and continued her career with the full support of her husband.

In 1992, Yalow stepped down from full-time work at the VA Medical Center to pursue what she calls a "separate mission." She has chosen to take on a broader role, becoming a national spokesman for the Radiation Society to help confront public fears about radiation and nuclear power.

INSTITUTION BUILDERS

J. PETER GRACE

Corporate Homesteader J. Peter Grace, chairman of W.R. Grace and Company, was for many years the longest-standing chief executive officer of a U.S. corporation until his retirement in 1992 because he had contracted cancer.

Grace was born into the family that founded his company (at that time simply a steamship firm), and he was given to understand early on that he would be expected to go into the company eventually.

Born in Manhasset, Long Island, on May 25, 1913, Grace lived there until the age of twelve, when he was sent away to boarding school. As with Milton Petrie, Grace's childhood passion was for sports, although he knew it was unlikely that he would be permitted to choose baseball as a career. Joining the Grace line wasn't entirely to his liking, however, because at the time "you had to live twenty years in South America to get anywhere in the company," and he already knew he didn't want to do that. But after his mother died he relented because of his father's grief, and he signed on with Grace and Company in October 1936.

At the time, even the son of the president started from the ground up. Grace told how he spent the first two or three years of his tenure in the mail room as an errand boy, carrying things around to people and being a "total clock-watcher." This changed when he was promoted to the next step, in the accounting department, a decidedly more substantive area. From accounting, Grace then spent six years as an assistant to a succession of top officials in the company.

There were two interludes in his early career. One was the dreaded stay in South America, which turned out to be brief because Grace developed stomach ulcers and had to return to the states. The second interruption was provided by World War II. Like many young men of his time, Grace was eager to enlist, and he did so the day after Pearl Harbor. But ultimately, wartime demands on the shipping industry got him reluctantly reassigned back to his own company for the duration of the war. After his father became ill, Grace was made the company's chief executive officer at the war's end and has remained in that position ever since.

An outspoken and energetic man, Grace has a fast-paced and highly condensed style. My interviews with him were interrupted by telephone calls, messages relayed through a secretary, scheduling adjustments, and requests for quick decisions from various officers of the company. He responded rapidly and then just as swiftly picked up the flow of the interview again, moving back and forth from the 1930s to the 1980s without missing a breath or a beat. Physically, his appearance and bearing suggest that he is at least fifteen and perhaps twenty years younger than his real age of seventy-nine. Grace is sturdy and compact, shorter than the norm but exuding vitality; he appears to be in peak physical condition.

Grace shows no indication of slowing down after his fifty-two years with the firm. "In the first place," he noted, "I've done a lot of other things, like a lot of government work. I served Eisenhower in the White House; served Kennedy and Reagan. So I'd say that I had a lot of outside interests."

"Number two," he continued, W.R. Grace "is a very dynamic company that has completely changed its spots, so I'm not sitting running a company with a steel mill and doing the same thing every day. So I don't think you could burn out. . . . It's a very exciting company. Constant change all the time."

Grace believes that whether a person continues to be productive or not depends entirely on the person and has little to do with age. He cited a number of people he had known on the Grace and Company staff who had had long tenure without a diminution in effectiveness or enthusiasm—including one man who was employed by the company for sixty-two years and died in office.

On the other hand, Grace also feels that people can go stale very young. "Some people are old and tired at fifty-five, and some people are wild men at seventy-two," he said. "I think a lot of people *should* retire at fifty-five. They've lost interest; they're thinking about what they're going to do when they retire and they've already retired mentally. . . . I think that just as a general answer nothing can be run by rule books that have no exceptions. I think anytime you say that sixty-five is the time to retire [for everyone], it's crazy."

GERARD PIEL

Creator of one of America's most popular magazines, *Scientific American*, Gerard Piel grew up with a strong interest in natural history, which he abandoned in high school because of ill-informed teachers. A voracious reader, he discovered the theory of evolution as he read his way through his family's *Encyclopaedia Britannica*. But when he tried to talk about evolution in his biology class at the Jesuit high school he attended, the teacher promptly said, "Sit down, doughhead!" As a senior in high school, Piel was further turned off from science by a physics professor who presented physics as a mechanical, closed-ended subject. "This old duddy taught us physics out of a thin little green book, one of whose authors was named Dull," Piel recalled, wincing. By the time he reached college, Piel did everything he could to avoid science, managing to graduate without having taken a single science course. Nevertheless, this nonscientist would one day create the most popular science magazine in the world.

Born in 1915 in Woodmere, New York, Piel grew up in a hard-working Catholic family that had originally owned Piel's Brewery. His first career ambition was to be a journalist. He worked on school publications in high school and as an undergraduate at Harvard. After earning his B.A., Piel went to New York, where he worked on the first four (and only) issues of a magazine called *Picture*. His experience there taught him a great deal about starting a magazine, knowledge that he would later put to good use. With his new professional experience, he won a position as an office boy at *Life* magazine, which he idolized. There Piel became an expert on finding photographs, both old and new, and soon began writing his own stories.

Piel's ambition to cover the impending World War II was dashed when the managing editor of *Life*, who was not happy with the existing science department and wanted a fresh approach, appointed Piel as the new science editor, despite Piel's apparent lack of interest in the subject. The managing editor's argument to him was: "If you can learn about science and explain it to me, then maybe you and I together can explain it to our readers."

Piel found himself completely intrigued by science reporting. He became aware that "very interesting people were engaged in working on deeply interesting questions and that this was an ongoing, live enterprise of our civilization." Constrained by the Life format and the use of photographs he produced the first authentic coverage of science in a mass-circulation magazine. He soon discovered that scientists were his most enthusiastic readers. He gained the respect and trust of scientists by allowing them to review and correct the articles, insistent that with science, above all it is important to "get the facts right."

By the end of World War II, Piel decided it was time to start a magazine that would make it possible for scientists to keep abreast of fields outside their own—in sum a magazine of science for interested lay readers. With the help of two partners, Piel scraped together the financing needed to buy and relaunch an ailing scientific monthly in 1947. Using shrewd marketing tactics, frugal management, and fine writing, Piel and his partners were able to increase the circulation of the magazine to one hundred thousand by 1950. By 1959, they were finally making a healthy profit. Piel attributes the success of the magazine to its unique writing style. "Sans-serif black—that's how science was supposed to look. Well, we made it look like poetry and art."

Today, *Scientific American* is translated into more than ten foreign languages, including Russian, and has a worldwide circulation of over one million. With the magazine coming under new ownership in 1986 and his son, Jonathan, assuming its editorship Piel retired from publishing in 1988. He remains active on the company's advisory board. *Only One World: Our Own to Make and to Keep*, published in spring 1992, is the first fruit of his new labors, Piel's new work on behalf of the U. N. Environmental Decade. Continually looking forward and engaged in his work, Gerard Piel has no intentions of retiring in the near future.

PEOPLE-ORIENTED HOMESTEADERS

"MOTHER" CLARA HALE

Clara McBride Hale, the founder of the Hale House center for child care in New York City, grew up in Philadelphia. Hale's family background is extraordinary and moving. Her grandmother was a slave on a North Carolina plantation and was made pregnant at a very young age by the slavemaster. As a child, Hale's mother apparently resembled the slavemaster very strongly, and he loved her more than he did his other, white children. However, neither Hale's grandmother nor her mother could stand the man. His behavior to the other slaves on the plantation was dreadful, even though he treated mother and daughter well. When Hale's mother was about eight years old, Hale's grandmother simply told her former master she was leaving, and she took her child to Philadelphia. By this time the Civil War had been over for some years and slavery had been abolished, so she was legally free.

Hale's career choice in caring for children was a natural one. Her mother had taken care of other people's children in her home to earn money, and Hale helped her as soon as she was old enough to do so. Hale's father died when she was about two, and she said that she had no memory of him. Her mother supported the family, supplementing income from child care by cooking food and selling it at the nearby Philadelphia docks. Hale's childhood, she said, was "a great life."

Hale was extremely close to her mother and was devastated when she died, at the age of forty-four, when Hale was sixteen. Hale finished high school the next year, but because she was black and had no training the only job she could find was as a domestic. At twenty-two, she married Thomas Hale, a man she met while her mother was still alive. After several years, Hale moved the family to New York, got a job as a building super—which came with a rent-free apartment—and started taking in children again.

When Hale's husband, who had suffered from "indigestion" for some time, became ill and died of cancer at the age of thirty-seven, Hale simply kept going. She took in more children to make more money, and continued raising her own two children.

One day in 1969 her daughter, Lorraine, saw a woman with a baby sleeping on the stoop of a neighboring house. The woman was high on drugs, and Lorraine, afraid that the woman might drop the baby and injure it, gave her her mother's address and telephone number. The next day the woman showed up, handed the baby to Mother Hale, and left. Three weeks later, the woman returned, told Hale the baby's name, and left again! Eventually the woman returned and brought Hale her other two children as well, two boys who were "real house wreckers," Hale added with a chuckle. Hale helped the woman get her life together and as a result she was able to remarry and take the children back.

Word spread, and soon Hale had a new vocation: taking care of the children of women who were addicts. But she was paying for it from her own pocket, and there were clear limits to how many children could be accommodated. By this time, Lorraine Hale had completed her Ph.D. in early childhood development and began to work with her mother. Lorraine incorporated their work as a not-for-profit agency, applied for government funding, and Hale House was born. Since its opening, over eight hundred children have come through its doors.

Hale House continues to care for infants of addicted mothers, although Mother Clara Hale died in December 1992. At the time that I interviewed her, in March, 1991, Hale was surprisingly resilient for a slender and seemingly fragile woman in her late eighties. She moved easily and quickly, climbing the five flights to her top-floor bedroom in one of Hale House's brownstones with a nimbleness that left me puffing away several flights below her. She had a delicate beauty, quite striking, with a regal carriage and long, aristocratic hands that gestured gracefully as she talked.

Like the other Homesteaders, Hale genuinely loved what she did in her life. She had a quality that children soaked up like sunshine, and the way she related to them was both brilliant and totally matter-of-fact. Hale's manner and actions when she was with her charges seemed like the most natural thing in the world to the observer. Only if you were aware of the complexity of the task of relating to young children and forging a bond with so many of them would the true nature of her genius become apparent.

ELEANOR LAMBERT

Founder of the world-famous "best dressed" list, Eleanor Lambert has built an almost-sixty-year-long career as a publicist in the art and fashion worlds. Born in Crawfordsville, Indiana, in 1903, Lambert went to New York in the early 1930s hoping to obtain a job with a fashion publication, *The Breath of the Avenue.* It was one of the lowest points in the depression years, and the firm's owner was able to give her only half-time work. She found another half-time job at Franklin Spear, a firm that did publicity for book publishers.

Mr. Spear noticed that Eleanor had a talent for calling people on the telephone and drumming up business. After several months, he suggested that she go into business for herself, using his office space until she was prosperous enough to rent an office of her own. She chose art publicity to start with and soon had enough clients to take an office for herself. Later she became the first director of publicity for the Whitney Museum and represented artists like Jackson Pollock and George Bellows. Lambert was so successful in promoting her clients that she was then approached by several dress designers who wanted her to handle their publicity.

Lambert's work came to the attention of Henri Bendel, who was interested in finding new ways to promote the U.S. fashion industry during World War II. Lambert decided that what was needed was a focus on personalities and stories rather than patriotic billboards. She was familiar with a "best dressed" list generated in Paris annually by French couturiers, and when the French list was discontinued because of the war, she claimed the list as her own and imported it to the United States. In 1940, after tabulating more than one thousand questionnaires received from style experts worldwide, Lambert released her first "best dressed" list.

This list rapidly became and has remained the most telling arbiter of style internationally; a spot on the list is coveted by thousands of men and women around the world. In fact, Lambert says that she has often had to turn down bribes by husbands eager to get their wives either on or off the list, depending on their social standing at the time. She acknowledges that the keys to being nominated for the list are wealth and visibility. But the people who make the final list also must embody a remarkable sense of style. Since its inception, numerous women over sixty-five have appeared on the list, including such notables as Estee Lauder, Mrs W. Vincent Astor, Pauline Trigere, Carmel Snowe (former editor of *Harper's Bazaar*), Diana Vreeland (former editor of *Vogue*) and Gabrielle "Coco" Channel, who was on the list every year from 1957 until her death in 1971 at age eighty-eight.

With her characteristically practical approach to life, Lambert claims that the reason she has never retired is because she has needed the income to keep the apartment she loves. "I was a widow and I needed to go and earn a living," Lambert explains. "And I love this apartment—it was our home. I'm going to keep it as long as I live, and in order to keep it, I have to work. But I've had no regrets about that; I love working, and I love the life here, being able to travel a lot." It's clear that, at age eighty-nine, Eleanor Lambert still enjoys her work immensely. Constantly on the lookout for that elusive and powerful quality of style, she remains a dominant presence in the world of international fashion.

ELEANOR BURNS

Born in Connecticut in 1903, Elizabeth Burns was the youngest of nine children in a close-knit family; only four survived to adulthood. Her father's death when she was eight meant that Burns, along with her siblings, took on new responsibilities in order to ease their mother's burden. This proved an important lesson in self-reliance for Burns, who had previously found herself, as the youngest, a little "spoilt." It also helped lay the seeds for the fierce independence she developed as an adult.

At age seventeen, after graduating from high school, Burns went to work for a real estate and insurance office. "I knew I was going to have to work for a living so I very carefully did every commercial subject I could find." Thus when she graduated she had a "complete education of the current office procedures."

Burns held a series of secretarial positions in an assortment of offices before taking a job at Connecticut General Home Office, an insurance company. She was to spend the next forty-four and a half years at the office. During that time, Burns says she "honed all her knowledge." She explains further: "I became a good all-round office worker. You may have met my counterpart in your travels—namely, the steady, reliable gal who could, would, and did do anything and everything necessary to keep the office on an even keel, whether or not it was part of her job."

Even at age eighty-nine, Burns is very self-effacing about her working life. "There obviously is nothing spectacular or even outstanding about my working career," she says. "However, it was important because then that type of work was required to keep the business world running." The duties of the girl Friday have always been underrated. In the comparatively primitive offices of the early twentieth century, the job required many hours of tiresome stenciling and collating to make multiple copies of any document. Skill and patience obviously had to go hand in hand.

Burns never married nor had children, although it was originally expected that she would work briefly until she got married. She found instead that she valued her independence too highly. "I figured if I was going to have to work I might as well have my money to myself. My independence really was a factor. I liked it then and I still do," she says candidly.

Burns retired at age sixty-five because she felt an obligation to look after her ailing sister. However, she admits, "if I had a choice I probably would have kept working." Fifteen years later, Burns returned to the work force, taking a job in the Travelers Insurance Company Job Bank. Her enjoyment of her newfound position is obvious. "I haven't decided who's nuttier—yours truly for having the colossal nerve for having applied when they opened up the job bank in the fall of '85, or them for taking me," she says. Her skills have created a steady demand for her services. Making no mention of future retirement, she instead says cheerfully, "They allow us to work 960 hours [a year] and I have hit that or exceeded it every year."

SUMMARY

What conclusions can be drawn from the experience of the Homesteaders? First, there are particular personality traits involved in the identity of this group. The Homesteaders are self-starters, people who generate their own change. Because so many of them are "creatives," a strong internal drive is thus indicated. "I am always thinking about the next painting while I am finishing the current one," said Françoise Gilot. "It isn't the subject of the painting that's important, it's the artistic problem I'm trying to solve in it." For some, having internal drive meant rising to the top of their company; for others it meant creating their own company or institution. For yet others it meant developing the highest level of skill at what they did and exercising that skill continuously. Once you have found the type of work that fits your own personality, you can generate your own change within many different frameworks.

Second, the Homesteaders are relatively independent. Many of them were not subject to the restrictions of a larger organization. Artists, designers, physicians, psychologists, writers, scientists, and entrepreneurs all have or acquire a great deal of freedom. Once they become established, they can do what they do for the rest of their lives with relatively little interference from others and without the stress imposed by being part of a close-knit or hierarchical organization. When these participants worked within a larger organization, either the system was compatible or its intrusiveness was manageable. In fact, many of them ran their own organizations, so they had a substantial degree of control over their circumstances.

Some of the Homesteaders developed parallel activities after they became established. As head of Grace and Company, J. Peter Grace did a great deal of work for the federal government during the 1970s and 1980s, chairing a federal commission on waste in government spending and turning up some striking abuses that cost taxpayers millions of dollars (like the Pentagon's $439 hammer, bought for its hardware-store price of $71 with an enormous $361 featherbed of additional charges.) William Greenough, as chairman of TIAA-CREF, accepted membership on a government commission that revised the Social Security laws.

The Homesteaders chose work that, in addition to being personally compatible, contained a high degree of variety. Not all jobs are alike in the degree of intrinsic change they provide. Some have very little; some contain a flow of continuous change as part of the job itself. The physician or dentist who sees a constant stream of new and old patients; the sales job that requires interaction with a steady stream of new people on a day-to-day basis; the lawyer who takes a succession of cases, all different; the psychologist or teacher who confronts a new dynamic with each new client or class; the office worker who gets to perform a variety of functions in the course of his or her daily work—all these offer long-term possibilities if you like the work itself.

We have grown so accustomed to the idea that change in itself is progress that we have forgotten that change can be negative as well as positive, and that development-in-place can be progress as well. Moving from one job to another or from one company to another is not the only way to grow, it is just one way. And it is not necessarily the best way for everyone at any given moment. It is possible to hone old skills and develop new ones within the context of the same job or organization, if the fit between worker and workplace is right. Lateral moves within a company or the shifting of responsibilities within the same job can offer new opportunities without having to uproot a family, rebuild job and friendship networks, and take on the financial risks of a move.

In summary, the most obvious lesson to be learned from the Homesteaders is simply that if you like your work—if it provides you with constant interest and a flow of activity that you enjoy— then as long as you continue to like it and to be good at it, there is no reason why you should change. In the current atmosphere of corporate shrinkage, where opportunities for upward movement are fewer than they were just a few years ago, this is an important message.

7

The Transformers

"Deep in the heart of everyone in their forties and fifties," mused an executive who was interviewed early in the Long Careers Study, "dwells the longing to change what they do for something more satisfying."

The image most people have of career change seems to be similar to this one: a deep restlessness in one's work brought on by "midlife crisis," a phenomenon that became a recognized part of adult experience as new research in the 1960s and 1970s deciphered the stages of adult development.

The Homesteaders' example makes it clear that not everyone wants to change work in midlife. But a great many people apparently do go through a period of feeling that they would like to transform their careers if they could find a way to do so. Some have quite specific goals they would like to pursue; others are simply dissatisfied with their current job or profession and have a strong desire to leave it, without having much sense of the direction they want to take. However, there are probably many more people who believe they would like to change careers than who actually end up doing so.

Forty-one of the Long Careers Study participants followed their feelings that the grass might be greener somewhere else and made one major change in their primary occupation. To our surprise, however, these Transformers did not make their shifts primarily at midlife. Instead, they clustered into three age groups, changing course at early, middle, and late stages in their careers. Furthermore, the division among the three periods is about equal. Fourteen of the Transformers changed what they did early in their worklife, within three to four years after they began working; sixteen made a change in midlife, somewhere between the ages of thirty-five and fifty-five; and the last twelve changed after the age of sixty.

The Transformers are not the only ones who changed jobs. Their distinction is that they changed only once. The largest group of participants, the Explorers, who will be discussed in the following chapter, changed their work periodically throughout their lives.

EARLY TRANSFORMERS

The early Transformers started their worklives in one occupation and within a very short period of time abandoned it for something else. This process seemed to be part of the trial-and-error process that accompanies most career choices. Several of the early Transformers got their dream jobs and then discovered that the reality did not match their expectations. Two people went into their father's firms, but then left for something that they liked better. One woman trained to be a lawyer but married a man whose family was in the bond business, so she switched from law to bonds at his urging. One woman got married and started a model agency because she could do the work at home after her first child was born. And several people changed careers purely as a result of chance occurrences. The majority, eleven, of the early Transformers were men; three were women.

In their general career pattern the early Transformers are very similar to the Homesteaders, because after their early career shift they stayed in the new career for the rest of their lives. In a sense, they are Homesteaders who needed one intermediate step, an experience in the working world, in order to find the work that was right for them.

REV. NORMAN VINCENT PEALE

Rev. Norman Vincent Peale's first choice for his career was something very different from the field in which he has become famous. Peale wanted to be a journalist. He had been the associate editor of his college newspaper and found he liked the atmosphere and challenge of the newspaper business. After graduating from Ohio Wesleyan, he got jobs first at the Findley Ohio *Morning Republican,* then at the Detroit *Journal.* Writing fascinated him, and he worked hard at it.

Peale's decision to join the ministry was completely unexpected. In fact, Peale's father was a minister, and Peale emphatically wanted a different profession. Nevertheless, he began to be haunted by the feeling, which he could not escape, that he was supposed to be "a messenger of the 'Good News' instead of the daily news." He resisted this impulse mightily, and probably would have gone on resisting it for some time. But a powerful incident in his workday life helped to push him across the line.

"I was sent out to cover a fire in Detroit," Peale said. "I pushed up through the fire line and showed my pass. There was a big, burly sergeant of police in charge of the situation. Then we discovered that on the sixth floor there appeared a girl about twelve years old. They said that the one elevator was filled with fire and smoke, and she couldn't get out; the stairways were also not negotiable. But somebody had pushed a plank out about a foot wide and it reached to the other building, the one that was afire. She was frightened, so she resisted the urge to crawl out on the plank. It was only about six or eight feet that she had to crawl. And everybody urged her to begin crawling.

"I shouted out, 'Honey, do you believe in God?' And she nodded. And I said, 'Do you believe he is right there with you?' She nodded again. 'Well, then he will guide you across that plank. Don't look down but look straight ahead and think of God.' She got about halfway across; we could see that she hesitated; so I gave her a little speech like the first one. And she got across! Eager hands reached up and pulled her into the other building. And this sergeant said to me, 'Good job, boy. You ought to be a preacher.' I said, 'I'm no preacher; I'm a reporter.' 'The hell you're not!' he said.

"About six months later I left the newspaper business. I couldn't get it out of my mind. I was in an indecisive state, and a thing like that can determine it." Within a year, Peale went back to school to study theology.

Peale used his journalistic skill later, in ways that he could not have foreseen. After he became a minister in the Methodist church, people began asking him for copies of his sermons. In trying to fill these requests, his wife, Ruth Stafford Peale, discovered that Peale did not write out his sermons but simply spoke from notes. So they set about devising a system through which the sermons could be transcribed, printed, and distributed to the list of twelve thousand people who wanted them.

Later, encouraged by the response to the sermons, Peale began work on a book. Articulate and possessed of a deeply caring nature, Peale had nevertheless struggled for years against shyness and had devised his own systems to overcome it. He thought some of these techniques might be valuable for others, too. Peale was also struck by the nation's recovery from the Great Depression, a decade so terrible that it seemed no deliverance was possible.

When Peale finished *The Power of Positive Thinking,* he took it to a publisher, who told him it was no good and wouldn't sell more than ten thousand copies. Discouraged, Peale took the manuscript home and put it on a closet shelf. One day when Ruth Peale was cleaning closets she found it, read it, and came to ask him about it. "That is no good," he replied with irritation. "Put it in the wastebasket, and don't you dare take it out!" Ruth Peale did exactly as she was told. She put the manuscript directly into the wastebasket. Then she took the wastebasket, manuscript and all, to another publisher, who liked it immediately. *The Power of Positive Thinking* was published in 1952 and has sold millions of copies to date.

The Peales also started a magazine, *Guideposts,* and began their own publishing company built around inspirational publications. Ruth Peale is its chief executive officer, and it has been tremendously successful. The aspiring journalist ended up reaching millions of people in a way that he never expected. Seventy years after he made the decision to go into seminary, his influence is still spreading.

Peale strongly believes that older people need to remain active and creative. Partly for that reason, he never formally retired from his position at the Marble Collegiate Church. One summer the Peales talked about the possibility of his retirement and decided he would simply not preach there regularly after the summer was over—and that is what he did. Even now, in his nineties, Peale says he doesn't think about retiring, not only because he loves his work, but because working has been a lifelong habit. "I've never been one to look forward to vacations much," Peale explained. "I continue to work because I have worked ever since I was a young boy. It's part of me, my work is."

John Forsythe

As Blake Carrington on "Dynasty," John Forsythe drew attention to the most attractive qualities of older men, with his commanding portrayal of experience, power, and sex appeal. His success in this role came after many years of film and theater experience.

But acting was not Forsythe's first ambition or career. Somewhere in his teenage years, John Forsythe formed a dream: he wanted a career in sports broadcasting. His special love was play-by-play baseball announcing. He attended college at the University of North Carolina at Chapel Hill planning to major in writing, so that he could do sports writing as well as announcing. In his junior year, however, he dropped out of college because he was offered a wonderful opportunity: Cincinnatian Larry McPhale had just bought the Dodgers and had installed a public-address system at Ebbets Field, and an announcer was needed.

"They wanted someone who knew the game," Forsythe said, "and I knew it very well; someone who loved the game, made a good appearance, and could handle himself on a microphone." Through a friend who knew McPhale, Forsythe applied for the job and got it. He was good at it, and he blossomed in it. It was a dream realized.

But baseball announcing had one disadvantage Forsythe had not considered: it was only a summertime occupation! Very quickly he realized that in order to survive, he would have to have another job for the nine months of the year when baseball was not being played. A friend who knew WYNC radio executive Ted Cott arranged an audition for Forsythe, which he promptly flunked. Determined, he asked for a second chance and turned in a much better showing. Cott gave him some announcing assignments—most of them without pay, but enough to get the feel of the profession, which he decided he really liked. Being able to have an impact on millions of invisible listeners gave him a sense of profound awe.

Radio announcing led Forsythe into acting. He sought out a job with a children's theater in Chappaqua; he played parts, acted as stage manager, and drove the truck that carried the troupe's equipment from town to town. Then he got a job with a Shake-spearean company for a year; next it was two jobs in Broadway shows and then a contract with Warner Brothers. Shortly afterward, he was touring the country in Moss Hart's wartime musical, *Winged Victory*.

Somewhere along the way, Forsythe got so fascinated by acting that baseball announcing simply disappeared from his list of priorities. He never went back to it. Today he remains one of America's most popular sex symbols, although Forsythe says that "it's been very amusing to me and my daughters and my wife, who just see me as an old shoe!" He has no intention to stop acting, and he stays in shape with rigorous tennis matches. "I don't believe in retirement. I'm never going to retire," Forsythe states emphatically. "I like what I'm doing." With several television projects both on the air and in the works, it is obvious that Forsythe means what he says.

SEN. MARGARET CHASE SMITH

The first woman elected to both houses of Congress, Margaret Chase Smith was born in 1897 in the small mill town of Skowhegan, Maine, the oldest of six children. Her father was a barber and her mother had done factory work before she had children. The family had to struggle to support itself, and as a teenager Margaret contributed by working in a five-and-dime store, as a telephone operator, on a local newspaper, and as a teacher.

An Early Transformer, she had become the business manager of a major textile mill in Skowhegan by 1930. There she met Clyde H. Smith, a prominent local and state politician, and they married later that year. She helped her husband campaign for Congress in 1936, and after he was elected she served as office manager, chief campaign coordinator, and executive assistant. In 1940 Clyde Smith had a fatal heart attack while campaigning for reelection. He had previously warned his constituents of his heart ailment and appealed to them to elect his wife in his place in the event of his death.

Smith ran in four consecutive elections in five months: a primary and an election to fill her husband's unexpired term, and then a primary and general election for the next term. She won all four elections and served in the House of Representatives for three more terms. Her greatest legislative achievement in the House was obtaining permanent status for women in the military, which directly affected military nurses serving in World War II.

In 1948 Smith decided to run for the Senate; no woman had

ever before been elected in her own right. She faced a difficult race in the Republican primary, without the support of the state Republican Party. She defeated her opponents by a margin of victory exceeding all other votes combined. She went on to defeat her Democratic opponent and became the first fully elected woman in the U.S. Senate. But Smith would not let the fact that she was a woman affect her career. "I never would be a 'woman' candidate. I was a *candidate*," she said emphatically. "Not that I objected to being a woman—I was proud to be a woman and doing what I was able to. But I think that women make the mistake of always apologizing and explaining that they are women; that's bad."

Smith held her Senate seat through six administrations, from Franklin Roosevelt to Richard Nixon's first term, for a total of four six-year terms. She held the all-time roll call voting record in the Senate until 1981, with 2,941 consecutive role calls. Throughout her political career, she maintained her interest in military affairs by her work in the Senate Armed Services Committee. But her most important contribution to American history was her opposition to the excesses of McCarthyism in the early 1950s. She gave a speech on the Senate floor denouncing Senator McCarthy for his ruthless tactics, which had paralyzed her colleagues with fear. Her speech was called the "Declaration of Conscience" and remains a testament to her stand against bigotry and injustice. Senator McCarthy retaliated by dropping her from a key committee and attempted to help defeat her in her 1954 reelection campaign. But her speech marked the beginning of the end of McCarthy's tactics, and she was reelected despite the senator's efforts.

Senator Smith's legislative interests were extensive and varied. She was extremely involved in space exploration as one of the original members of the Senate committee that dealt with the space program. The then–director of NASA later remarked, "If it were not for a woman—Margaret Chase Smith—we would not have put a man on the moon." She was also committed to legislation promoting the expansion of medical research.

In 1954 Smith personally financed a trip to twenty-three countries to better inform herself of the conditions in a rapidly changing postwar world. She met and conferred with many world leaders, including Churchill, de Gaulle, Franco, Adenauer, Chiang Kai-shek, and others. The trip, filmed by Edward R. Murrow, helped establish her as a respected world figure in her own right.

In the fall of 1963 Senator Smith decided to seek the Republican nomination for the presidency (she had received consideration in the past as a possible vice presidential candidate). Although she did not win, she became the first woman in U.S. history to have her name placed in nomination for the presidency by a major political party.

Smith retained her Senate seat for ten more years, until she left politics in 1973, at the age of seventy-six. After her retirement from politics, she became a visiting professor and lecturer and has continued such work until the present day.

In 1989 Smith received the highest national honor, the presidential Medal of Freedom. Her hometown of Skowhegan has created Margaret Chase Smith Day and proudly exhibits her many awards in the museum portion of the Margaret Chase Smith Library, which was built in 1982. She recently received her ninety-fifth honorary doctoral degree from Colby College in Maine.

When asked why she didn't retire at sixty-five, Smith said she never even thought about it. "Age never meant anything to me. I never think of myself in connection with years. I ran always on my record, and my phrase was always, 'Don't change a record.'"

MARVIN BOWER

Marvin Bower, founder of the management consulting firm McKinsey and Company, is another participant who got the job he longed for and then discovered that it didn't fulfill him as much as he had expected. Bower had put years and years of preparation into landing the job he had set his heart on, getting two graduate degrees in order to qualify. But that effort wasn't wasted; it enabled him to conceive of a new field, management consulting, and later to succeed in establishing it.

The son of a Cincinnati land surveyor, Bower had gone to Harvard Law School at his father's suggestion because he had no clear feeling about what career path he wanted to pursue. A summer job between law school terms helped him to decide that he wanted to work for the best corporate law firm in Cleveland—Jones, Day, Reavis, and Pouge. But when he graduated, the firm declined to hire him because he hadn't made the *Law Review*.

Bower was disappointed, but not discouraged. He reasoned

that since he wanted to go into corporate law, he would be better equipped if he went to the Harvard Business School and got an M.B.A. in addition to his law degree. He applied, enrolled, studied hard, and made the *Business Review*—and when he graduated he got the job he originally wanted at Jones, Day.

This story sounds like it could end here with, "And he lived happily ever after," but Bower's journey was only beginning. After several years at Jones, Day, Bower realized that he didn't really like the practice of law as much as he had thought he would. About half of his work was interesting, and the other half was as dull as dishwater. He wasn't sure what to do about this, if anything, but it certainly was not what he had expected.

Bower had entered the work force during the depression, when law firms were busy with defaulting bond companies. One of his assignments within the firm was to help either salvage or close down companies in trouble. He soon realized that many companies had no access to professional advice on how to manage their affairs. He conceived of the need for a professional firm that could give companies sound management advice, one that would have the highest ethical and educational standards.

Through pure chance, while on a trip to Chicago for one of the bondholder's committees, Bower met James O. McKinsey, the founder of a small management consulting firm. The older man obviously sensed a kindred spirit in Marvin Bower. "McKinsey asked me how I liked my work," Bower recalled. "I said, 'I like half of it very much; the other part of it is boring.' He said, 'Why don't you join our firm and like it all?'"

It was an appealing idea and sounded like a great opportunity, but it also entailed high risks. Moving to Chicago meant giving up the considerable security of his job at Jones, Day, and the Depression was still in full force. Bower talked with his wife, Helen, at length about the idea. Even though the family had no financial reserves, Mrs. Bower felt that he should go with McKinsey. And so he did.

In 1934, Bower was transferred to New York to replace the manager of the office there. Later, part of the company was sold to a New York businessman. Then, in 1935, McKinsey got pneumonia from a tiring visit to several southern textile mills, and he died at the age of forty-eight. Bower took over the company and began to develop his innovative management ideas. More than

half a century later, McKinsey and Company has forty-three hundred employees at fifty-one offices in twenty-five countries
around the world.

Bower stepped down as managing director in 1967, but he
continues to work for the firm as a consulting director, spending
most of his time on client work and training new members of the
firm. He is especially interested in mentoring younger people and
takes great pleasure in that role. At age eighty-nine, Bower is still
fascinated by his work. "It's harder to get bored and to burn out
in a professional firm," he says, "especially in a managing firm
because there is a constant change of scene all the time."

EDWARD L. BERNAYS

Edward L. Bernays's career is described in Who's Who as "public
relations counsel to government, industry, corporations, professional and trade organizations, and individuals from 1919–." The
founder of the field of public relations, Bernays has been actively
engaged in that field for more than eighty-three years.

Born in Vienna in 1891, the double nephew of Sigmund
Freud, Bernays celebrated his first birthday on the ship that
brought him and his family to America. His family settled in New
York, where his father became a successful grain exporter.
Because of his father's interest in agriculture, he sent young
Bernays to Cornell University, where he graduated with a degree
in agriculture in three and a half years at the age of nineteen.

Not surprisingly, Bernays got his first job working on the
Commodities Exchange in New York. But it paid very poorly, not
enough to live on even for a young single man. An old school
friend whom he ran into on the elevated train offered him a job at
a newspaper his father had just given him, and Bernays accepted
because the salary was much better.

This job editing the Medical Review of Reviews changed
Bernay's life, and ultimately led to his creation of the field of public relations. One morning Bernays saw an article in the Times
about a controversial play on sexually transmitted diseases that
had just been banned as a public production. Bernays decided
that, as editor of the Review, he would help to get the play produced as a private venture because it was educationally valuable
for the public. He was brilliantly successful and thus discovered
that he had a natural aptitude for publicity and promotion.

Bernays next took his savings and went to Europe, staying first in Paris and then in Vienna with his famous uncle. On returning to New York, he brought with him his uncle's book, *Introductory Lectures in Psychoanalysis,* for which he found a publisher. The revenues from this book supported the Freud family for several years (pre–World War I inflation had wiped out the family's savings and left them in financial difficulties).

Bernays's feat in producing the originally tabooed play had made a reputation for him. He was promptly hired by Claus Erlanger, a powerful Broadway producer, to do theatrical publicity. During this time, he worked with performers as diverse as opera divas, Broadway stars, and dancers in Diaghilev's Ballets Russes. During World War I he worked for the U.S. Information Agency in New York and in Paris, making the world safe for democracy through propaganda ("as opposed to improper-ganda," Bernays adds. "The Germans did improper-ganda").

When he left the federal position, he decided it was time to start his own agency: Edward L. Bernays, Inc., founded in 1919. He didn't want to use the word *publicity,* so he came up with the term *public relations* and cemented his authority by writing the first book on the subject, *Crystallizing Public Opinion,* the seminal work in the field. He defined a public relations consultant as "an applied social scientist who advises a client or employer on the social attitudes and actions to take to win the support of the public upon whom the viability of the client or the employer depends." Bernays convinced New York University to offer a course in this new field to establish it more solidly, and he taught it for some years. He has since taught public relations in dozens of classes and seminars all over the world.

Bernays's firm remained in New York for forty-two years, until 1962 when he and his wife moved to Cambridge, Massachusetts, where Bernays would write his autobiography. He continues to do consulting work from his office in Cambridge. Although his fee is a steep $1,000 per hour, people still come to consult him, and his schedule is always full.

EILEEN FORD
Founder of the Ford Model Agency with her husband, Jerry Ford, Eileen Ford had a succession of career objectives when she was growing up, as well as several short jobs at the beginning of her

work life—all different from the career she eventually created for herself out of luck and her own tremendous ability to respond creatively to unexpected events.

Born in 1922, she grew up on Long Island (with the exception of three years during the Depression when the family couldn't afford heating oil for their home and moved into a New York apartment). An adored child, Ford always knew that she was going to work, because her mother told her that she would be a lawyer. However, Ford's own ambitions were more flamboyant. First she wanted to be a movie star, with bleached hair, plucked eyebrows, and a white fox fur stole. Then she was going to be a show business agent. She tried out for the Billy Rose Aquacade, but her mother wouldn't let her accept.

After she graduated from Barnard she worked for a photographer as a secretary and stylist and did volunteer work nights at the Navy League. Through a friend she met Jerry Ford and fell instantly in love with him. When he graduated from midshipmen school, he was sent to San Francisco before he was shipped out to the Pacific. Eileen borrowed money from everyone she knew to buy a train ticket to San Francisco so they could get married.

When she got back to New York, Eileen got a job as a stylist for Constable's, a rather large department store. She got to know a number of models who worked there. After the war was over and Jerry returned, Eileen became pregnant and realized she would need to find work that could be done at home. Several of the models from Constable's needed an appointments secretary, so she took them on. By the time the baby was born, Eileen was managing eight models, and Jerry took over part of the work. The couple has headed the agency together for over forty-six years.

Neither Eileen nor Jerry Ford intended to start a model agency; it "just happened." And once established, it "grew like Topsy," Eileen says. "You have to be in the right place at the right time to do what we did." They started a children's agency because Terri Shields came to them in quest of an agent for her daughter Brooke, who at age eight was getting too tall for the taste of her current agent. Their men's agency was launched when they bought out a rival firm started by Huntington Hartford.

There were two other widely known model agencies in New York at that time but they functioned poorly. One owner went to jail, while Eileen and Jerry were just the opposite: a "family-style" model agency, as they were billed in *Life* magazine. Models had typically been considered fair game by every unscrupulous type in the book; Ford's was the first model agency that protected its models from unsavory advances and had truly professional standards.

Eileen Ford sees her work essentially as "helping people," and she is still as passionate about it as she was forty-six years ago. "I work because I like to work, and also because I am driven. I know that; I'm restless," she acknowledged.

"If I retired, I wouldn't sit around and wait to die," she continued. "I would write a book. I would work as a volunteer for the Humane Society. Even if I were just a surrogate grandparent at the New York Family Hospital, there are so many things you can do to help people."

HENNY YOUNGMAN

Comedian Henny Youngman astonished both himself and his family with an early career change that made use of a trait that his family considered a behavioral problem serious enough to ruin his life: his irresistible impulse to be funny.

Youngman's natural talent for comedy as a youngster was unfortunately regarded as disruptive everywhere he went. What was worse, the older he got, the funnier he became. Finally, he got expelled from Manual Training High School for consistently breaking up the class. Youngman's parents did not find this amusing. Depression-era families took their children's future prospects extremely seriously; without a high school degree, it was difficult to get a job that paid enough to support a family.

When her son was much younger, Youngman's mother had thought that music might be his ticket to fame and prosperity, and she made him take violin lessons. "She wanted me to be Jascha Heifetz," Youngman quipped. "But I couldn't, because Jascha Heifetz was already Jascha Heifetz." As Jack Benny had done, Youngman would later capitalize on this musical ambition by putting it into his comedy routines, carrying a violin and playing it badly. The humor resulted in part because many of Benny's and Youngman's listeners had had similar experiences, getting pushed into music by well-meaning but overassertive parents.

When Youngman was forced to make his way in life without a high school diploma, the violin unexpectedly turned into an asset. Years of lessons had given him enough musical education to start a small band, which he developed into a kind of comedy routine.

"People would pass by and I would comment on them," he says, "make jokes." He developed a facility for short, pithy comments that later won him the title "King of the One-Liners."

One night, at a club where his band was playing, the main attraction for the evening didn't show up. The club manager, desperate for an act to draw customers, came to Youngman and begged him to go on as a replacement—but without the band. He accepted. Afterward, he went to the manager and asked him, "How did I do? Was it OK?" "Fire the band," the manager replied. Youngman did. Later he became nationally famous after being hired as a regular on the Kate Smith radio show.

Youngman's voice still holds a touch of anger and bitterness when he recalls the way he was mistreated as a child for his comic talent. In retrospect, it seems quite remarkable that his family did not perceive his talent; but the modern occupation of a comedian, in all fairness to them, is a fairly recent invention. Be that as it may, Youngman feels extremely lucky to have found a career that he enjoys so much; he thinks that the most important factor in choosing a career is that "you've got to find a business you like." Because he likes his work, Youngman can't imagine retiring. "Why should I retire? Where would I go? What would I do? . . . If you've got something going that's good and you're wanted, you're in demand, and you're healthy enough to do it, why retire?"

At eighty-five, Youngman has lunch every day at the Friar's Club, a private club for actors and comedians, where he has a telephone on his customary table. Over lunch he wheels and deals, makes engagements, and always answers his telephone calls. Are there advantages to his age? "I'm treated nicer, I'll tell you that," he says. "I get standing ovations when I just walk out on the stage! I don't know if it's for my age or for the jokes—but who cares?"

MIDLIFE TRANSFORMERS

The second cluster of Transformers shifted careers in the middle part of their lives. There were sixteen midlife Transformers, nine men and seven women. The reasons for their changes ran the gamut. One woman was forced to find a new career because she married a co-worker and was required to resign from her job. One man got fired in a financial crunch and, in his effort to help others who were losing their jobs, became the nation's foremost career expert. Another man rebelled against a bureaucracy and ended up leaving his job and launching into a new career. Three women went back to work after raising families and made exceptional careers for themselves. And one man deliberately changed jobs because he saw that once he passed the age of fifty he would probably get fired because of his age.

JULIA CHILD

Julia Child's career has been the result of a wonderful combination of creativity and luck. Her midlife career change ended up ultimately changing an entire nation's attitude toward food and cooking. Born Julia McWilliams in Pasadena, California, in 1912, she graduated from Smith College in 1934. When World War II broke out she joined the Office of Strategic Services, the fledgling intelligence organization that subsequently became the Central Intelligence Agency. In Ceylon, her first overseas assignment, she met Paul Child, her future husband. Later in the war both were transferred to China; after returning to the United States, they were married.

In those days, Child said, if two people in government service got married, one of them was expected to quit—and it wasn't the man. Dutifully, she resigned, and then began looking around for another career. Nothing sprang up immediately, however, and the search dragged on for several years, to her frustration. Only when Paul Child was assigned to France by the U.S. Information Agency, where he was employed after the war, did the light dawn. "I stepped off the boat," Child remarked, "took one mouthful of French food, and I was hooked for life."

She enrolled at the Cordon Bleu, studying continuously for the next six or seven years, and made two friends who would become important collaborators, Simone Beck and Louise Bertholle. The three women decided to open their own cooking school in Paris, and they began writing a book on French cuisine for an American audience. Ultimately it became *Mastering the Art of French Cooking*.

Child's career has been marked by several chance events that subsequently resulted in huge changes in her life or circumstances. The first was the discovery of French food, which she had never been exposed to before nor had any interest in. She had not considered becoming a chef at any time in her career search; it was simply not on her list of possibilities, although one other study participant, Louis Hector, who knew her during the war remembered that she was always very enthusiastic about food. "In China, she used to organize the most fantastic dinners," Hector said. "She'd choose the restaurant, order the food, everything. And it was always wonderful." But when the moment came, she recognized it instantly and moved toward it without hesitation. Perhaps, like Henny Youngman's consideration of his enjoyment, she hadn't thought of her enjoyment of food as something on which you could base a career.

Another important coincidence presented itself when *Mastering the Art of French Cooking* was published in 1961. Publishing a French cookbook was a rather daring thing to do; the American public was not particularly interested in "foreign" food. Knopf had ordered five thousand copies, and clearly the company was worried about selling such a vast quantity. Child felt obliged to fill every publicity engagement they made for her, in the service of selling the cookbooks.

The Knopf publicist set up an interview for Child on a very popular television book review show at WGBH in Boston. The problem was that the show lasted an hour, and Child was publicizing a *cookbook*. This posed a crisis. "What was I going to do?" she exclaimed. "Read recipes for an hour?"

In her anxiety to please the publisher, keep the engagement, and find something more interesting than reading recipes, Child hit on the notion of taking along something edible that she could just "whip up" on camera as a demonstration. She would make an omelet, which required only a dozen eggs, a wire whip, an omelet pan, a copper bowl in which to beat the eggs, and a hot plate to cook it on. This would fill a substantial amount of time, perhaps even the whole hour.

The omelet was a tremendous success. The station got a large number of letters afterward, commenting on Julia's "review," and as Child tells it, a few days later she received a phone call from WGBH asking if perhaps she might be interested in doing one of those shows every day. Even with her husband helping her to manage the process, she now wonders how they could have kept such a schedule. "I guess we just didn't know any better," she says with a chuckle.

In a very real sense, Julia Child's creative response to a sticky professional problem changed American cultural history. Up until that point, Americans had been surprisingly jingoistic about food, unimpressed by the potential variety offered by foods available in other cultures, and unfamiliar with most of it unless one lived in a large urban area and went out to relatively sophisticated restaurants regularly. There were few restaurants serving such food— French, Italian, Chinese, Japanese—and the thought of making dishes such as omelets had never occurred to most Americans.

Child changed all that. Suddenly French cooking became both accessible and entertaining, because of Child's engaging and light-hearted manner. People loved it when, for example, if she dropped a turkey on the floor while on camera, she would simply pick it up, dust it off, and plop it back in the pan, ad libbing that she hoped the viewer's kitchen was as clean as hers. Americans bought her book, used it, and watched the TV show. And Child is still going strong at the age of eighty, having published a new book five years in the writing, *How to Cook,* and put together a new TV series, "Dinner with Julia."

WARREN ROBBINS

Warren Robbins, founder of the Smithsonian's National Museum of African Art, spent the early years of his career as a teacher and then as a cultural attaché in the U.S. foreign service, stationed in Germany and Austria. During his final two years there, he rose to a position of great responsibility as head of all American cultural operations in Germany, in which capacity he was in charge of twenty-five America Houses (cultural information centers for the United States).

At that point, Robbins had been in Europe for about ten years and, according to U.S. foreign service regulations, had to go back to the United States for two years of domestic assignment. His return to home turf was not exactly the kind of welcome he might have expected, however.

"I had the attitude of most foreign service officers regarding Washington, which was to do your two years of 'penance' and then get back into the field where the work was exciting. Interesting jobs in Washington were in short supply and although I had been running the largest U.S. cultural program in the world," Robbins said, "they wanted to put me in some broom closet, reading and reporting on what was in East German newspapers. In the foreign service, you are not supposed to refuse an assignment, but I said, 'This is ridiculous.'"

His protests came to the attention of someone in the secretary of state's office, and he was appointed as assistant staff director for the U.S. Advisory Commission on Education and Cultural Exchange. Among his duties, he worked on a lengthy report from the secretary of state to Sen. J. William Fulbright, chairman of the Foreign Relations Committee, and also drafted the report's cover letter. When the report was received, Fulbright's office called upon Robbins to draft the senator's reply to the secretary of state. "I was writing letters to myself!" Robbins exclaimed.

Things would undoubtedly have gone on in this vein for some time had Robbins not gone in to work one day to discover that his parking space in the department's cavernous basement garage was being reassigned to a political appointee. In Washington institutions, parking spaces are the most sought-after perks. Robbins quickly informed his superiors that if they took away his parking space, he would quit. Apparently they thought he was joking. But when they gave his parking spot to someone else, Robbins made good on his claim. The administrators then spent a week trying to talk him out of it, without success. There were deeper, more serious reasons for his resignation: Robbins wanted to become involved in the civil rights struggle then coming to the fore in the United States.

While in Germany, Robbins had bought thirty-two objects of traditional African art for about $1,000—a risky thing to do, he said, since he did not know very much about African art, which was little known then in the United States. Robbins felt that greater awareness of the art could contribute to a better understanding of what he calls "the African facet of American heritage." In art as in music, Africa has had a great impact on modern culture.

Having made the leap out of the State Department, Robbins decided that the time had arrived to create a museum of African art in the nation's capital. He bought a house on Capitol Hill that had been the home of the great nineteenth-century black abolitionist orator and publisher Frederick Douglass, and he moved into it with his collection.

Surviving without a salary was a problem for Robbins. He collected unemployment compensation for the maximum period of time, got various consulting and teaching assignments, and began to sell pieces from his collection of contemporary European and American art in order to sustain himself. But his belief in the need for an African art museum never faltered. He recognized the significance of African art and knew that public understanding of these extraordinary art objects, so unlike anything the "civilized" world had produced, could make an important contribution to the growing sense of positive cultural identity among African-Americans, as well as to the education of all Americans. That was in 1964.

By 1979, the Museum of African Art had grown in size and complexity from a local museum to a national institution with an international reputation. Robbins, with congressional support (particularly from Hubert Humphrey as senator and then as vice president), entered into negotiations with Smithsonian officials and eventually worked out arrangements to give the museum (with its collection of five thousand objects that he had amassed) and the real estate (which had grown to encompass thirteen properties) to the nation.

Today, Robbins remains a founding director emeritus and senior scholar at the museum. Without the burden of museum administration and fund-raising, Robbins devotes his time to lecturing around the country, consulting, and writing. In addition to having written numerous articles and essays, he has finished one major book that has sixteen hundred illustrations, the most comprehensive photo survey ever done on African art, and is working on another book, *Unmasking Picasso,* about the influence of African sculpture on twentieth-century art. He also has worked to secure funding for public school students to paint fourteen Mondrian murals on highway overpasses in Washington.

Robbins, who at age sixty-nine has no intention of retiring, believes that "it is energy that is the secret of effectiveness in life" and that he derives his own energy from work that he loves.

ELIZABETH JANEWAY
Writer Elizabeth Janeway made a shift of a less radical kind than perhaps that of the other Transformers, but it was one that nonetheless changed the character of her career and gave it a second phase in many respects more powerful than the first.

Janeway was for twenty years a highly successful novelist. She grew up in a large, slightly eccentric family whose immediate history stretched back to her grandfather in the early nineteenth century. Early in her life, Janeway became accustomed to the idea of writing as something people did all the time. "Most of my family had a kind of capacity to write," she said, "the way some families can sing or have musical talents."

Janeway attended Swarthmore for a year but had to return to New York because of the depression. She wrote advertising copy for Abraham and Strauss's *basement* (emphasis hers) and attended Barnard, where she earned a degree in history. She then took a job with the Book-of-the-Month Club, negotiating an agreement that allowed her to work half-time so she could work on a novel she had in mind, *The Walsh Girls*.

"I wrote it over seven years and I wrote it three times," Janeway says. "I didn't know how to write a novel; I had to figure out how to do it and I am a rewriter by nature. I finally finished it because I was about to have a second child, and I sort of thought, you can have one child and still think of yourself as a writer, but if you have two children, you are a housewife, dear, and you'd better face up to it. And I didn't want to. So I finished it very fast the winter I was pregnant with Bill. I completed it about two weeks before he was born."

The Walsh Girls was published—and was featured on the first page of the *New York Times Book Review*. Well launched by her persistence and this piece of good fortune, Janeway subsequently wrote six more novels and four children's books.

In the 1960s, in the middle of what was an extremely successful career, Janeway began to take stock of the massive upheavals occurring in the society around her. "It came to me that it was going to be hard to write fiction, because so much in the world was changing," she said. "Not just the outer things, but the basic premises fiction takes for granted. During most of this century, for example, if you had an unmarried girl who was pregnant, you had a big problem—and the basis for a plot. Suddenly that wasn't true any more.

"So I decided to turn to nonfiction, and wrote *Man's World, Woman's Place*, which presented a view of the changes in those fundamental assumptions—what they had been, how they had affected men and women, and how we looked at the world. Again, I had to write it three times—learning how to write nonfiction is very hard if you have been used to the advantages that fiction gives: characters and dialogue and suspense and narrative that hold people's attention. Fiction is much easier to write: you just make everything up!"

Man's World, Woman's Place did very well, and Janeway was

able to make a lateral career change, from being a fiction writer to being a social commentator. She has written a number of other books on the women's movement and on other social issues. For example, *The Powers of the Weak* examines how subordinate groups in any society use their powerlessness.

HERBERT WEST

Of all the Transformers, the only person who made a conscious, planned career change—one that was mapped out and then carefully implemented—was Herbert West, the late president of the New York Community Trust. But West's move was planned only up to a point. The process he went through shows that even the most careful thinking about a transition may inevitably leave out vital aspects of the real process.

West, who grew up in Birmingham, Alabama, worked for thirty years in advertising in New York, most of it at the then-well-known firm of Batten, Barton, Durston and Osborne. He was extremely successful. But in his late forties he became aware of something quite troubling.

"I began to notice that the people in their fifties in the agency seemed to disappear," he said. "Some died, some drank themselves to death, some others said that they always wanted to run a corner store in a little town in New Hampshire or an inn in Vermont. Or they got fired, or something else happened to them. And I thought, this is very strange. Nobody ever reaches sixty-five and retires. So I said to my wife, 'We had better do something about this, because we have five children and I'm going to need a second career!'"

West and his wife decided they wanted to stay in New York. They blocked out three fields that they thought might be possibilities: educational television, teaching, and foundation work. West set out to explore them. Teaching was eliminated right away: West had only a bachelor's degree, so despite his gift for advertising, he wasn't qualified to teach at a level that would interest him without going back to school for another degree. Next came educational television: he discovered that jobs there didn't make much money and were rife with internal politics. That left foundation work.

West was in the process of sifting ideas for foundations when an odd thing happened. A man he had never heard of before named Ralph Hayes came to see him, having heard his name

through the grapevine, and gave him a long, confusing monologue about something called the New York Community Trust.
West assumed that the job would entail working for Hayes, and
because they weren't at all on the same wavelength, he listened to
Hayes politely and thought no more about it.

Hayes came back, however. On the third visit he mentioned
that the job was as Hayes's replacement, not his employee. West
suddenly got very interested. In 1967 he became president of the
New York Community Trust.

Again, this sounds like a happy ending—except that it wasn't
the last episode. West's negotiations had included the usual dis-
cussions about salary. However, when West reported to work,
Hayes told him in an offhand manner that there was one little
problem: there was no money to pay his salary. Hayes would
put enough money into the administrative fund to pay West's
salary for two months, he said; after that, he was sure a smart
man like West could figure out ways to solve the little problem of
how to pay himself, like selling historical plaques to put on buildings and wallet-sized who-to-call-in-emergency-cards to insurance
companies.

West was horrified. Neither one of Hayes's ideas would raise
enough money to buy peanuts to feed the pigeons, much less support a foundation staff. But he had already left the advertising
agency and accepted the trust position, so he was stuck. He had
to try to find some kind of solution.

Once Hayes had left, West did find a solution, which turned
out to be much more elegant and practical than Hayes could have
imagined. The New York Community Trust at that point was the
fourth largest community foundation in the United States, but its
money was still being held in trust by various banks, instead of
being turned over to the trust itself to be used in the normal way.
West had the money transferred, accomplishing this change with
a maximum of diplomacy and a minimum of fuss, and there was
never any more problem about paying the staff.

West stayed on as the trust's president for twenty years. He
increased its endowment many times over, broadened the scope of
its programs, and drew many individuals into its sphere who had
not previously been interested in philanthropy. About a year
before his seventieth birthday, he began making plans to retire
and become a consultant to the trust, working only on special
projects and doing a lot of writing. On the surface, he seemed

very much to be looking forward to this; he was full of plans for things he was going to do. His successor was chosen and a year's transition period was provided for.

Halfway through the transitional year, West began having disturbing symptoms—which, after a long diagnostic period, turned out to be lymphatic cancer. He lived through the end of the transitional year and died several weeks later.

West's experience, along with those of a few other participants, raises the question of the role that life change and stress play in health. West had chosen to retire, and to all appearances he was looking forward to it. But research indicates that all major changes are stressful, even if they are positive ones. Theoretically, it is possible for any significant stress to trigger physical changes that could lead to illness or tip the balance in favor of an illness that is already present but has not yet overwhelmed the body's defenses.

LATE TRANSFORMERS

Twelve people in the Long Careers Study made their career changes relatively late in life, after the age of sixty. These people were well established financially and personally, enabling them to turn to other interests comfortably. Four of them had changed to a field that had been a lifelong interest; their stories follow, with the exception of William Kirby who is presented at the end of the chapter. The others formally retired from their first careers and then began second careers that in several cases were more satisfying and more distinguished than the original ones; these will be discussed in chapter 11, "Retirers and Returners."

JANET JEPPSON-ASIMOV

Janet Jeppson-Asimov grew up wanting to be a writer. It was an interest that she first formed from telling stories to her younger brother, for whom she had to baby-sit for long periods of time when she was about six. Her stories kept him quiet, and, like Celeste Holm, Jeppson was enthralled by the stories' effect on the audience: her brother's saucer-round eyes, his surprise at a new twist in the plot, his eagerness for the next installment.

Jeppson nursed this ambition through high school but was discouraged by an unsympathetic English teacher. At the same time, she had a wonderful teacher in biology, a subject she thoroughly enjoyed. She decided in college to become a physician chiefly because she realized she would have to make a living somehow; medicine was familiar to her because her father was a physician. The moment of decision was completely spontaneous. She was filling out a form and saw that one of the questions was, "Are you premed?" She looked at the question and thought, "Why not?" So she checked yes. She graduated, enrolled in medical school, and became a physician, doing a residency in psychiatry. Over a twenty-year period she built up a substantial private practice.

In 1973 she married writer Isaac Asimov. About ten years later, she experienced a period of personal strain after certain health crises for several family members, including her husband, who had suffered a heart attack. Gradually she found that she was not able to spend the entire day listening receptively to the problems of other people anymore. Over a period of about a year, she closed her practice and took up her lifelong dream of becoming a fiction writer.

Jeppson had continued writing on the side during all her years of practice as a psychiatrist and in the previous two or three years, encouraged by her husband's example, had begun to sell a few stories. Today she is a full-time writer, has published many books and a number of short stories, and is extremely happy with her new career. "It's an absolute miracle that I have had sixteen books published with more coming, with something interesting to do," Jeppson commented. "I've had the marvelous experience of being a doctor and a psychiatrist and now a writer. And," she added, "I'm very lucky to have met the most wonderful man in the world."

Helen Breed

Actress Helen Breed made an even later change than did Jeppson. A housewife and mother for her entire life, up to her early sixties, she had always nurtured a desire to be an actress. Her passion for the theater drew her into amateur theatricals, where she acted, produced, and directed for over thirty years. But because she was married and had children, she could not take on anything more than part-time, amateur involvement.

When Breed was sixty, her husband died. Unexpectedly freed of her day-to-day family obligations, Breed decided to make the best out of a bad turn of events and pursue seriously her ambitions as an actress. By this time she knew she would be a character actress, not a romantic lead—but that didn't matter. She gave herself five years to get a paying job in a stage production and set out to work toward that end as hard as she could.

Exactly five years later, she got her first paying role in a little theater production of *The Holly and the Ivy*. But what happened next was a total surprise. Someone apparently saw her in the production and passed favorable comments along to the producers of the upcoming Jack Nicholson film, *The Witches of Eastwick*. Breed got a call asking if she would be interested in auditioning for the film. The role she played is small: Mrs. Biddle, who owns the gift shop where Cher sells her clay figurines. But it gave her career a great boost. Next she was asked to play the "chairman of the board" in the Madonna film *Who's That Girl?* She has been in a number of other films as well, most recently *Passed Away*, starring Maureen Stapleton.

Breed looks aristocratic and rather austere, and the parts she gets reflect those qualities; they are parts made for someone who is a presence. She has an exceptionally expressive face, which stands her in good stead in serious parts, and great comic aplomb as well, demonstrated in her hilarious scenes from the Madonna film.

Her latest project is doing voice-overs for television commercials. When I interviewed her, she had recently finished a course at a voice-over school and was beginning the process of sending out demonstration tapes and résumés to agencies that hire actors for voice-over work.

I had heard about Breed occasionally through mutual friends for some fifteen years before I interviewed her for the Long Careers Study, and I remembered some of the reactions people had had to her career aspirations. The general consensus was that she wanted very much to be an actress, but her work in amateur theatricals was as far as she would get; it was considered impossible to become a "real" actress at her age. Some people thought it was sad that she was so fixed on what to them was such an obviously impossible goal, others that she was a little obsessive to want to be an actress "at her age." I never heard anyone say that they thought she had a chance of genuinely realizing her dream.

But she has realized it, and she derives enormous satisfaction from it. "I am having the time of my life!" Breed exclaimed. She sees herself as having "retired from being a wife and mother" so that she could make her childhood dream of being an actress come true. For Breed and many other study participants, reaching "retirement age" gave them the courage and the motivation to realize these kinds of long-cherished plans.

NORMAN COUSINS

Perhaps the most celebrated example of a person who has made a career change after sixty is the late Norman Cousins. His first career was spent as editor of the *Saturday Review,* a magazine he bought in December 1940 at the age of twenty-four. At that point its circulation was only about fifteen thousand. "There was a convention at that time—almost a rule," Cousins said, "that no quality magazine could surpass a circulation of thirty thousand. The theory was that there weren't enough educated people in the country to read such a magazine."

Cousins found backing to increase the circulation to thirty-five thousand and went on to make the *Review* one of the most popular magazines in the nation. By 1957, when his original backer died, the magazine had a circulation of two hundred thousand.

The 1960s and 1970s brought several unpleasant episodes for the magazine, involving corporate takeovers and buybacks. To get access to more economical printing and paper, Cousins affiliated the magazine with *McCall's.* But when he sought to buy out of the arrangement after the death of *McCall's* chairman, Norton Simon, Simon's successor sold the *Review* to someone else on the sly. Within eighteen months, the buyers went bankrupt. Cousins took over the magazine's debts to get it back and paid off more than $6 million of obligations. By this time he had published his famous book, *Anatomy of an Illness,* an account of his recovery from a normally fatal disease of the connective tissue, and was beginning to receive invitations to become an associate member of various medical school faculties. A friend who had been on the board of McCall's Corporation with him told him he should go out to UCLA and talk with Dean Mellencamp at the medical school there.

"I rather liked the idea of shaking up the format of my life, of putting new chunks into my subconscious," Cousins said. "Trying something entirely new in every respect. Not just a new career. I wanted to go to the other side of the continent, make new friends, everything."

Cousins made a trip to Los Angeles to talk with Mellencamp and, shortly afterward, at the age of sixty-four, moved to UCLA as adjunct professor in the School of Medicine. His special role was to help create a group that would study the interrelationship of the mind and the body in maintaining health and recovering from illness. Cousins's work at UCLA flourished, developing into a "more than full-time" career.

At the time of Cousins's interviews for the Long Careers Study, he had just received computer print-outs for a project that capped his ten years of research at UCLA. The project involved one group of melanoma patients who had been taught coping skills and received special training, including "being taught confidence and how to enjoy life despite the illness, and being liberated from the depression that is almost universally characteristic of a serious diagnosis," and another group of patients who received no such training.

The print-outs showed that at the end of one year the group that had been taught how to think about problems and about the essential robustness of the human body had "up to twenty times more immune cells than the other—up to twenty times! Then we saw direct correlations: as people were lifted out of depression, there was a corresponding rise in interleukins in all categories. . . across the board. That was thrilling," Cousins exclaimed.

The results of this project and many others were presented in *Head First: The Biology of Hope,* which Cousins published in 1989. He also co-wrote a play addressing similar issues in a dramatic medium. Cousins continued writing, lecturing, and doing research at UCLA up to his sudden death from cardiac arrest in November 1990.

ANALYSIS

Absence of the midlife crisis: It is striking that none of the Transformers made their career changes because of the traditional midlife crisis. However, the midlife Transformers did have a harder time making their shifts than did the early and late Transformers. Robbins was made so unhappy that he quit; West moved to avoid an uncertain future in an industry where nobody lasted until retirement. Richard Bolles (who will be discussed in chapter 16) was fired.

A few of the midlifers changed easily. Samuel Allen Williams, a Chicago stockbroker, spent almost thirty years (from his early twenties until his early fifties) in the office supply business, building up his firm with two partners. By the time he was in his early fifties he was ready to take a year off to travel around Europe with his wife. When they returned, he intended to go back to work in the office supply company, but he got a chance call from a friend who owned a brokerage firm, suggesting that he join him and try being a broker for a change. Williams had always been interested in finance; he accepted, not expecting that he would spend the next forty years as a broker.

By contrast, the early Transformers made much smoother transitions. They were not burdened with large families, mortgages, and the responsibilities that people commonly acquire after twenty years of adult life. Young and relatively unencumbered, they were free to spend time looking around or to start over at the ground level in a new career without great sacrifice.

The late Transformers had far more economic security than the midlifers, so their path was easier. They also had the benefit of years of experience in managing their lives and their professional careers, and they had a self-confidence derived from the successful navigation of previous life events. Most of them made their shift at an age when, according to what has been the popular wisdom, they were too old to do so, but they used their considerable know-how and networks of friends and acquaintances to either create or find a new position. And chance and circumstance played a very large role in all their changes. (That is a phenomenon we will see repeated in the experience of the next group, the Explorers.)

The percentage of women in each group rises as we move from early to midlife to late Transformers, and their changes are in large measure related to their marital status. All three women in the early Transformers group changed their career plans because of marriage; the women in the midlife group were all going back to work after a change created by their marital status; and two of the six female late Transformers went back to work because they were widowed or divorced. There are a few women in the study whose marital status apparently did not affect their careers at all; but for most of the Transformers it was a factor.

Picking up abandoned interests: Two of the midlife Transformers and over half of the late Transformers used the second part of their career to follow through with a prior interest that had been a subtheme in their adult lives until that point. In this change of focus, a combination of factors was involved. For one thing, many had had their secondary interest since childhood, and for some it would have been their first choice of career if things had worked out differently. Even though they did not pursue it as a career, they had maintained the secondary interest in some way throughout their primary careers. As a result, they built up a history of activity and interest in the secondary field. At a certain point this secondary interest became substantial enough to allow them to shift. Norman Cousins's interest in health led him to become involved in managing his own illness and recovery and to write the book that made him an appealing candidate to medical schools. Janet Jeppson's persistence in writing short stories on the side during her career as a psychiatrist made it possible for her ultimately to become a writer. But most of the Transformers who, like Jeppson and Cousins, changed to a field that they had loved since childhood did not consciously plan that move. It was triggered by external factors that hadn't been foreseen.

For Helen Breed, on the other hand, the event that left her free to choose her own directions may have come out of left field; but from that point on she deliberately set out to create a career. She had always wanted to be an actress but had never been able to break free of her family responsibilities and become a professional. She always nursed the dream, however, of becoming a "real actress" when her family was raised. When she became a widow at sixty, leaving her with no need to work to support herself, she decided it was now or never—and she made good on her commitment.

Other midlife and late Transformers moved to an area of interest that had developed during their adult lives. While it was not the fulfillment of a childhood dream, it was an interest as real and substantial as their primary careers, which had somehow reached a dead end. For some, there was a specific incident that triggered the change, like the State Department's hunger for Warren Robbins's parking space. For others it was a gradual development: during a period of years, Robert Popper, the vice president of a dairy firm, became so interested in health care issues that he ultimately retired so he could work full time as a volunteer on the board of Blue Cross/Blue Shield.

A few, like Chicago lawyer William Kirby, were given the focus of their change and pushed into the shift by circumstances. Kirby was a tough and brilliant litigator who made his reputation defending maverick automobile maker Tucker just after World War II. Later, after Kirby became the attorney for Chicago insurance magnate John D. MacArthur, he was asked for a commitment to help form MacArthur's new foundation at whatever point MacArthur might die. Kirby did not think much about what this would mean, and while MacArthur was alive there was no occasion to do so; he assumed that it would be a simple legal matter. It turned out, of course, to be anything but simple. After a lifetime spent as a contentious, street-smart trial lawyer, his promise to MacArthur pushed him into a new career as a philanthropist, where he had to develop qualities that in many respects were the exact opposites of those required in his courtroom work. Instead of trying to get or keep more money for a company, he was now engaged in giving its money away. Not an easy shift to make—but an enormously educational one—it led him into a completely new world of research and the dissemination of knowledge. It engaged him in constant growth and learning until his sudden death at the age of eighty in 1991.

In short, it is literally never too late to change, and never too late to learn something new.

8

The Explorers

An image of discovery similar to the image of the Transformers describes the third career pattern that emerged from the Long Careers Study. The Transformers remade their careers once; the Explorers changed careers periodically throughout their lifetimes. Contrary to what anyone might have expected, because of the idealization of the one-job/one-career Homesteader pattern during most of the twentieth century, this third category is the largest. A few more than 40 percent (sixty-one) of the study participants were Explorers. During the course of their careers, they often changed what they did—from as few as three to as many as ten times.

In several ways, the Explorers were the most complex of the three groups. First, because of their many changes, their careers were more intricate than those of the Homesteaders or the Transformers. Second, the incentives and reasons for the Explorers' changes were varied, although they generally responded to seven types of motivation. Most Explorers made changes for several of these reasons at different times in their careers:

• Unmet Expectations: Some changes, as was true for some early Transformers, were made because the real experience of the job did not match the external image it presented before the person took it.

• Lack of Fit: Some shifts occurred because the job's requirements or conditions did not match the person's abilities and needs as closely as had been expected.

• Internal Drive for Growth: Some participants reached a point when they knew everything there was to know about the job and felt the need for a different kind of work.

• External Factors: Some changes were made in response to outside events, like a change in the company's management, an offer of another job somewhere else, the death of a boss, or local or national political events.

• Short-term Opportunities: Some people took positions (often in government service) that were attractive but intrinsically limited in duration, requiring another change in a few years.

• Family Considerations: Some changes were triggered by the unexpected needs of a sick child, sibling, or spouse; for men, the need to earn more money to meet certain responsibilities; for women, the desire or obligation to stay at home while their children were small, or the expectation that they would tailor their work to their husband's career moves.

• Pure Chance: Finally, some changes were initiated by coincidental events that could never have been foreseen or planned but that changed the course of the person's entire life.

The Explorers include eleven people who had careers in public service and two-thirds of the study's lawyers (twelve out of a total of eighteen lawyers in the entire study). Two additional Explorers graduated from law school but never practiced (Max Lerner and Studs Terkel). The category also includes five businesspeople, four research scientists, four administrators of nonprofit groups, and a number of smaller categories containing only one or two persons, such as filmmaking, journalism, management consulting, farm/ factory work, and secretarial work.

The Explorers fall into two general categories based on the nature of their career changes. The first group are the type-A Explorers; they account for roughly two-thirds of the group (forty out of sixty-one). Although no analogy is intended to the famous classification of heart disease personality types, the type-A Explorers were extremely active: they made the most radical career shifts. Like a person crossing a stream by stepping from stone to stone, sometimes moving in one direction, sometimes in another, these people moved from one job to another as a result of the different factors present in their lives at the time of each change. Not only did they change jobs, but often they changed fields as well. Sometimes it was one aspect of their interests or personalities that led them to a particular job, sometimes another. Whatever the stimulus, the type-A Explorers kept moving.

Within the type-A Explorers, there was a small subgroup of people who changed jobs periodically until they hit one particular field that was an unusually good fit. Then they stayed in that field for the rest of their work life. They were settled Explorers. Only three people fit into this category: radio talk show host Studs Terkel; opinion research expert Dan Yankelovich; and advertising magnate David Ogilvy.

The second cluster of Explorers, the type-B Explorers, is much smaller than the first, with twenty-one individuals. These participants had career patterns with a continuous central track and many branches off to one side or another—a configuration something like that of a road with many side loops. The type-B Explorers stayed connected to the same field, always using it as a point of reference; but periodically they made changes in the nature and orientation of their work. When they had exhausted the possibilities for personal growth in one job, or conquered a particular problem, they would branch out in some other direction. Although some of these changes involved taking on very different functions than those of earlier jobs, each position was related to the person's original career identity.

THE TYPE-A EXPLORER

John W. Gardner

Because there were so many type-A Explorers, it was extraordinarily difficult to single out those who were the most characteristic. Perhaps the clearest example of the type-A Explorer in the study is John W. Gardner, author of *Excellence* and *Self-Renewal;* former secretary of the U.S. Department of Health, Education and Welfare; and founder of Common Cause. Gardner has changed careers frequently throughout his working life. In 1992, by his own count, he was engaged in his eighth career.

Born in California in 1912, Gardner lost his father to "pernicious anemia" (probably leukemia) when he was only one year old. His mother then took him and his older brother to a small, remote, lima bean farming community named Beverly Hills, where she built the nineteenth house in town. Gardner's recollections of rural Beverly Hills and its struggle to persuade more people to settle there are funny and ironic, given the community's current incarnation as the glitz capitol of Tinseltown, the site of some of the most expensive and highly desired real estate in the country.

As a youth, Gardner wanted to be a novelist. In the 1920s and 1930s there was a tremendous flowering of English-language fiction both in the United States and in Europe—Hemingway, Fitzgerald, Lawrence. None of the writers whose work he so admired had finished college; they had educated themselves. So at the end of his sophomore year, John Gardner decided to take a year off from his studies to try his hand as a writer.

Gardner went to live with two uncles in the Klondike who had been prospecting for gold (with little success) for many years. He wrote and wrote, accumulating piles of rejection slips. One night, near the end of the year, Gardner went to the movies. On the Pathé newsreel (a short film about current events) there was a report about two brothers who were still trying to make a plane that flapped its wings, a quarter of a century after the Wright brothers' first flight.

"They looked like the mountaineers in the old *Esquire* cartoons," Gardner said, "and when the camera rolled up to this dilapidated old barn, they opened the huge doors and out rolled a moth-eaten plane—the machine that was supposed to flap its wings. They said, 'You know, someday it's going to work.' As I came out of that theater," Gardner continued, "I was thinking that maybe there ought to be some kind of statute of limitations on dreams. And I set out to reassess." Gardner returned to Stanford and majored in psychology "because psychology was more like the study of literature than any other subject."

After earning his Ph.D. at Berkeley, Gardner accepted a teaching position at Connecticut College. But he was soon drafted into World War II. Sent to Washington to work on propaganda analysis, he was put in charge of a group of six people and began getting unexpectedly positive comments about his gift for management. This came as a complete surprise, since Gardner had always considered himself something of a loner.

Gardner's perceived talent would become a shaping factor for the rest of his life. "There is a curious thing I've tried to explain to people interested in human development," Gardner said, "that the gifts you have tend to determine the course of your life. Sometimes quite tyrannically. Mozart is an example. How much time did he have to find out what other gifts he had? So the fact that I had really quite a lot of management ability determined a series of assignments one after the other."

Later Gardner served in the marine corps and the Office of Strategic Services, ending up as executive officer of the agency in Austria after the war. At that point he received a letter from Henry A. Murray, a professor at Harvard, saying that a job was waiting for him at Carnegie Corporation of New York. Gardner had never met anyone from Carnegie and thought the letter was a joke. But it wasn't; there really was a job waiting for him there, and after an interview he accepted it.

Gardner remained at Carnegie for nineteen years; for the last decade of that term he was its president. His work there gave him the opportunity to engage in an intense learning curve. He devoured everything that came across his desk, systematically working his way through each subject that came up on the corporation's agenda. Foundation work was something that he did well and enjoyed enormously. Among the foundation's many outstanding achievements during Gardner's presidency was the creation of a different kind of educational television program for children: "Sesame Street."

At Carnegie, Gardner began using his writing ability again in an unexpected way. As a result of taking part in a Rockefeller commission on the future of the nation, he wrote a slender book called *Excellence,* which has shaped the American debate about quality versus equality for almost thirty years. It was followed within a few years by *Self-Renewal,* a book that also quickly became a touchstone of American business.

In 1965 Gardner received an offer from President Johnson to become secretary of Health, Education and Welfare. He debated the offer briefly. Gardner was fifty-three. It meant leaving a job where he was comfortable, polished, and knew how to do everything, and moving to what everyone saw as the treacherous political thickets of Washington, D.C. Because of that, it appeared to be a very risky move. Gardner consulted his friends and was strongly advised against taking the position. "Don't do it," James

Conant, the president of Harvard, told him. "That town will eat you alive. You're too civilized. You're too nice. That's a mean crowd down there. They play rough. The country will lose a good educational leader and Washington won't gain a thing."

Gardner's intuition told him to take the job; the position intrigued him, despite the warnings of his friends. Ultimately, he decided to follow his instincts and accept the position. His feelings were right: the years in Washington were exhilarating, enormously fruitful, and full of new experiences and discoveries.

After stepping down from HEW in 1968, Gardner decided to take an even greater risk: he founded an organization for the American citizen, Common Cause. Next he started an organization for nonprofit organizations, Independent Sector, providing a forum where such organizations and donors could come together under the same umbrella and communicate more easily. Both organizations continue to flourish today.

In 1990 Gardner made another career change: at the age of seventy-eight he left Washington to return to Stanford University. As centennial professor of business, he is sharing what he has learned with a generation of students more than half a century behind him in their educational lives. Gardner has had a lasting impact on American business through *Excellence* and *Self-Renewal,* even though he himself has never been a businessman nor attended business school.

Outgrowing a position—knowing how to do everything the job required, leaving no further sense of novelty or personal challenge, and wanting to move into work that provided more opportunity for growth—ranked high on the list of reasons for the shifts that Explorers made. The amount of time it took to outgrow a job varied from person to person and situation to situation. When a job was particularly challenging or had special advantages, finding the internal motivation to leave it could take a long time, as was the case with John Gardner's twenty years in foundation work.

Gardner realized he was ready for something new when chance brought him an offer to leave the presidency of Carnegie. Explorers who sought a new challenge without a boost from coincidence often had a harder time of it, as in the case of Betty Furness, who became nationally famous as a spokesperson for Westinghouse and then had trouble breaking out of that highly visible, but extremely limiting, role.

BETTY FURNESS

Betty Furness was nudged into her career when she was fourteen; her father told her to find a job instead of sitting around for the summer. An actress friend of her mother's introduced her to John Robert Powers, a modeling agent, who was quite impressed with Furness's voice. "Sound had just come in," she recalled. "Stars were dying like flies in Hollywood because no one could talk— and I could."

In 1932, at the age of sixteen, Furness signed a two-year contract with RKO. With her mother's help she remained in Hollywood six years and made thirty-five movies. She married songwriter Johnnie Green, author of "Body and Soul," and moved back to New York; but the couple's careers stalled, and they divorced.

Furness returned to California and got remarried, to a man who did not want her to work. But by 1948, his own professional life was not going well. They returned to New York and Furness took any job she could find—a principle she has found very useful in her life.

"I followed my nose at that time into television," she said. "It was just beginning. In the spring of 1949, I did a commercial for Westinghouse. They were brand new at this, and they were hiring radio actresses who couldn't remember lines and panicked looking at a camera. I could remember lines and I knew how to look at a camera. I did the show once, and they said come back next week—and eleven and a half years later I left."

Furness became famous almost overnight, a vivacious and sophisticated brunette who demonstrated the fine points of refrigerators and other kitchen appliances in an era when being an efficient housewife was serious business. She enjoyed the celebrity and wore her role easily. But by 1960, Furness was forty-four years old, had been with Westinghouse for eleven years, and had become restless. Although she did not talk about it in those terms, her description of her experience is the closest in the study group to the conventional midlife crisis.

"I wanted to find out if I could think," she says. "I had spent my entire career doing what people had told me to—learning lines and saying lines. I had become very interested in government and politics at the political conventions; I had done three sets of them. I decided that I didn't want to be around show business at all anymore. I wanted to deal with the real world."

Furness decided that she wanted to be a television journalist. But her association with Westinghouse, her lack of experience, and the fact that she was a woman made finding a job impossible. "It took me about six years of taking, again, any job I could get, trying to fight my way toward something that might have some meaning," she said.

As one step, since she could not find a paying position, she did some volunteer work for Vista and Project Headstart in 1965–66. This must have extended her reputation, because in February 1967 she got a call from the White House asking if she would like to be President Johnson's special assistant for consumer affairs. "I was totally stunned," Furness said. "I went to Washington a couple of days later, and said, 'Would you say that again?'" They did, and she took the job.

Inwardly, Furness was concerned because she felt she knew nothing about consumer affairs. "I figured that although I didn't know anything about it, I'd better do it right, as I didn't want to embarrass the president of the United States. I did not know the consumer world at all. What I didn't appreciate then was that neither did anybody else!" Furness worked very hard in the position and by the time she left felt that she had earned respect from professionals as well as the public.

After leaving the White House, Furness wrote a consumer column for *McCall's* magazine. A year later she accepted a position as first executive director of the New York Consumer Protection Board. But it soon became evident that the New York State legislature's commitment to the board was minimal. Furness resigned. Six months later, Mayor John Lindsay called and asked her to fill out Bess Myerson's term in the New York Department of Consumer Affairs.

During this term, a television executive saw Furness on a televised news conference and called to ask her if she would be interested in being a consumer affairs reporter on television. So when Lindsay's term was over, she signed with NBC—and remained there for eighteen years.

Furness began working for NBC when she was fifty-eight.

From the time she first began looking, it had taken her fourteen years to find a job as a television journalist.

For a while after arriving at NBC, Furness aspired to become an anchorperson on the "Today Show," and when Barbara Walters left NBC Furness longed to be her replacement. She wasn't chosen because of her age; she was considerably older than the other candidates interviewed. "But what I didn't realize," she says now, "was that because I had my subject, age had nothing to do with what I was doing. So I sat there and kept my mouth shut. Pretty soon my sixty-fifth birthday was coming up and I didn't say a word, I just went on working. Then my sixty-fifth birthday was past and I was still working. I was delighted that I had gotten away with it. Before long I was seventy, and the same thing happened." By this time, she realized that she was the oldest reporter of either sex working on network television. Eventually she brought up the subject, and the station manager even began to brag about it, saying, "Nobody can accuse us of age discrimination—we've got Betty Furness, and she's seventy-two!"

In 1992, NBC redefined Furness's job so that she no longer fit its criteria, and at the age of seventy-six she retired. Her feelings about this were mixed. On the one hand, she wanted to continue working, and there was the appearance that she had been gerrymandered out of her job. On the other hand, she found the idea of taking a few months off intriguing, because she had had so little time for leisure or a social life during the previous twenty years. She had just successfully fought off cancer, and that gave her a heightened sense of the preciousness of time.

"I am torn between thinking that I don't want to fall into dry rot by retiring," she said, "and realizing that there are other things in life. Maybe I would like to go to a museum one day, on the 'smell-the-roses' theory. I think I will sample it; let's see what it's like. Then a few months down the road I'll say, 'Let's go back to those offers that were phoned in and see if any of them look any good.'"

Furness's and Gardner's careers provide an interesting contrast. Gardner's family placed an emphasis on education, which was lacking in Furness's upbringing; that parental interest and the awareness of education's importance was clearly an advantage for Gardner. Furness's parents simply did not think about education as an investment in their daughter's future. Furness herself did not really expect to have a career and didn't think about going to college. In addition, her career was heavily influenced by her gender. Her role at Westinghouse was one that fit traditional concepts— she was an attractive woman demonstrating household appliances for other women. Once she left Westinghouse she was working in fields in which women were only marginally accepted, and she had to wait longer and work harder for the opportunities to come. On the other hand, being married provided her with some measure of support between one job and the next, which worked to her benefit.

During Gardner's early career, a kind of mentoring network existed among men through which they recruited talent, shared names among each other, and "brought along" younger men whom they saw as promising. Partly because of this network, many of Gardner's jobs came to him in a way that today seems enviable. And Gardner's education opened to him a number of familiar career paths, from which movement to other jobs was comparatively easy. By the time he went out on his own, founding Common Cause, he was so well established in reputation and in his wide network of professional friends that his chances of success were greatly enhanced.

STUDS TERKEL

Chicago radio talk show host and oral historian Studs Terkel began his career by achieving his two strongest career ambitions and then discovering he didn't like either one of them.

The son of a tailor, Terkel was born in New York in 1912. His father became ill when he was about seven, and the family moved to Chicago, where they had relatives. There, his mother ran a rooming house and later a hotel, the Wells Grand Hotel (which is still standing).

Terkel grew up around the working men who lived in the hotel, and he had a great time there. But his dreams were larger. His first career ambition was to be a lawyer. "I thought I'd be Clarence Darrow, attorney for the underdog. And I get to law school, and I get things like 'Contracts,' and 'Real Property.' It drove me out of my mind." He attended both college and law school at the University of Chicago and passed the bar exam, although not without a cliff-hanger: "I flunked the first bar," he said, "which was yes and no questions, and I didn't know them from Adam. The second bar, which was harder, was essay questions; how could I miss?" His new dream was to be a civil servant because of the tremendous security it seemed to offer—"because during the depression, you have a job, nine to five." Armed with his law degree, Terkel went to Washington to take the civil service exams. "I got a wire saying, 'You're among the cream of the crop. The job pays $1,260 a year.' Treasury Department, the second lowest [grade], CAF2. But I wanted it."

But when Terkel started work, he discovered that the job consisted solely of putting bonus coupons in envelopes so they could be mailed to World War I veterans. "It drove me nuts, of course," he said.

Having discovered that his first two career choices were jobs that he couldn't stand, Terkel quit the civil service and went back to Chicago, with no idea of what direction to take. Essentially, he changed tactics: his planned careers hadn't worked, so he decided to do whatever he could find and see how it worked out. He joined a WPA project, and one of the other men in the project, Charlie, had a (labor) theater group. Charlie invited Terkel down to see a play; the next thing he knew he was on the stage, acting.

Charlie then suggested that Terkel try out for radio soap operas—"Ma Perkins," "The Guiding Light." "And I tried out," Terkel says, "and I had that perfect gangster voice. I was the guy who said, 'Get in there, you guys.' That was me. I was threatening good ol' middle Americans all the time."

Later Terkel had a succession of other jobs: he became a disc jockey; a sportscaster, re-creating sporting events; and then a commentator, "a sort of liberal pro-Roosevelt guy. Most commentators were anti," he added, "so I got kicked off the air a lot, back and forth."

When television appeared in Chicago in 1950, Terkel became part of Chicago-style TV, along with Dave Garroway and Kukla, Fran, and Ollie. His program, "Studs' Place," was very popular. But his success didn't last long: the McCarthy era had begun, and Studs was already well known for speaking out too bluntly. He refused to say that he had been misguided in his opinions, and he was blacklisted.

Eventually an FM music station, WFMT, contacted Terkel and offered him a job. He took it because he had once heard the station play Woody Guthrie records. From his talk show came several interviews for magazines, and then Andre Schiffrin, publisher of Pantheon books, read one of the articles and called him up. Schiffrin had published Jan Myrdal's book, *Portrait of a Chinese Village,* and thought there should be an American version. "You're crazy, you're out of your mind," Terkel replied. "You can't compare a small town in China with something that happens to a big industrial city with revolutions going on at this moment." So Terkel wrote *Division Street, America,* which received much favorable attention. Schiffrin and Terkel took up the same dialogue periodically, and other books followed—*Hard Times,* written about the Great Depression for the baby-boom generation, which was growing up without knowing anything about it; *Working,* a book about working men and women and how they feel about what they do; and, most recently, *Race.*

Terkel's newest book idea wasn't given to him by Schiffrin but by "an old radical, a friend of Maggie Kuhn's, an old New England scrapper who's about seventy-five. He pins me to the wall one day and says, 'I know your next book; you're not moving until you give me your word the next book will be on old people who are troublemakers.' The idea of old people—who are often thought of as passive, quiet, dependent, and ill—being troublemakers delights Terkel and has fueled a rocket blast of enthusiasm under the project.

Terkel's saga is particularly interesting because, despite the sizable number of changes he made in the first twenty-five years of his working life, once he found the combination of being a radio talk show host and a chronicler of twentieth-century American oral history, he stayed with it and reveled in it. He derives enormous satisfaction from his work.

ROBERT MCNAMARA

The women in the Long Careers Study were not the only ones whose careers were shaped by family considerations. Robert McNamara, former secretary of defense and director and president of the Ford Motor Company, changed careers from academia to corporate management in midlife because of his wife's illness.

McNamara was born in San Francisco in 1916 and grew up in a poor neighborhood. His parents, neither of whom had gone beyond a high school education, encouraged him early on to achieve at school. McNamara excelled, graduating Phi Beta Kappa from the University of California at Berkeley in 1937. In college he developed a passionate interest in economics, and two dynamic teachers encouraged him to apply to the Harvard Business School, which he entered in 1938.

At Harvard, McNamara married a former Berkeley classmate, Margaret Craig; they would remain married for forty years until her death in 1978. After business school, McNamara worked as an instructor at Harvard, but with the outbreak of World War II he was asked to go to Europe as a civilian consultant to the War Department. There he earned a Legion of Merit award in the Air Force.

When McNamara returned in 1945, both he and his wife fell ill with polio while McNamara was stationed at Wright Field on inactive service after his discharge. McNamara suffered only a light illness, but his wife became seriously ill and would remain hospitalized for eight months. Faced with mounting hospital bills, McNamara soon realized that his teaching job at Harvard, which he hoped to resume, would not cover these debts. Fortunately, an entrepreneurial colleague of McNamara's had thought up an idea to help save the Ford Motor Company (which had been experiencing large financial losses at the time), by sending a group of ten economists along to help run the company. McNamara was reluctant to take on this new position, but with his friend's encouragement and his concern about his wife's health, he accepted the role of assistant director of the group. He began work at Ford in 1946. It was the beginning of a long and distinguished career with the company; in 1957, he was elected director, and by 1960 he would become the first person in the history of the company who was not a member of the Ford family to be elected as the company's president.

Five weeks after he was elected president of Ford, the president of the United States, John F. Kennedy, asked McNamara to be his secretary of defense. McNamara accepted, but the decision to leave Ford was a difficult one. "I recognized my responsibility to the Ford family and to the company," he explains. "But it was very difficult to put personal or corporate considerations above those of the national interest." He took the oath of office on January 21, 1961, and served as secretary of defense until March 1968. Later that year, he became president of the World Bank Group of Institutions, eventually retiring in June 1981.

Since his retirement from the World Bank, McNamara has served on the boards of numerous corporations and is associated with a number of nonprofit associations. He is also the author of *The Essence of Security,* which he wrote while serving as defense secretary, and has written four other books to date. He often speaks publicly on global issues, such as world peace and the environment, and is the recipient of numerous honorable degrees and prizes worldwide, including the Albert Einstein Peace Prize.

McNamara attributes his achievements to a "sense of social responsibility," which developed from vivid childhood recollections of the Depression. "The memory of that economic environment is with me to this day," he says. Now in his mid-seventies, McNamara is not daunted by the aging process but instead sees it as "a function of the mind." He explains: "I think the mind is a muscle. Therefore, the exercising of the mind is a way to maintain the strength of the muscle." Aside from his mental pursuits, he is an avid skier, tennis player, mountain climber, and runner. "I enjoy physical exercise," he says. "Exercising the mind and the body is important to maintain both physical strength and mental capability."

"I am seventy-five, but I don't feel physically or mentally old," he continued. "I have an intense interest in the learning environment; it is fun for me. I don't feel any desire to retire to Palm Beach or go to the baseball games."

Sen. J. William Fulbright

Chance and circumstance played far more important roles than we had imagined for both Explorers and Transformers. Even for a man with the stature of former senator J. William Fulbright of Arkansas, a man whose legislative genius has changed the lives of millions of people, the most significant shaping factor in his career was chance.

Fulbright is a type-A Explorer who had four different jobs before he found the career that was most compelling for him: public service. First he was a businessman; then an antitrust lawyer; later a law professor; and then a university president. He served one term in the House of Representatives before becoming a senator. After leaving the Senate he became a practicing lawyer once again. Most of these shifts were the product of coincidence. Fulbright himself did not foresee any of the major turns in his career and says that he could not have done so. "None of it was anticipated," he said.

Fulbright was born in Missouri on April 9, 1905, and grew up in Arkansas. In his senior year of college at the University of Arkansas, he was awarded a Rhodes scholarship to study for three years in England at Oxford University. After returning from England, Fulbright ran into a fellow Rhodes scholar, who invited him to Washington, D.C., for a visit. During his stay, Fulbright suddenly decided it might be interesting to study law at George Washington University. He enrolled, completing his law degree in 1934. After a year at the Department of Justice, he began teaching law, first at GWU and then back home at the University of Arkansas.

In 1939, the president of the University of Arkansas died unexpectedly. To Fulbright's utter astonishment, he himself was elected to the position, becoming at thirty-five the youngest man ever to serve in that position. After three years, Fulbright returned to teaching law after having been ousted from the presidency by a vindictive politician. In 1942 a former student suggested he run for Congress against the very same politician. He followed the suggestion, was elected, and two years later decided to run for the Senate. Not only did he win, but he held his Senate seat for the next thirty years, becoming one of the nation's greatest legislators.

One of the reasons Fulbright decided to run for the Senate was the positive reaction that greeted a resolution he introduced in the House to revitalize the concept of the League of Nations. That resolution led ultimately to the creation of the league's modern successor, the United Nations.

The achievement for which Fulbright is known throughout the world was the creation after World War II of the Fulbright Fellowship program, funded by postwar loan repayments to the United States by foreign countries. It was a brilliant solution to the dilemma raised by these loan repayments, which would have bankrupted the recovering nations if they had been made in U.S. dollars. Instead, the payments were made to U.S. students in the debtor country's own currency and within its borders, providing the students with money for travel, tuition, and living expenses. Equally as important, the Fulbright scholarships initiated a new era of U.S. understanding about other nations; the United States had not previously had an active tradition of educational exchange with other countries. Today the scholarships still exist, although the loans have long since been repaid. The funds are appropriated from our own budget, and thirty foreign countries make contributions.

Another great accomplishment was Fulbright's idea for a national performing arts center in Washington; his bill was before the Senate when John F. Kennedy was assassinated. Fulbright renamed the center in honor of the slain president and, after the bill was passed, raised all the money for the center's construction from private donors.

Since leaving the Senate in 1974, Fulbright has had of-counsel status at Hogan and Hartson, a powerful Washington, D.C., law firm. He is also the honorary chairman of the Fulbright Alumni Association, which boasts thousands of members all over the world.

"I never had any idea of being a politician; nobody in my family was," Fulbright said. But although he did not plan his career in the sense we normally understand, he met opportunities more than halfway when they appeared and kept going even when he encountered obstacles. For many of the Long Careers Study group, these two qualities have been of singular importance in the shaping of their lives.

THE TYPE-B EXPLORER

DR. JONAS SALK

While the type-A Explorer (the pure explorer, if you will) changes fields and professions as he or she progresses, the type-B Explorer retains an identity based in one specific field, using that as a starting point for a number of other activities related to his or her primary profession. Dr. Jonas Salk is a strong example of the type-B Explorer.

Salk, a medical scientist and immunologist, spent the first twenty years of his professional life creating vaccines. After the splendid achievement of his polio vaccine in 1955, Salk decided that the nation needed a biomedical research institute where basic research could be housed and nourished. With the backing of the March of Dimes Foundation, he set about finding a site and gathering support for what became the Salk Institute for Biological Sciences in La Jolla, California.

After the institute was up and running, Salk turned his attention to the basic ideas connecting science and the humanities. He wrote and published several books focused on his concept of human beings as the only biological form that can consciously participate in and change the course of its own evolution. Meanwhile, he had been tapped to be a member of the board of trustees of the newly organized MacArthur Foundation in Chicago and began a period of deep involvement in the board's efforts to bring shape and purpose to the huge, but still unformed, new foundation, concentrating particularly on research programs in health, the sciences, and medical research.

After four years of intense work with the MacArthur Foundation, Salk began to take note of another new development: the appearance of AIDS. It was perhaps inevitable that the man who created the vaccine for the most feared disease of the 1940s and 1950s would become deeply fascinated by the AIDS virus and its devastating impact on human life. Because of the many contacts he had in France through his wife, artist Françoise Gilot, Salk became acquainted with the major figures in a transatlantic quarrel over who first isolated the virus: French researchers or American researchers. He played a key role in mediating that quarrel, which had threatened to disrupt research on both sides of the Atlantic for years to come, and his signal contribution was explicitly described and acknowledged with gratitude in the written accords that laid the controversy to rest.

Meanwhile, Salk's own work on the AIDS virus appeared more and more promising. In September 1987 the state legislature of California passed a bill allowing California physicians to test experimental substances within the state on residents of the state, with permission required only from the California Food and Drug Board, rather than from the national Food and Drug Administration. As this book is being written, Salk's immunotherapeutic preparation is still in the process of testing in both animals and in a number of human subjects.

Liz Carpenter

Liz Carpenter is a type-B Explorer in the field of journalism. Reading and writing were part of her heredity. Her ancestors had brought an entire town library from Tennessee to Salado, Texas, where she grew up, and she retains fond memories of days spent devouring the stories in those musty books. Writing became a natural form of expression for Carpenter almost from the moment she entered school.

"It never occurred to me to do anything but go into journalism and newspapers, because I'd enjoyed so much working on the high school paper and I excelled at it," Carpenter explained. She entered the University of Texas School of Journalism and wrote for the Austin paper and the *Daily Texan,* as well as for the university paper. She also was the first woman to run for (and win election to) the office of vice president of the student body. After graduating in 1942, she went to Washington, D.C., with a scrapbook full of clippings and literally knocked on doors at the National Press Building.

As a young reporter in Washington, Carpenter attended several of Franklin and Eleanor Roosevelt's famous press conferences. In 1944, she married a former classmate from her high school newspaper days, Leslie Carpenter, and moved with him to Philadelphia, where she worked for the United Press while he was stationed at the Naval Yard. When the war ended, the Carpenters moved back to Washington and formed their own news bureau in 1952, representing twenty newspapers in the Southwest.

In 1960 Carpenter's career experienced its first change in course. After attending the Democratic convention that nominated Kennedy and Johnson, Carpenter was asked to join the campaign as Ladybird Johnson's press liaison. Carpenter accepted and was soon hard at work all over the country—though she concentrated her efforts on Texas. After the election had been won, Robert Kennedy told her that it was Ladybird who had carried Texas.

Carpenter found it fascinating and exhilarating to be on the other side of news stories for the first time in her life. She never returned to her full-time partnership in the Carpenter News Bureau. Johnson appointed her as his executive assistant, the first woman to hold the position; from 1963 to 1969 she served as Ladybird's press secretary and chief of staff.

After leaving that position Carpenter wrote a book about her years in the White House, *Ruffles and Flourishes,* which became a best-seller, and then became vice president of the public relations firm Hill and Knowlton. In 1971, she became actively involved with the women's movement and was a founding member of the National Women's Political Caucus.

Today, Carpenter continues to be actively involved in women's political issues. She has recently written another book called *Getting Better All the Time;* and she is the lead singer of a decidedly informal singing group, the Bay-at-the-Mooners.

"I think one of the most aging things is to have no sense of purpose. When you work, you have a sense of purpose," Carpenter emphasizes. Her sense of purpose was given a new focus when her dying older brother asked her to take on his second family of three children in the summer of 1991. At the age of seventy-one, Carpenter readily accepted the responsibility for three adolescents. "Maybe grandparents should have been the child-raisers all along," she says. "I think God should have let us have kids later in life, instead of when we were young and ambitious and had to hire baby-sitters. Because I think you learn more from them now."

In Carpenter's career, each position led to another, different but related, position. "It happened without my setting any goal. None of that went on; it just happened," she said.

DR. JAMES DUMPSON

Dr. James Dumpson's career was influenced in large part by a series of mentors who advised, encouraged, and assisted him in the development of his career. Dumpson, for many years vice president of the New York Community Trust, has based his career in social work, serving his community in a number of different but related capacities, in the pattern defined by the type-B Explorers.

Born in 1909, Dumpson grew up in a tough and very poor district of Philadelphia that was largely segregated. He believes now that his must have been a low-income family, although at the time he thought they were middle class. He lived in a brownstone tenement and went to school in a settlement house.

Dumpson had two main early mentors. The first was his mother, who had been a teacher before her marriage. The second was a high school teacher who assigned him to write a paper on Alain Locke, the first black Rhodes scholar. After high school, when he was working as a butler and cook, his employer suggested he attend the University of Pennsylvania and work only part-time for her. He then worked as a waiter for Richard Beamish, who later became secretary of state in Pennsylvania and hired Dumpson to work in his office for a year after his graduation from Teachers College.

Dumpson then taught at a Pennsylvania public school for four years before returning to Philadelphia in 1937 to work in the Department of Public Assistance. His supervisor there encouraged him to get a degree in social work. He enrolled at the Pennsylvania School of Social Work, where he met yet another mentor, Dorothy Kahn. He credits Kahn as one of the people most responsible for his going to New York, where he worked for seven years for the Children's Aid Society before joining the Welfare Council of New York City in 1947.

Since then, Dumpson has had a brilliant career as a consultant to several United Nations delegations on welfare and social services issues; executive director to many federal and state agencies; commissioner of welfare for New York State; and dean at the schools of social work at Fordham and Hunter. He was instrumental in reforming New York's social services network in the 1950s, including setting up the foster care program as a replacement for the dismal and depressing orphanages that had been the only refuge for abandoned children. He is currently a special assistant to Mayor Dinkins and is the health services administrator of the New York City Health and Hospitals Corporation.

Mentors often played a significant role in the careers of the minority participants who had to combat more overt discrimination than they might today. Though all his mentors other than his mother and Alain Locke were white, Dumpson says he never questioned their motives for helping him at the time and firmly believes, in retrospect, that their motives were personally, not racially, based.

LOUIS HECTOR

A number of explorers made at least one change to a position that was intrinsically short-term in nature. For example, people who had begun their careers in business or law and then took government positions in Washington, D.C., usually knew when they accepted the job that they would not stay in that position beyond a certain term. A number of short-term changes were associated with war, particularly with World War II.

Miami attorney Louis Hector is one of the most flexible of the Explorers. By his own count, he has changed tacks ten times in his career so far. Hector attributes this diversity in part to his legal background. "Since a lawyer's life consists of taking up new problems constantly," he said, "problems that often involve a new type of business or subject matter, new people, I think lawyers are particularly flexible."

Hector was born in 1917 and grew up a native of Florida, but his parents sent him to traditional northeastern and European schools: Phillips Academy in Andover, Massachusetts; Harvard and Williams colleges; Oxford University, England (as a Rhodes scholar); and Yale Law School. He recalls his first career aspiration at the age of twelve was to be an architect. "I like planning things," he adds. It wasn't until he was a student at Oxford that he became interested in law.

After serving in the Department of Justice, the Lend-Lease Administration, the State Department, and the Office of Strategic Services during World War II, Hector returned to Miami in 1946 to work for an established law firm.

Hector was thirty-three when he made his first major career change. In 1947, he stopped practicing law to run a family agricultural business, Hector Supply Company of Miami. Eight years later, he returned to the practice of law and formed his own firm. Three years after that, he took another new direction to work in Washington at the Civil Aeronautics Board for two years until 1959.

"The Civil Aeronautics Board controlled the airlines," he recalled. "By that point, it was clear that the city of Miami in South Florida was heavily dependent upon civil aviation for tourism. . . . I knew our two senators and several other civic people in town thought it would be important to get someone from Florida who understands Florida's particular aviation problems on the Civil Aeronautics Board. They approached me and asked me if I would do it, and it sounded very interesting. Which it was!"

Two years later, he returned to his practice in Miami for another seven years, during which time he took off a year to serve, for Howard Hughes, as trustee of Northeast Airlines and arrange for its sale. Then in 1968, he became chairman of the executive committee of Southeast Banking Corporation.

Once again in 1974, Hector went back to law. And since 1983 he has been the chairman of the Lucille P. Markey Charitable Trust, a private foundation whose sole interest is basic medical research. He continues to sit on various boards and to practice law.

Hector believes that law firms generally value the presence of older lawyers. "They encourage the older lawyers to come down and have lunch with the younger lawyers, and they encourage the younger lawyers to ask the older lawyers for advice. I don't think that corporations operate that way. When you're out, you're out." He also mentioned that he thinks it can be very useful for lawyers to take time away and work in business or government. "One of the reasons why it is so interesting—and so much fun— for a lawyer to become a businessman or a banker for a while is that he becomes a client who employs other lawyers and sees how the relationship works from the other side. When they do go back to practicing law, I'm certain they are much better lawyers for having the experience of being a client."

Hector is one of the many study participants who told me they simply never thought about retiring at sixty-five. He insists that today, at seventy-seven, he continues to be much too busy to consider retirement. "If you're part of an institution or if you're practicing law or administering an estate, you have to keep busy," he said. "If you've been an officer of a corporation and you retire [you've been living in a big city, probably, and you move to a sub- urb], there's no institution that keeps you involved in new, fresh problems and in contact with younger, busy people. I find I get the greatest pleasure out of the younger lawyers because they are so active and they're so interesting. They're enthusiastic and that's contagious."

SUMMARY

There is a discernible set of patterns underlying all of the Explor- ers' career changes. A large percentage of Explorers went from being employees in their early jobs, to becoming managers, and finally to becoming entrepreneurs, creating their own business or nonprofit organizations. This *employee-manager-entrepreneur* sequence held true for both type-A and type-B Explorers.

Most Explorers showed some version of this pattern. A typi- cal employee-manager-entrepreneur sequence was that of pro- ducer David Brown, who started his career alternating between free-lance and employee jobs, climbed his way to a vice presi- dency of Twentieth Century–Fox, then became disillusioned with destructive corporate politics and launched out on his own. He has since thrived on running his own production company, the Manhattan Project.

Some Explorers went from employee to manager and then remained at the managerial level for the rest of their careers, as did Dr. James Dumpson. He has changed managerial posts a number of times but has always worked in an institution or government organization.

Others skipped the manager phase and simply went from employee to entrepreneur. Robert Schwartz, an Ohio-born journalist, spent a number of years at the beginning of his career working for Time-Life. One day a corporate friend suggested he open a conference center to serve the many companies that wanted to give training seminars and other types of conferences but were having trouble finding appropriate, well-run hotels or conference centers. Schwartz built the Motel on the Mountain, a Japanese-style hotel outside New York City that became famous for its beauty and efficient operation. Next he bought the old Harriman mansion in Tarrytown and renamed it Tarrytown House. It not only attracted corporate clients but became a thriving intellectual center, attracting a board with nationally known figures like Margaret Mead and developing the concept of entrepreneurship into a School for Entrepreneurs. Eventually, Schwartz sold Tarrytown House and has since shifted his focus again, to a different kind of entrepreneurship: he is writing a book on innovation in contemporary society and developing a role as a freestanding magnet for ideas and people, without the setting of a conference center around him.

The fullest version of the employee-manager-entrepreneur pattern was found in John Gardner, who went from teacher, to employee, to manager, to entrepreneur, and back to teacher again in his most recent move. A few Explorers (such as former secretary of labor Willard Wirtz, former TIAA-CREF chairman William Greenough, and Gray Panthers founder Maggie Kuhn had a teacher phase at the start of their careers but did not return to it. Another common sequence of pattern was a *change in the focus of the person's work from narrow to broad*. Dr. Jonas Salk, for example, began his career with a narrow focus as a medical scientist, although his natural interests were always much wider. Success as a research physician enabled him to broaden his career activities: to found the Salk Institute, then to write about the ideas that undergird science, next to become involved in philanthropy, and finally to return to medical research while retaining the other activities he had developed along the way.

Other Explorers changed the *order of magnitude* of the issues they dealt with. They began by dealing with local, grass-roots, microlevel problems and then progressed to the regional, national, and finally international levels. Esther Peterson, whose career is described in more detail in chapter 11, started her work at the most individual grass-roots level, teaching in summer schools for union women and doing union organizing. She moved up to successively broader work for unions, eventually representing an entire union as a lobbyist. Then she moved on to a still larger, national scale as a consumer advocate and an official in the Department of Labor. After a detour working for a large regional corporation, the Giant Food chain, she went back to the national level and then moved to the international level, where she is currently the consumers union representative to the United Nations.

Some participants changed both focus and order of magnitude. Dr. W. Edwards Deming, the management expert whose ideas triggered the Japanese quality revolution after World War II, moved both from a narrow focus (in one field, mathematics) to a broad one (the use of statistics in quality control), and from the grass-roots (the management of employees in one organization) to the collective (organizational management and quality control) level. He began his career as an engineer and a mathematician, spending a number of years working for manufacturing companies and for government agencies that made heavy use of statistics, such as the U.S. Census Bureau. Invited by the Japanese to help them rebuild their census bureau after the war, he became fascinated with the quality control difficulties faced by their industries and began to work with them on that problem. He then developed a consulting clientele among companies that wished to improve their quality, in the United States and elsewhere. Statistics was an important tool in his system of quality control, but its boundaries encompassed other types of knowledge as well. Now internationally famous, he consults for individual corporations and teaches his methods—to an estimated ten thousand people each year.

The most provocative question raised by the Explorers is: why is theirs the largest group? Judging from what was thought to be typical of work practices during the first half of the century, the largest group should have been the Homesteaders. The group that made only one change, the Transformers, should have been the next largest; and the smallest group should have been the Explorers.

There was essentially no difference in the level of talent

among the three groups; indeed, some of the most visibly talented people (writers, artists, and actors) were Homesteaders. There were equivalent percentages of professionals in the Homesteader and Transformer categories.

One exception to the relatively even spread of professions through the three groups seemed to be law. As I mentioned earlier, two-thirds of the study's attorneys were Explorers. A law degree seemed to provide an unusual amount of flexibility and opportunity in career development. It enabled the person to have a base in a law firm if they wished and to leave periodically to do other things, returning to the firm when each short-term assignment was over. A partner who was successful outside the firm became an asset in new ways, drawing favorable public attention to the firm, making valuable contacts for it, and bringing the prestige earned in outside assignments back to the firm with them. In firms where attorneys were required to take of-counsel status at the age of seventy, the individual was still able to use the firm as a base while doing other things.

Although there does not seem to be a single reason for the differences between the Explorers' job patterns and those of the other two groups, and for the Explorers outnumbering the Homesteaders and the Transformers, there are two possible explanations that might be valid. First, the study did not include many people in midlevel and low-level industrial, manufacturing, or corporate jobs. Because work in these categories may have been more physically demanding or less interesting, it may be that people in those categories had a greater tendency to conform to the one-job/one-career pattern and then retire. Because of age bias, many people who might have liked to continue working might not have been able to. It could also be true that there *are* just as many Explorers at those job levels, like Ollie Thompson and Louise Brown, but we did not have any way of finding them. It would be an interesting question for other researchers to consider.

The second possibility is that we have simply underestimated the amount of change in people's careers during the early part of the twentieth century. There was a great deal of social upheaval during the first half of the century, of a kind that typically results in work-life changes for millions of people: World War I, World War II, and the Great Depression and several minor depressions (one in 1921 immediately following World War I and one around 1950 just following World War II). Perhaps corporate America endorsed the Homesteader as an ideal but that it was never the pattern of even a majority of workers throughout their work life because of economic and historical factors.

In a sense, the Explorers are especially relevant for contemporary readers because the Explorer pattern has become so much more widespread in the post-1960's United States. As we near the beginning of the twenty-first century, loyalty and stability have become relatively unimportant qualities in the marketplace, while adaptability and flexibility have become more desirable. The Explorer, with his or her constantly expanding horizon, is a highly contemporary figure. The ability to adjust well to change may allow the individual to fill multiple roles at work, adapt quickly to rapidly evolving technology, and absorb the stresses and strains of recessions, plant closings, corporate downsizing, and early retirement, while still retaining enough self-esteem and energy to function well despite the shifting work environment.

The Census Bureau predicts that children born in the 1990s will have, like John Gardner, an approximate total of about eight jobs during their lifetimes. As society absorbs the massive changes wrought by the 1980s in the job market and the economy, Explorers will probably continue to outnumber any other career pattern for the foreseeable future.

The Many Paths to a Long Career

Contrary to what might be expected, adding length to careers does not necessarily mean that they will be more likely to follow a particular pattern. Two of the three oldest people in the study, Michael Heidelberger and Theresa Bernstein Meyerowitz, were Homesteaders, and the third, Edward Bernays, is an early Transformer. An examination of the career patterns described in the previous chapters revealed that there was no single decisive factor that caused a person to become a Homesteader, a Transformer, or an Explorer. Career patterns were not based strictly on age, gender, or field. Each participant had developed his or her career through a unique combination of personality, talents, background, changing circumstances and interests, luck, and determination.

Although traditional thinking about careers might lead to the hypothesis that certain fields dictate a particular career pattern, that idea was contradicted as often as it was supported by the participants' experience. Some fields did tend to cluster in a particular career category. For example, that many of the artists and scientists were Homesteaders; that a career in law lends itself to developing an Explorer-style career, and to various kinds of public service, because of the way law firms are organized and the huge variety of ways in which legal training can be applied.

Career patterns were independent of generational differences: there were Explorers who were in their nineties and Explorers who were in their sixties. Even the career patterns themselves weren't entirely exclusive or linear in structure. There were a few participants who had multiple-track careers, maintaining two or more separate careers simultaneously throughout their work lives.

MULTIPLE-TRACK CAREERS

The possibility of multiple-track careers was first pointed out to me by Peter Drucker, who described an example that he had heard about from his father in his youth. An English banker who wrote the first book on banking (which was used as a textbook for many years afterward) died in 1912. At the man's funeral, Drucker said, an odd thing happened. The man's banking colleagues were present, but there was another large group of mourners also in attendance, whom the bankers had never seen before although they seemed to be well acquainted with the deceased. It turned out that the strangers were classicists. Unbeknownst to his colleagues, the banker was the world's greatest living expert on Homer and had been recognized as such for many years. His banking colleagues knew nothing about his "other" professional identity as a classicist. And his classicist colleagues didn't know of his prominence as a banker. In fact, Drucker says he thinks it is possible that no one whom the man knew, until his funeral, was aware that he had had two simultaneous careers, both distinguished, in widely different fields.

This man's two careers were exceptionally compartmentalized. Most double or triple careers are not as stringently separated from each other as his were. There are also double and triple careers that interlock in some way, each reinforcing the other.

Six of the Long Careers Study members had careers that appeared to be double or triple (or even quadruple) in form: Cyrus Vance, Françoise Gilot, Arthur Schlesinger, Jr., Max Lerner, Shelby Cullom Davis, and Charlotte Zolotow. The criteria we evolved to describe a multiple-track career were that the person had to be perceived as a full-fledged professional in that field and that the interest had to persist throughout the person's work life. There were many people in the study who went through periods of doubling in brass in some respect, but they didn't do it consistently throughout their lives.

CYRUS VANCE

Former secretary of state Cyrus Vance developed two interests in childhood that persisted into his adult life and shaped his career in an exceptional manner. After his father died in 1925, when he was eight years old, Vance and his younger brother were taken to Switzerland for a year by his mother. The two boys lived with a Swiss family, went to Swiss schools, and learned to speak French. The trip may have been, on Mrs. Vance's part, a way of distracting her sons from the enormous loss they had suffered. But it gave Vance an unusual education about other cultures, which he found fascinating.

Vance attended Yale University both as an undergraduate and a law student. Next he served for almost five years on a navy destroyer, first as a gunnery officer and late in the war as acting executive officer. When he returned home, he briefly considered a career in business and worked for six months for the Meade paper company. Through that experience he reaffirmed that he really wanted to be an attorney, and he joined the law firm of Simpson, Thatcher and Bartlett as a litigator.

In 1957, Vance was asked by a colleague to act as cocounsel for a set of hearings of the Senate Armed Services Subcommittee, chaired by Lyndon Johnson. During the several years when he was involved in the hearings, Vance met many politicians and became known in Washington. When Kennedy was elected, Vance was asked to serve as general counsel to the Defense Department and special assistant to Robert McNamara. After a year and a half, he was appointed secretary of the army, and two years later he was appointed deputy secretary of state, a post he held until 1967. Vance then returned to his practice as a trial lawyer. One issue for many of the study participants who performed public service was the decrease in their earnings that they had to accept in order to spend time in a government job. Vance, like many others, addressed this problem by alternating time in Washington with work in his profession.

Even during times when he was back at his firm, Vance occasionally was asked to take on special projects. One such instance arose the day before Thanksgiving in 1967. Vance got a call from Nicholas de B. Katzenbach, then the deputy secretary of state, on behalf of President Johnson. "He said, 'The President wants you to go to Cyprus this afternoon,'" Vance recalled. "I said, 'Nick, you're kidding.' He said, 'No, he said he absolutely wants you to go.'"

"Subsequently, the president and I talked," Vance said. "He told me that it looked like there was going to be a war [between the Greeks and the Turks] and he wanted me to get myself damn quick on a plane that he had already sent up. He said, 'It's on its way to Kennedy. I want you to go over there and stop these people from invading and see if you can work out a solution.' I said, 'Mr. President, what are my instructions?' He said, 'Use your best judgment. If there is anything I can do to help, let me know. Otherwise, you are on your own.'"

Vance and his team were successful. An agreement was reached among Greece, Turkey, and Cyprus, using the United Nations as a mediating agent.

In 1968 Vance was asked to go to Korea to prevent the resumption of hostilities between the South and the North, and then to Detroit to represent Johnson when race riots broke out after the assassination of Martin Luther King. Vance's critique of what the country needed to do to be better able to handle problems of that kind became a kind of bible for how military forces should handle themselves in the event of civil disorder. Subsequently, Vance was asked to play a role in quelling the riots in Washington, D.C. He used everything he had learned in his previous experience to help restore order to the city.

After Carter was elected, he asked Vance to serve as Secretary of State. The Carter administration achieved several very important goals, restoring international affairs to public attention and highlighting the importance of human rights. Perhaps the most important of these was the Camp David accords, which ended open hostilities between Israel and the Arab countries.

Vance continues to pursue his interest in controversial legal issues, being a proponent of, for example, mandatory pro bono work, court reform, and minority participation. He is also serving as the chairman of the Federal Reserve Bank of New York. In 1991 he was asked by President Bush to go to Yugoslavia as personal envoy of the United Nations Secretary-General. He has also played a role in mediating between warring sides in South Africa.

At age seventy-five, Vance has not retired and has no immediate plans to do so. He expects to continue working indefinitely, and he reels off a list of international, national, social, and legal problems still to be solved. "There is so much to be done," he says. "There are more things than I could have dreamed of."

Like many other lawyers in the study, Vance, a type-B Explorer, has had a pattern of alternation between his legal career and outside assignments. Unlike most of the other attorneys, however, Vance's outside assignments have been almost exclusively in diplomacy and mediation, giving him a second, parallel career, connected in many ways with his primary occupation.

What is curious and somewhat provocative about the remaining five participants with multiple-track careers is that each had writing as one main career track. These people had a compelling drive to translate into writing the experiences and concerns of their other activities. Because writing is a flexible pursuit in terms of scheduling, these participants were able to find time for their writing projects either during or after other work.

For all of these participants, their writing has brought them equal or greater success than their other career tracks, which often provided them with the material or the environment necessary for writing their books.

FRANÇOISE GILOT

Although she identifies herself more as a painter than a writer, Françoise Gilot has had careers in both fields. Like Celeste Holm, Gilot became aware of what she wanted to do very early in life. When she was about one year old she woke up one morning to find that it had snowed. She was utterly astonished that everything had suddenly become white and beautiful. She also remembers, shortly after that day, cutting her finger accidentally and being transfixed by the bright red color of the blood. These intense early memories of color showed very directly her early artistic inclinations.

The only child of a demanding mother and a difficult father, Gilot had to face a number of hurdles before she was free in adulthood to follow her dreams. Despite her long fascination with art, her father decided that she must go to law school in order to acquire a practical skill that would enable her to earn a living. She did so, and even passed her bar exam; then she moved out of her parents' home and went to stay with her grandmother so she could paint.

Around this time she met Pablo Picasso, who was attracted to her both for her exceptional beauty and intelligence and because her training as an artist enabled them to communicate as equals. They lived together for ten years and had two children, Paloma and Claude. Meanwhile, Gilot continued to draw and paint, receiving a good deal of favorable critical attention and mounting several shows. As her career bloomed, Picasso became more jealous because it distracted her from him, and he began to be unfaithful; in 1954 Gilot left him. Returning to Paris, Gilot tried to reestablish herself on her own. Eventually she began to seek a wider audience, coming to the United States several times to work at Los Angeles Tamarind Workshop. On one such visit, mutual friends introduced her to polio vaccine pioneer Dr. Jonas Salk. They were married some six months later, and they now make their home in La Jolla, California, not far from the Salk Institute, with regular visits to New York and Paris.

As a girl, Gilot had written poetry; she branched out into essays when she began to be established as an artist. She has always been interested in the ideas underlying art as well as in the act of painting and the object of art itself, and her writing reflects these themes. After breaking up with Picasso, she decided to write a book about their life together. *Life with Picasso* was published in 1964 and became an international best-seller. She has published a number of other books, including several volumes of poems and the recent memoir *Matisse and Picasso: A Friendship in Art*. She continues to paint, to write, to lecture on art and on her writing, and to exhibit widely.

There is no sense of conflict in Gilot's double-track career. Painting and writing are two very different ways of recording and shaping experience, although she does say that she finds painting the more relaxing of the two activities. For major projects she alternates between the two; when she writes she paints very little, and when she paints she does not work on major writing projects.

What Gilot has struggled with most has been the special professional difficulty of being a woman. In her case, an early committed relationship with a world-renowned colleague was both an advantage and a handicap: it made her famous, but it also made her seem less of an artist in her own right in an era when women were universally viewed as second-class citizens. Rebuilding her career after the relationship ended took extraordinary strength and determination, even though ultimately she succeeded. Almost forty years later, she is one of the greatest living woman painters;

at seventy, she is starting a new career peak as her reputation continues to ascend.

ARTHUR SCHLESINGER, JR.

Despite his formidable career as a historian, Arthur Schlesinger, Jr., sees himself first as a writer. He has also spent time as a public servant, and has earned his living as a university teacher. The son of a historian who taught for several years in Iowa before moving to Harvard University, Schlesinger was born in Iowa and grew up in Cambridge, Massachusetts. He went to Harvard, where he wrote a senior honors essay that later became his first book, published in 1939. Three years of postgraduate work as a member of the Society of Fellows provided the opportunity to write his second.

Although he does not remember a particular point when he became aware of it, Schlesinger had a sense early on that he wanted to be both a writer and a historian. "I grew up as the son of a historian in a house filled with history," he said, "and I suppose the alternatives are either to acquiesce, or to rebel against fate and become a broker or something. I have always been fascinated by history. It was a natural evolution."

After Pearl Harbor, Schlesinger worked first for the Office of War Information and later for the Office of Strategic Services. His second book, *The Age of Jackson*, came out in 1945. After the war ended he stayed in Washington for a few years doing freelance writing assignments for *Life, Colliers,* the *Saturday Evening Post,* and "other extinct magazines," as he puts it. Finally in 1947 he returned to Harvard and taught there until 1961, when he was asked by President Kennedy to serve as his special assistant.

After Kennedy's assassination, Schlesinger again stayed in Washington for a time. *A Thousand Days* was written in 1964 and published in 1965. When Schlesinger resigned from his White House job, he didn't want to return either to Cambridge (where he had already spent forty years) or to full-time teaching, which left him too little time to write and think. At that point, City University of New York offered him one of its Schweitzer professorships in the humanities, so in 1966 he moved to New York, where he has lived ever since.

Schlesinger is not a conventional academic. "I always found

the larger life, nonacademic and so on, more fun than academia," he said. And, in fact, his engagement with the "larger life" has enriched both his writing and his understanding of history. "The years in the White House confirmed certain impressions I had about the way the world is governed," he said. "That is, historians tend to tidy up the past, impute plan and premeditation to situations—whereas most things happen much more casually and with much more improvisation and accident."

Schlesinger has been married twice. With a historian's penchant for measuring time, he told me that the fall of 1991 was the first time since 1942 that he had lived in a house without children—he had had children in his house for fifty years! (He has six in all, including one stepson.) "Which I think is wonderful," he said. "It's kept me young. I've had children every decade; it's kept me abreast of everything that's going on." And the empty nest "hasn't been as much of a shock as I expected."

Schlesinger is just now beginning to draft the fourth volume of *The Age of Roosevelt*; the first three volumes were published in the late 1950s. When I asked him why he did not retire at sixty-five, he replied, "Writers never retire. Historians never retire. I saw my dear friend Ken Galbraith the other day, and he said (I forget what this was a propos of) 'The trouble is, I just can't stop writing! Every morning!' And I feel the same way."

MAX LERNER

Columnist Max Lerner had what is essentially a double-track career, but it was the most complex of any of the people in this category. Throughout his career, he alternated between teaching and writing, interweaving these two activities in many different ways.

Lerner was born in 1902 in a small village in "Polish Russia," as he called it, and was brought to the United States in 1907. Eventually his family settled in New Haven, where he went to Yale from the elementary level to his undergraduate studies. He majored in literature and wanted to become a college professor but was discouraged by a senior faculty member who told him, "Impossible! You're a Jew and no good college will take a Jew in literature." So Lerner chose instead to attend Yale School of Law, which he didn't particularly like. He left law school to pursue graduate work in economics; ultimately he earned first a master's degree from Washington University and then a Ph.D. from the Brookings Institute in Washington, D.C., both on fellowships.

Over the next few years, Lerner worked on the *Encyclopedia of the Social Sciences,* taught at Sarah Lawrence and Harvard, and became an editor at the *Nation.* He subsequently taught at a number of other colleges and universities, wrote many books on American culture and political life, and undertook various editorial positions. In 1948 he became a columnist for the *New York Post,* a role he filled with great enjoyment until his death in the spring of 1992.

In 1990, Lerner completed a personal memoir of his two bouts with cancer and his recovery from a heart attack, *Wrestling with the Angel: A Memoir of My Triumph Over Illness.*

A colleague of Lerner's described him as having five lives: his teaching life, his columnist's life, his lecturing life, his book-writing life, and his personal life. Despite the illnesses he suffered in his eighties, Lerner at almost ninety still kept up all five interests. "You can't retire from life—or from work, in a true sense," he said. "A job is something you get paid for—you need that. [But] work is something you do because you have internal needs. I can no more help working than I can help breathing. . . . It is one way to keep your energy going. I have found my work saw me through my two cancers."

Like Studs Terkel, Lerner went to law school, didn't like it, and never practiced. Instead he studied economics and political science, both social sciences that resembled his original love, literature, more than they resembled law. He found a way to use his passion for literature through writing, and then wrote on the subjects he had ultimately chosen in college, politics and economics. In his later life, when illness struck, Lerner believed his work actually sustained him; it gave him a way to continue to be active in the outside world and a motivation to recover. Indeed, when he died he was on his way to recovery from his third bout with cancer and looking forward to taking up his regular schedule again in the not too distant future.

SHELBY CULLOM DAVIS

Another multiple career is that of Shelby Cullom Davis, a historian, businessman, and former ambassador to Switzerland. Born in 1909, Davis grew up in Illinois and received his under graduate degree from Princeton, earning first honors in history.

In the summer of 1930, following his graduation, an event took place that had a major impact on the rest of Davis's life: he was chosen to be a delegate to a mock League of Nations meeting held in Geneva, Switzerland. This was his first venture into international affairs and diplomacy, a field that would be an important strand of his later life. The trip had one other important result: on the train to Geneva, Davis met a young woman who was the Wellesley delegate, Kathryn Wasserman, and the two fell in love.

When he returned from Geneva, Davis attended Columbia University and earned an M.A. in foreign affairs. The next question was employment: the Depression was in full force, and finding a job specifically for a historian seemed at first an impossible task. As it turned out, one of Davis's professors at Columbia knew Frederick William Wyle, the chief Washington broadcaster for CBS, who was being sent to Geneva to cover the World Disarmament Conference. Wyle was looking for an assistant to go with him—and Davis seemed heaven-sent, since he spoke French and had already spent time in Geneva. Davis and Kathryn Wasserman were married on January 8, 1932, and immediately afterward sailed for Europe.

Although the World Disarmament Conference is all but forgotten today, in 1932 it was a major news item; high hopes rode upon its deliberations. The Western nations were determined to prevent another world war and saw the conference as the main instrument for doing so. In addition, Wyle's mission was a technological first.

"Transatlantic broadcasting had never been done before," Davis said. "No one was even sure whether it would work. [The first broadcast] was such an occasion that Mr. Wyle said we must do it in black tie. So we put on black tie." After a great deal of deliberation about how to structure the broadcast, they decided that Davis would go on first and introduce Wyle, who would then begin the actual broadcast. When the moment came, Shelby Cullom Davis spoke the first words ever uttered on transatlantic radio: "This is Shelby Cullom Davis speaking from Geneva, Switzerland. I now have the pleasure of introducing Mr. Frederick William Wyle." On this first broadcast they had one guest, the foreign minister of Italy.

The conference wore on, without the quick conclusion that the organizers had hoped for. Wyle went back to the United States after four months; the Davises stayed on. Their two and a half years in Switzerland were eventful. Davis traveled to Berlin and heard Goebbels speak. He heard Hitler in Hessen and sensed the rising threat of the Nazis to European and world peace. He also wrote his first two books. Both Davises earned their Ph.D.'s while in Geneva; Kathryn Davis's was in international affairs.

When the couple returned to Philadelphia in the fall of 1934, Davis went to work for his brother-in-law's investment firm for five years to learn the financial business. His first book, on World War I, had been written in Europe. In 1938, he began work on another book, *America Faces the Forties,* addressing the country's agricultural, employment, and other social and economic issues. Partly because of his publications, Davis was drafted for the Dewey campaign as a speech writer and economic adviser. He worked for the War Production Board during World War II and later served as first deputy superintendent of insurance for New York State, stimulating his interest in insurance.

In 1947 Davis was asked to take over a firm, F.L. Brokaw and Company, which specialized in insurance stocks. He renamed the new firm Shelby Cullom Davis and Company, and he has run the company for forty-two years, with one exception: from 1969 to 1975 he served as ambassador to Switzerland.

Today his main track is running his business. He has taken considerable pride in the growth of Shelby Cullom Davis and Company. At the age of eighty, Davis said: "I am up at 6:00 A.M., leave the house at 6:30, take the 6:40 train into New York, and I am in the office at a quarter to eight. . . . I enjoy more this way. I say it is the best game in town!" As a businessman he has enjoyed great success, so much so that he became a philanthropist in his own field of history, providing the funds for the Shelby Cullom Davis Center for Historical Research at Princeton and many other smaller projects.

This type of multiple career requires a certain breadth of interests and talent to maintain. Davis was able to pursue his professional interests sequentially and often simultaneously. He maintained his career as a historian by writing articles for journals, remaining active in professional associations, and becoming involved philanthropically, while pursuing other career paths. His identity as a diplomat was sustained even while he earned his living in business through his involvement in international affairs organizations and his political network.

CHARLOTTE ZOLOTOW

Children's book author Charlotte Zolotow has had a double career as a writer and as an editor; she briefly added a third role, being a publisher, to the mix, not because she wanted to but chiefly to support herself. Alternating between two, or even three, occupational spheres may have been comfortable and natural for Gilot, Schlesinger, Lerner, and Davis, but Zolotow did not find the process of doubling and tripling herself professionally to be an easy one. "*Schizophrenic* would really describe it," Zolotow said. "They are each totally different functions. If I had been financially able, writing would have been my only choice. But I never tried to earn a living by my writing, because *that* is creatively constricting. I have to be free for the kind of writing I can do."

Zolotow grew up in Norfolk, Virginia, the daughter of a lawyer father and a restless Baltimore Southern belle who moved the family's residence frequently. After attending a series of schools all over the Eastern seaboard, she enrolled in the University of Wisconsin, where she met her future husband, Maurice Zolotow. She returned to New York, found an entry-level position with a publishing house ("practically a scrub-lady at Harper Brothers," as she puts it), and married Maurice. The job at Harper paid $12 a week.

Zolotow worked her way up and into the editorial structure, ending up as the assistant to Ursula Nordstrom, who started the company's children's books division. Although Zolotow had been writing since she was in the fourth grade, she hadn't yet tried to get anything published. Nordstrom was extremely skilled at drawing people out, however. One day Zolotow sent Nordstrom an idea that she thought would be perfect for a picture-book author of theirs, Margaret Brown. Nordstrom wrote back, saying, "I don't know what you mean. Expand it further." Zolotow wrote a longer memo and submitted it. After reading it, Nordstrom came over to her and said, "Congratulations! You just wrote your first children's book."

From 1944 to 1962 Zolotow took time out from editing to raise two children; meanwhile, she wrote constantly and published a number of books. She also went in twice a week to have lunch with Nordstrom and follow the department's development. Once her children were grown, Zolotow went back full-time and resumed editorial work. But at home she continued writing. Because she was so successful as an editor she was made a vice president and put in charge of the Harper Children's Book Division, a position she held for some years. Her heart simply was not in administrative work, however, and in 1989 she resigned as publisher to go back to editorial work, with her own imprint.

However, even that proved too much for her growing urge to write. Zolotow tapered off her editorial duties over a period of about a year and a half, taking six months to assign all her projects to other editors and to make sure the relationships between authors and their new editors worked. Then she was given a gala retirement party by the company (now called HarperCollins Publishers) at the New York Public Library and presented with the gift she wanted most in the world: her old manual office typewriter (with a big red bow tied to it), which was wheeled into the party to a fanfare of applause.

"It's a wonderful feeling to wake up in the morning and know that what I've got to do is all invested in my own life and work, rather than in other people's," Zolotow explained. "The other people are a part of my life, but this is really an in-depth investment in all the years I've lived." The move from double to single track is clearly the right move for Zolotow at this point in her life. Her choice to "retire" from editing was based not on burnout but on the burning desire to focus on her own creative work.

The question was raised by several participants as to whether they would have had double-track careers had they been able to make a living, or acquire the other perquisites they wanted, from simply being writers. Schlesinger and Zolotow both consider themselves writers who had to earn a living doing something else—teaching in Schlesinger's case and editing in Zolotow's. Schlesinger, when asked why he hadn't retired, replied, "I would love to retire, and the reason why I can't retire is that I can't figure out any other way to get an office and a secretary, and any other place for books. I have [two offices filled with books]; I have a house filled with books. If I would bring all these books home, a couple of thousand, there'd be no room for them in the house—or for my wife Alexandra and me!"

Zolotow commented: "I never wanted a career as a publisher

anyway, or as anything except as a writer. But natural necessity and other things started me in it, and I was lucky to find something I loved as much as I do love editing. It's a way of knowing people very intimately through their writing. So I do love it. But this [work of my own] is what I've been wanting to do, waiting to do it and pushing aside."

Max Lerner, on the other hand, liked both teaching and writing and would have done both even if he hadn't had to. Shelby Cullom Davis became a businessman principally to make a living but enjoyed it as much as he enjoyed history, writing, and diplomacy. He is highly people-oriented, a characteristic reflected in his periodic involvement in diplomacy. Françoise Gilot was always intensely drawn to both painting and writing, even though she sees her primary identity as a painter. She would have done both even if monetary considerations had not been a factor.

Finally, Cyrus Vance has held a genuine passion for both law and international affairs since childhood; chance and his own substantial talents enabled him to make careers in both. His training as a lawyer enabled him to pursue his double-track career by giving him the flexibility and versatility necessary to maintain a law practice and outside diplomatic assignments.

In short, this small cluster of people with multiple careers had at least two simultaneous interests throughout their lives and who managed to find a way to pursue all of them. A particular kind of mental focus was required to maintain two or more career tracks at once; their success also benefited from a measure of luck in the practical world.

SAME FIELD, DIFFERENT PATTERN

In the Long Careers Study, participants' choices of what field to work in did not always determine career pattern. In fact, it was quite the opposite: there were participants in the same field with very different career patterns. A good example of this diversity is provided by three distinguished survey experts who took part in the study: Louis Harris, founder of Louis Harris and Associates; and Florence Skelly and Dan Yankelovich, two of the three founders of Yankelovich, Skelly and White. Each of these participants falls into a different career typology. Skelly is a Homesteader; Harris is an early Transformer; and Yankelovich is one of the study's three Settled Explorers. Because two of the three remained in the same firm, I have changed their usual order, putting the early Transformer, Louis Harris, first followed by the Homesteader (Skelly) and the Explorer (Yankelovich).

THREE POLLSTERS

LOUIS HARRIS

Founder of the famous polling firm Louis Harris and Associates, dean of American pollsters Louis Harris was the son of a successful businessman who lived in New Haven, Connecticut. His father died suddenly in 1928, when Harris was seven; a week later, during a pre-Depression bank run, the family lost everything they had.

The family's only source of income during the Depression was the rent on a commercial garage; however, the renter rarely paid. Harris found work selling magazine subscriptions to help support his family and save money for college (at the time, most magazines were sold only by subscription through private agents).

Like Dr. Jonas Salk, Harris initially wanted to be a lawyer, and he dreamed about how far he would go. "I had a picture of myself as a justice of the U.S. Supreme Court. . . . This was probably when I was eight or nine. I could see the door for some reason: 'Justice.' Never 'Chief Justice,' just 'Justice Louis Harris.'"

That aspiration evolved into a desire to enter the world of journalism. "I always thought I would have something to do with journalism, with expression," Harris said. "I had a yen to communicate. That's been a thread all through my life." He won a spot as a journalist on his extremely competitive high school newspaper, then got a paying job as a high school correspondent for the New Haven *Register*. Later he became editor of the school's magazine and associate editor of its newspaper.

Harris used much of the money he saved from these jobs to buy himself a secondhand typewriter so that he could teach himself to type; it cost $8.75, a small fortune in 1933. "That was blood money," Harris said. He still has the typewriter, which is now a prized memento (and an antique to boot).

After "a wild but very formative college education" at the University of North Carolina at Chapel Hill and a stint in the Navy for which he received a commendation, Harris went to work for the American Veterans Committee as its research and program director, even though it was not, strictly speaking, a journalism job. One day he noticed an article in the *Herald Tribune* about a poll that had been done on veterans. Harris went to see the man who had conducted the poll, Elmo Roper, and before he left Roper's office he had been offered a job as Roper's assistant, which he accepted soon thereafter.

In 1956 Harris left Roper's to set up his own firm in New York. Because he had very little savings, he started the business on a wing and a prayer. His clients had encouraged him to open his own office, and they supported his business in the early days of the firm. Soon the business was doing extremely well, polling for a variety of political candidates and for the AFL-CIO. Eventually, the accuracy of his polls made him famous, and in 1960 he became the chief pollster for John F. Kennedy's presidential campaign.

Harris has advanced the field of polling dramatically by initiating such changes as the use of computers to assist the CBS Vote Profile Analysis. He is also the author of six books on contemporary American issues and writes a syndicated weekly column called "The Harris Poll."

Among the most important contributions made to the field of aging are two polls that Louis Harris and Associates conducted for the National Council on Aging: "Myth and Reality in Aging in America," in 1977, and "Aging in the Eighties: America in Transition," in 1981. They showed an astonishing difference between society's view of older people and the image older people have of themselves. The general perception of older people and their lives is far more negative than their personal experience. (Some of the results of these surveys are cited in chapter 5.)

Although he is in his seventies, Harris looks far younger than his chronological age. His unlined face glows with vitality, and he moves with the speed and grace of a man in his forties. He constantly generates new projects. Recently, he sold Louis Harris and Associates and formed a new firm, LH, Inc., through which Harris and former public servant Robert Wagner are developing market research in Russia as one of their first projects.

Despite this new direction, Harris still keeps on top of national trends and attitudes. He believes he has a natural affinity for polling. "Data is always talking to me. I have a feel for what people are trying to say. I try to glean it out. I always work hard. I've always thought nothing of working until three in the morning and going to work later that morning and working hard all day. It's always been work, work, work for me." At the same time, his great vitality has allowed him to maintain a deep involvement in family life. Like so many of the participants, Harris's passion for his work fuels his energy and drive.

FLORENCE SKELLY

A founder and partner in the polling firm Yankelovich, Skelly and White, Florence Skelly has pursued her interest in market research steadily since the age of nineteen. She started working when she was thirteen, in 1937, as a sales clerk in a hat store. Her early career ambition was to be a writer—either a playwright or a novelist. As a senior at Hunter College in 1944 she wrote her honors paper in social psychology on a survey of a YWHA operation on the Bronx.

"I loved the survey," Skelly said. "I just thought it was wonderful. I was so excited about it that I wanted to go into survey work. I said to my professor, 'I love doing this. Can I get a job where I can do this kind of thing?'" Her professor suggested a company that had a survey branch; Skelly went for an interview, got the job, and started working before graduation. This job involved market and public opinion research, areas in which she would continue to work for the rest of her career.

Skelly spent two years at that company, then worked for another market research company, Stewart Dougall, for four years. In 1950 she got a job with the U.S. Census Bureau in Washington working on the new census. She spent two years as the administrative assistant to the head of the housing census before returning to Stewart Dougall as a senior associate. Working with her there was Arthur White, who headed the retail research branch while Skelly handled the consumer research division.

By 1961 Skelly had decided either to move into management of a company using market research as a tool or to start her own market research firm. That year she met Dan Yankelovich, who was starting a firm with their mutual friend Arthur White. She joined them, and the three of them founded Yankelovich, Skelly and White the same year. By 1986, when Skelly left the firm, it had been twice sold to larger companies, and all three partners became dissatisfied with the changes in administration. They left and formed the Daniel Yankelovich Group, a market research and survey operation, of which Skelly serves as vice chairman. At the same time, Skelly started a small, wholly owned subsidiary of US West called Telematics and is currently president of that company as well.

Since survey researchers are always hired as outside consultants, Skelly said she rarely was subject to gender discrimination in her work. In fact, she feels that being a woman actually helped her in the market research business. "Because the consumer market is so heavily skewed toward women, there was a mystique about having a woman interpret what women were doing. Now I did not know the first thing about housework. I still don't. But there was an illusion that I understood women because I was a woman." However, there were still occasional obstacles, as, when giving a presentation at the Milwaukee Athletic Club, Skelly was forced to enter the club through the back entrance where the garbage dumpsters were kept because women were banned from the club.

One of the younger members of the Long Careers Study, Skelly (born in 1924) does not plan to retire. Because she has always been so deeply fascinated by her work, she believes it would be hard for her to make a transition to something else; in any case, there is nothing else that interests her as much. "I dread the idea of all that idle time—idle, unstructured time." So she has kept on at her work. "I think as long as I am able, I will go on doing what I'm doing now: trying to help [Daniel Yankelovich Group] and primarily run Telematics," she said. She then added, with some levity, "Now there could be a time when I'm just not able to do it, if the traveling becomes too hard, for example. Then I guess I'll stay in bed late! There might be some rewards—I wouldn't mind that!"

DAN YANKELOVICH

Dan Yankelovich, the principal founder of the firm Yankelovich, Skelly and White, is a man of wide-ranging interests, centered especially on individual values and how they are reflected (and supported or weakened) by the society as a whole.

Yankelovich's childhood, like Harris's, was shaped by the Depression and presented many obstacles that had to be surmounted. Born in 1924, he lost his mother to cancer when he was seven. Yankelovich's father, overwhelmed by his wife's death, lost everything in the Depression, and the three children were sent to foster homes because he could not care for them. "So what had been a very happy childhood in a very sudden and mysterious way became a difficult period of wandering from one foster home to another." He finally settled in one home at age fourteen, staying there until he went into the army after his freshman year at Harvard. As a serviceman, he spent three years in Europe.

After his discharge in 1946 he returned to Harvard and finished his undergraduate degree. His dream was to be a philosopher; he saw philosophy as a means of understanding life and its vicissitudes. But the Harvard philosophy department at the time was dominated by mathematical logic, an extremely technical branch of academic philosophy that tenaciously avoided all of the deeper questions about the nature and meaning of the human experience.

Yankelovich abandoned academic philosophy and spent several years working on a graduate degree in Harvard's celebrated Social Relations Program. Ultimately, he left and went to Paris, where existentialism was in full array, and the life of the mind was at an extraordinary peak. It was a lively and vital time. Yankelovich worked for the *Paris Review,* made friends, took courses at the Sorbonne and started to write a philosophy book. In 1952 he came back, settling in New York instead of Boston.

Instead of returning to graduate school, Yankelovich found a job with an industrial design firm where his research experience was useful: the firm's founder wanted to do consumer research on the design of the company's new products. In the late 1950s he left to establish his own firm, Daniel Yankelovich, Inc. Shortly after setting up the firm, he was joined by his old college roommate, Arthur White, and White's associate, Florence Skelly.

The firm developed an excellent reputation in the marketing research field, but Yankelovich was eager to extend it into more societal concerns. It evolved, said Yankelovich, "to a point where it had one foot in the marketing research field and another in the social research field."

Yankelovich's professional life has been a constant balancing act between his need to make a living and his intense curiosity about values and social trends. It was the first half of this equation that led him to create the first modern, design-conscious, low-cost furniture company. One night in the late 1950s, he was having dinner with a friend in the lumber business who mentioned that he had four hundred slightly damaged doors on his hands and didn't know what to do with them. "I knew that people were looking around for these things to use for tables, couches and desks," Yankelovich said. "So I took the four hundred doors from him on consignment. I rented a store in Greenwich Village and this friend of mine who was handy. . . joined me to make the wrought-iron legs that we attached to the doors to make tables and couches and so forth out of them." That was the birth of the Door Store, a firm that has become a landmark in the home-furnishings market in this country.

"I thought if I could get this business going it would give me enough money to buy some time for myself to finish the book I had started in Paris," Yankelovich reflected. "It didn't work out exactly that way. I found myself twice as busy." When he found another opportunity to finish the book, he sold the store to his friend, who continued to run it; the firm is still thriving.

Yankelovich wrote his book *Ego and Instinct* with philosopher William Barrett. In 1975, Yankelovich and Cyrus Vance created a nonprofit organization called the Public Agenda Foundation. Yankelovich is still its president and Vance its chairman. "I found it was hard in a profit-making firm to do the kind of public-policy research that I felt was needed," he said. "So this nonprofit entity helps to serve that purpose. My managerial time has been divided between the firm and the Public Agenda. It's dedicated to enhancing the quality of public debate."

In the 1970s Yankelovich wrote a series of books on the revolution in social values that had incubated on the nation's campuses in the 1960s culminating in his 1981 book, *New Rules: Searching for Fulfillment in a World Turned Upside Down.* It described the shift in values from the World War II generation to that of their children, the baby boomers. He published his sixth book, *Coming to Public Judgement*, in 1991; in it he develops a new seven-stage theory of how public opinion evolves from raw mass opinion to mature judgment.

"For the most part, I'm an outsider," Yankelovich says. "Independence is what moved me to stay in that role; I guess a certain orneriness also. I think I always had certain convictions about the way to do things and the way to look at understanding and to gain experience. It is hard to do that in a sheltered environment."

In his late sixties, Yankelovich has finally created the freedom he wants to participate more actively in the ongoing national dialogue of what direction society should take as it moves into the twenty-first century.

The example of these three pollsters is fascinating. All are in the same field; all are outstanding. But each has had a distinct career pattern. Skelly decided what she wanted to do in college and has never deviated from it, nor has she grown tired of it. Harris wanted to be first a lawyer and then a journalist, but he couldn't find a good entry-level job, so he took an administrative position and through it found survey research, which he loves; at this point in his career, it seems like part of his very nature. Yankelovich yearned to be a philosopher, worked for a variety of enterprises, and got into survey research for practical reasons—to make a living—but also because he enjoyed it and was good at it. In a way that could not have been foreseen, it has enabled him to continue searching for the mysteries of meaning that drew him at the beginning of his career, yet from a much stronger base.

CAREER CHOICE AND THE HUNDRED-YEAR LIFE SPAN

Within one lifetime the oldest participants in the study went from a society in which gaslights were common, horses were the major means of transportation, motion pictures had no sound, and a telegram was the most sophisticated means of long-distance communication to a society in which human beings have traveled to the moon, the trip from the United States to Europe can be made in three hours on the Concorde, television programs are relayed around the world by satellite, and documents can be faxed anywhere in the country within minutes.

Dr. Michael Heidelberger
When Dr. Michael Heidelberger was a child in the early 1890s, his family lived on East Ninety-first Street in New York City, in a recently built, walk-up apartment building. One block away, on Fifth Avenue between Ninety-first and Ninety-second streets, was a farm, which occupied about half a block and kept chickens and cows. When anyone in the family was sick, Heidelberger recalled, his mother would send him over to the farm to buy a fresh egg or two for the sufferer at the price of a nickel apiece.

Around 1897 the farm was bought by a millionaire immigrant

Scotsman named Andrew Carnegie; on its site he built a splendid house known as the Carnegie Mansion, where he and his family lived for the rest of his life. Today the building is the Cooper-Hewitt Museum of American Design, part of the Smithsonian Institution. Its tranquil manicured gardens are protected by tall wrought-iron fences, through which the mansion's elegant lines can be admired by passersby.

Heidelberger was the oldest member of the Long Careers Study, and the differences between the world of his childhood and the world of today are the most extreme. His account gives a fascinating glimpse of the wide spectrum of change that people can experience within a long lifetime, along with the radical social and technological transformation that can take place during a century.

The phases of Heidelberger's career (also the longest in the study) are particularly interesting. A Homesteader, Heidelberger decided when he was eight that he wanted to be a chemist, even though he had no real concept of what a chemist did. He was to realize his dream and become known as the father of modern immunology for his work in deciphering the basic mechanisms of the immune system.

After earning his bachelor's degree in science and doing some graduate work at Columbia, Heidelberger was told that he should go to Europe to study because the best chemists were there. He spent a year working with a famous chemist in Zurich, where, Heidelberger said, he "really learned what hard work chemistry was." In 1912, on returning to the United States, he took a position at Rockefeller University, exploring the chemistry of immunology and what was then called "chemotherapy," the development of chemical substances (drugs) that could be used to treat illness (remember that at that time there were almost no drugs for medical use). He also developed a vaccine for pneumonia, a major cause of death at the time. When I interviewed Heidelberger, in 1988, he was still taking an injection of pneumonia vaccine every year.

Heidelberger left Rockefeller to become the clinical chemist at Mt. Sinai Hospital, but he found the job so overloaded with work that he did not have time to continue his own research. A year later he went to Columbia Presbyterian Hospital, where he remained until 1955. There he was faced with mandatory retirement but instead of retiring he took a year's leave of absence; in

1956 he accepted an appointment at Rutgers University. While still at Rutgers, he was invited to be a member of the faculty of New York University's School of Medicine, where he remained until his death in 1991.

The course of Heidelberger's career thus looks something like this:

Rockefeller University	15.5 years
Mt. Sinai Hospital	1 year
Columbia Presbyterian Hospital	9.5 years
Rutgers University	27 years
New York University	26 years

In one lifetime, Heidelberger had the equivalent of two or three careers of "ordinary" length, depending on where "retirement age" is pegged. If you begin working in your early twenties and retire early, around fifty, you will have spent roughly twenty-six or twenty-seven years in the workforce, the length of two of Heidelberger's three career segments. If you begin working in your early twenties and work until sixty-five, you have worked a little over forty years—whereas Heidelberger's total career length was seventy-eight years, almost double that amount of time.

Heidelberger never lost interest in his field; he worked at five different universities but he was always a research chemist and he consistently did research on the immune system. During his lifetime, Heidelberger was also married twice (each time for thirty years, and very happily); had children; and received a number of awards for his contribution to the development of chemistry as a science, including two Lasker awards, the National Medal of Science, and the Louis Pasteur Gold Medal of the Swedish Medical Society.

As Heidelberger aged, he modified his aspirations and his goals; he closed his laboratory, no longer performed experiments, and turned to writing about many of the things he had not had time to set down earlier. He also edited the scientific writing for the other members of the chemistry department, since his 1890s education in the use of the English language was far superior to the training of his younger colleagues.

This gradual reshaping of the boundaries of activity is a pattern identified by Dr. O. Gilbert Brim, head of the MacArthur Foundation Research Network on Midlife, and is described fully in his book *Ambition*. "We have a basic drive for growth and mastery that is expressed in a variety of specific ambitions," Brim writes. "This is a universal characteristic of humans." In pursuit of this growth we instinctively tend to keep our tasks at "a level of 'just manageable' difficulties," easy enough to be possible and hard enough to test our abilities.[1]

Working on tasks at this just-manageable level is one of the major sources of human happiness, Brim says; so if our physical condition becomes less vigorous as we age, we tend to revise our levels of aspiration to keep the tasks manageable. Brim's father did this in relation to his farm, going from maintaining the whole farm in his younger years, to tending large gardens around the house, and later to planting window boxes. Then, in his 102d year when his sight was failing, he contented himself with listening to books on tape and tending the window boxes by touch. Dr. Heidelberger similarly worked at manageable tasks—from doing research to mentoring and editing the work of his younger colleagues.

David Ogilvy

As the hundred-year life span becomes more common, there will be more careers like Heidelberger's that constitute the equivalent of two or three conventional careers. David Ogilvy, advertising executive and one-half of the advertising giant Ogilvy and Mather, remarked on this career phenomenon: "If you work to age eighty-five or more, you have, in effect, two careers, one after the other. Your normal career, which lasts forty years until you're sixty-five, and then your second career, which is another, say, twenty years. You outlive your competitors, and you achieve more. And when you finally give it up at eighty-five, you're famous."

Ogilvy is a settled type-A Explorer who is still active at eighty-one as the chairman of WPP, the conglomerate that purchased Ogilvy and Mather. Like Studs Terkel, Ogilvy had a wide assortment of experiences before discovering his genius and passion for his career. He believes that those early experiences gave him the education he needed to succeed in advertising.

Born in Surrey, England, in 1911, he grew up in a difficult family with a Scotch father and a mother who "hated men." During his youth, he wanted to go into advertising and at seventeen applied for a job in London in the field. "Thank God they turned me down," he exclaimed. "I would never have gotten the education [that] taught me two things: . . . to have exorbitant standards, to try and do everything you did better than anybody's ever done it or will ever do it again; and secondly, to work myself to death. Well, not to death, to life!"

Ogilvy attended Oxford University, but it was an unhappy experience; he dropped out without getting a degree and went to Paris, where he took a job as a chef at the Hotel Majestic. Its prestigious kitchens attracted a glamorous crowd, including the president of France, whom Ogilvy saw twice. Although he feels that his early training as a chef taught him the importance of maintaining high professional standards, he found the sixty-three-hour workweek and the low pay discouraging. After several years he returned to Scotland and took a job as a salesman for Aga cookers.

Ogilvy proved a natural at the sales business. Indeed, he was so successful that he was asked to write a sales brochure to teach the other salesmen how to sell. The success of the brochure spread around the advertising world, and Mather's, the highly successful advertising company, offered to send Ogilvy to New York to set up an American office.

Ogilvy moved to the United States in 1938, but it was to be another ten years before he founded Ogilvy and Mather. Rather than become part of the fast-paced advertising world of New York City, he went instead to Princeton, New Jersey, to work as associate director of George Gallup's Audience Research Institute. Three years later, with the outbreak of World War II, he moved to Washington to work for the British Intelligence Service at the British Embassy. Next, in a sudden and odd change of pace, he moved to Lancaster County, Pennsylvania, where he worked as a farmer, living with an Amish family.

Four years later he returned to New York and founded Ogilvy and Mather, in 1949. The company was immediately successful, largely because of Ogilvy's creative genius. Ogilvy feels that his talent is not due so much to imagination but rather to his ability to use his life experiences, such as his sales career, along with the knowledge he has gained through study. "I've read every book that's ever been written about advertising," he says.

Over the next few decades Ogilvy dazzled the New York advertising world. He was chairman and director of Ogilvy and Mather until 1973. During that time he dedicated a substantial proportion of time to nonprofit activities, in addition to his work. He also found time to write several books: *Confessions of an*

Advertising Man in 1963, followed by *Blood, Brains and Beer* fifteen years later, the very successful *Ogilvy on Advertising* in 1983, and, most recently, *The Unpublished Ogilvy*.

Ogilvy now lives in a nine-hundred-year-old French chateau, the upkeep of which he says, humorously, is another career. A strong proponent of the abilities of aging people, Ogilvy has had several outstanding older clients, such as cosmetics queen Helena Rubenstein, who worked until she was ninety. "When she died she was still the prime mover in her company, all over the world," Ogilvy delights in pointing out. Ogilvy also mentioned that the people in the "Business Hall of Fame" in *Fortune* magazine are all older people. "If they'd stopped working at a normal age, nobody at *Fortune* would ever have heard of them, nor would anybody else. They're the opposite end from child prodigies; they're sort of . . . mature prodigies."

SUMMARY

The profiles of participants in this chapter clearly demonstrate that there is tremendous variety and flexibility in career patterns. There is no one element that dictates the path a career will take. But the most important factor among many is that each participant found work they enjoyed, and a few found they could enjoy several careers simultaneously because each career fueled the others in a significant way.

The lesson to learn from their experiences is that pursuing work that truly engages us may or may not take us on a straight path; it may even take us on several paths at once. To find a career that provides us with the greatest range of expression and satisfaction, we must be willing to explore opportunities as they present themselves, and we must be persistent in seeking whatever goals we choose.

PART III

BREAKING THE BOUNDARIES

Long Growth Curves and Late Bloomers

During the Long Careers Study interviews, an unusual pattern began to emerge from some of the life histories. Although all the participants continued working past the age of sixty-five, some sustained a remarkably high level of achievement in their careers beyond that point. These participants had growth curves that either showed a high level of accomplishment after the age of sixty-five or peaked later in life than they should have according to widely accepted ideas about age and career development. Moreover, a few participants did not really begin their careers until after the age of fifty. Not only did these people continue to work beyond age sixty-five but many of them had outstanding accomplishments to their credit after that age. For some, the greatest achievements of their careers came after they passed what we consider retirement age.

More than one-third (fifty-seven) of the Long Careers group either had long growth curves or were "late bloomers." The career development of those with long growth curves continued to rise after ages when common wisdom assumes that people are "winding down." The late bloomers fell into two types: those who started their careers later in life and those who reached their highest career peaks later in life.

LONG GROWTH CURVES

Our society has held firmly to the idea that most achievement comes in youth, and as a result we have steadfastly insisted that older achievers are exceptions. When we encounter people with long growth curves we tend to explain them as rarities. Often we add, as Harvey Lehman did in *Age and Achievement,* that the base for their work was probably laid much earlier than sixty-five, so we believe that their late-life accomplishments are just fallout from earlier career phases.[1]

C. DOUGLAS DILLON

One of the participants whose career has had an especially long, sustained growth curve is C. Douglas Dillon, a type-A Explorer who has been a businessman (in investment banking); a diplomat (ambassador to France); and a public servant (secretary of the Treasury). Then, at the age of sixty, he became president of the board of the Metropolitan Museum of Art (he later became the board's chairman).

Dillon was born in August 1909 into a well-to-do New Jersey family. His father was head of the New York banking firm Dillon Read and Company, and Dillon went to work there after graduating from college in 1931. He was not settled on banking as an exclusive career, however. After serving overseas in the navy during World War II, he returned home and became involved in New Jersey Republican politics. Later, in 1953, he was made ambassador to France, returning to Washington in 1957 to run foreign economic policy for the State Department.

By the time of the 1960 election, Dillon had earned such widespread respect in Washington for his understanding of finance and international markets that president-elect John F. Kennedy went to his home to ask him to disregard his affiliation with the Republican Party and become Kennedy's secretary of the Treasury. Dillon accepted, holding the office from 1961 to 1965 and drafting many improvements in fiscal policy during his term.

Dillon left the Treasury in 1965 and began to lay plans for retiring from the financial world to begin new projects. At the time, he chaired the boards of both the Rockefeller Foundation and the Brookings Institute, an important policy research organization in Washington, D.C. He was deeply engaged by policy research and felt very involved at Brookings, so he assumed that he would spend most of his time on its affairs. But, as he pointed out in his interview, fortunately he had been exploring a variety of possible activities, because the things he had planned unfolded in a very different way, which he had not foreseen.

In 1970, at the age of sixty, Dillon was elected president of the board at the Metropolitan Museum of Art. Over the first few months in office he found that "the Metropolitan just became more and more engrossing." Brookings, on the other hand, never developed into a major interest, for complex reasons that could never have been foreseen. Eventually Dillon's work on behalf of the museum became "more or less full-time," to the exclusion of other board commitments. He became particularly interested in Asian art and focused his efforts on expanding the museum's Asian holdings, which resulted in his collaboration with Mrs. W. Vincent Astor on the construction of the Astor Court and Dillon Gallery to house a growing Chinese art collection. After 1976, when the museum established a full-time president, Dillon became chairman and remained actively involved with the museum's governance and continuing growth.

During the fifteen years when Dillon was president and chairman of the board, the museum doubled its gallery space. Many new collections and exhibition areas were added, including the famous Temple of Dendur and the new American wing. Dillon proved to be one of the greatest leaders in the Metropolitan Museum's history. In his role he was able to use all the abilities developed in his previous positions: his financial acumen, his reputation for exceptional intelligence and honesty, his diplomatic skills, his love of entertaining, his fine taste, and his ability to relate well to other people and to command respect.

One of Dillon's first acts after he had joined the museum was to institute mandatory retirement rules. Although the museum begged him to stay on, he preferred to honor the new system. In 1989, Dillon retired voluntarily from the chairmanship at age seventy-four and gave the board ample time to find a successor.

Dillon was not an attorney, but his career had the same pattern as many of the attorneys in the study: he alternated between work within his firm or his original field—investment—and outside work. His financial independence enabled him to continue using his talents at a nonprofit institution after retiring from business. By the time he retired a second time, from the Metropolitan, he still had more than enough affiliations and projects to stay occupied at a less hectic level. In his eighties, he continues to be active in the museum, in a more limited role that leaves him time for other personal interests. He remains a trustee emeritus and devotes his efforts to the Asian collection.

Dillon's entire term at the Metropolitan took place after he turned sixty, and the most brilliant part of it occurred after the age of sixty-five. One could look at Dillon's achievements at the Metropolitan and contend that because he was always exceptional, his accomplishments there are attributable to his being an unusually talented individual. This is a clear reinforcement of the message that it is ability that is the most important factor in a successful career, not chronological age, and that chronological age does not present a biological barrier for talent.

PAULINE TRIGERE

Designer Pauline Trigere is another participant whose career curve has continued to rise into her sixties and seventies. Indeed, in 1992 it was still rising: in October 1992 Trigere celebrated the golden jubilee of her fashion house; a few weeks later she presented her next collection and won praise for its originality and continuing elegance.

The daughter of a dressmaker and a tailor, Pauline Trigere was born in the heart of Pigalle, a section of Paris famous for its artists, performers, and authors. In her father's tailoring shop she learned to cut and fit, and at an early age she made her first "toiles" at the then-celebrated house of Martial and Armand, Place Vendome.

In 1937, en route to Chile, Trigere arrived in New York with her husband, her brother Robert, and her two infant sons, for a brief stopover—or so she thought. New York City and its people captured her heart immediately, and she stayed. Shortly afterward, she decided to try her hand at making up a few dresses. They were an instant success. As a result, with the collaboration of her husband and brother, she took steps to set up her own business in 1942, starting with a collection of eleven styles.

Trigere still does most of the firm's designing herself. In the great classic tradition of Vionnet, Lanvin, and Chanel, Trigere does not sketch; she cuts and drapes directly from the bolt of fabric. Through this technique she has pioneered an extraordinary number of fashion themes, innovations that inevitably enter the vocabulary of Seventh Avenue. The cornerstone of Trigere's art is her artistic, intricate cut, always flattering to the wearer and pure enough to withstand fads and uncertainties. Her clothes are time-less, a quality that was demonstrated remarkably in her retrospective; dresses forty and fifty years old could not be distinguished from contemporary creations. She has been the recipient of every major American fashion award, as well as the Silver Medal of the City of Paris, awarded to her in 1972 at the Hotel de Ville.

In her seventies, Trigere is as trim as any of her models, a perfect size four. She does yoga exercises every morning, spending two minutes each day standing on her head. She believes that this upside-down posture "bathes the brain. . . . It is like shaking a bottle."

The rank she has attained in the world of fashion is a matter of great pride to Pauline Trigere. What gives her equal pleasure is her influence on new emerging designers. "Their fashions are original, individual—and yet, my faithful clients come back to tell me that these fine new designs are 'à la Trigere.' Could any creative person ask for a nicer tribute?"

HUME CRONYN

For more than sixty years, Hume Cronyn has developed his career as an actor while expanding his interests to other related activities, extending the growth and achievements of his career through many decades. He has contributed to the entertainment world also as a producer, director, playwright, screenwriter, and lecturer.

A Homesteader, Cronyn was born in 1911 in London, Ontario, Canada, in what he calls an "Edwardian" family. Though he never planned on becoming a professional actor when he was growing up, he spent his childhood days in "some sort of mad fantasy world," where he played both the cowboys and the Indians—and even the horses.

He graduated from Ridley College in 1930 and entered prelaw studies at McGill University. "I went through my first two years and found I was doing absolutely nothing about law, but I was in every amateur theatrical project that was offered to the community." With his family's support, he left his legal studies and went to New York City. The first casting director he met told him frankly that "you don't look like anything." What she meant, fortunately, was that he couldn't be easily typecast. This quality turned out to be an enormous advantage for Cronyn in his career, allowing him to play a broad spectrum of roles.

In New York, Cronyn enrolled at the American Academy of Dramatic Arts, graduating in 1934. He made his professional stage debut in Washington, D.C., in 1931. His Broadway debut soon followed in 1934 in *Hipper's Holiday*. Since then Cronyn has appeared in more than eighty plays. He made his screen debut in Alfred Hitchcock's *Shadow of a Doubt* and has appeared in thirty-two major motion pictures as well as numerous television productions. He has garnered nominations and awards from all three entertainment mediums.

In 1942 he married actress Jessica Tandy. Tandy and Cronyn have enjoyed performing together throughout their careers and have become America's favorite entertainment duo, working together in hit plays like *The Gin Game* and on screen in the landmark film about aging, *Cocoon*. Together they were honored by the Kennedy Center for their lifetime achievements in the arts.

As Cronyn describes the actor's life, "to go on being an actor, you need sheer animal energy. If you can't restock your energy, you have to hide your lack of it." He continues to be involved in several projects at once and exhibits no lack of energy, finding sufficient fuel in his work. In person, this energy communicates in a very direct way: in his eighties, Cronyn looks easily much younger than his chronological age and is still very handsome—a feature that does not show up much in his screen performances because now he plays mostly older characters who aren't supposed to be magnetic and attractive.

Cronyn's career has grown continually over the years as he has expanded his efforts and interests into new areas such as writing, directing, and producing. His greatest successes have come in the last ten years, during which time he has directed Broadway hits and starred in films. The arc of his career is still rising. Recently he wrote his autobiography, and now he is working on new scripts for future television productions.

"There is a quotation I'm very fond of by I. J. [Israel Joshua] Singer," Cronyn said. "He was changing careers, giving up journalism and becoming a professor of classical languages. He learned to speak both Latin and Greek. And somebody said, 'Mr.

Singer, what do you have to look forward to?' And he said, 'I hope to die young, as late as possible.' Isn't that marvelous?"

EVELYN NEF

Evelyn Stefansson Nef, a type-A Explorer, has had a diverse career that culminated in her decision in her early sixties to train as a psychotherapist, thus beginning the first phase of her most satisfying career peak.

At the time Nef decided to become a therapist, she had recently married her third husband, John Nef, and was living in Washington, D.C. She knew that since John was older than she, she was likely to outlive him, and she needed a profession of her own. Evelyn had enjoyed a stint of volunteer work she had done with Dr. Paul McClain, the inventor of the concept of the triune brain, at the National Institutes of Mental Health.

Nef was concerned that because she was in her early sixties, institutions would not be enthusiastic about admitting her as a student. But she secured an interview in New York with the director of the Institute for the Study of Psychotherapy, who admired her knowledge of Eskimo child-rearing practices gained through an earlier career as wife and assistant to Arctic explorer, Vilhjalmur Stefansson. She was admitted to the program even though she did not have the required master's degree in social work. She commuted to New York from Washington for three years while pursuing her degree.

After she graduated, Nef set up her own practice in Washington. When her husband contracted Parkinson's disease in his eighties, she dedicated herself to keeping him engaged and active for the duration of his life, which her flexible schedule as a therapist made possible.

Nef is still delighted with her decision to become a psychotherapist, and by all accounts she is an unusually successful one. She credits her unorthodox education with allowing her to look at situations from a different perspective—a quality that she believes makes her a better therapist. "I've found a use for everything I have ever learned," she says. "I think it was an advantage for me to start very late, because I have the feeling I don't have seven years on the couch to give to somebody. If I'm going to do this, I have to do this quickly. My patients solve their problems and move on."

Nef finds her work energizing. "At the end of a day when people say, 'Aren't you exhausted and depressed when you had six or eight patients?'. . . I'm exhilarated, because I've resolved, because I've helped, because the feedback is very good when you are successful as a therapist. Somebody who was unable to face something suddenly says, 'Ah, I found a way.'"

Nothing in Nef's life up to her sixties had indicated that she would someday find her greatest career satisfaction in being a psychotherapist. The daughter of Hungarian immigrants, Nef grew up in Brooklyn. Her father, a successful fur designer, was preparing her to work with him when he suddenly died of a heart attack; as Nef puts it, "his business died with him," and so did her budding career opportunity. Almost overnight the family went from being well off to fighting for survival. Her mother slid into a depression from which she never recovered. Nef, thirteen at the time, and all of her siblings went to work to support the family. She worked in a dress shop on weekends; later she sang in a nightclub and became a photographer's assistant; she also sold chintz at Gimbel's and thread at Macy's for a commission of a penny or two a spool. Eventually she escaped this struggle by developing her interest in marionettes. Through this work she met a gifted young marionette maker, whom she married when she was nineteen. The marriage lasted three years.

Later she met and married a polar explorer, Vilhjalmur Stefansson, who had discovered large landmasses in the Canadian Arctic and had written twenty-seven books on his explorations. Thirty-three years her senior, he became not only her husband but her mentor, encouraging her to write, sending her to make speeches for him when he was unable to. She considers her first real job to have been her position as the librarian for Stefansson's personal collection of books, which was the largest library of polar information in the world. Encouraged by Stefansson, she wrote two books of her own, *Here Is Alaska* and *Within the Circle*. Later Stefansson gave his library to Dartmouth and the couple moved there, both teaching at the college.

Stefansson died when he was eighty-two; Nef was forty-nine. Nef soon discovered that "widows were not invited out the way couples were, and without the famous husband, life was a little more restricted." Despite her twelve years at Dartmouth and the presence of the Stefansson Library, she did not have a future at Dartmouth. The head of the school's sociology department was moving to Washington to set up the American Sociological Association's national office and wanted to bring an executive assistant. He offered Nef the job, though she was neither a sociologist nor an administrator.

In a very real sense, at this point in her life Evelyn Nef felt that she had lost everything: her husband, her career, and their life together at Dartmouth. Her life seemed to be over. Since she believed she would just be marking time until her death, from that point forward, she reasoned that she might as well accept the position in Washington—and she did, determined to do a good job despite the unfortunate term of her life. Nef moved to Washington and plunged into her new job.

Then something quite unexpected happened. A couple she knew in New York introduced her to John Nef, a history professor at the University of Chicago who was working in Washington. He proposed to her five days after they met. They honeymooned in Europe for five months, dining with his stellar collection of friends, such as T.S. Eliot and Marc Chagall. It was a spectacularly happy marriage.

When they returned from the trip and moved into their new home in Washington, Nef first began to consider the idea of becoming a therapist. After forty years of exploring a truly eclectic range of interests and abilities, she finally found a career that was perfectly suited to her talents.

DAVID BROWN

"I became more productive in my seventies than I ever had been before in my whole life," says blockbuster film producer David Brown, another type-A Explorer. He has achieved his greatest successes in the ten years after age sixty-five. With careers in journalism and publishing behind him, Brown shifted his focus to Hollywood in the 1960s and has since produced such hit movies as *Jaws* and *The Sting*. In the last five years, he has produced several Broadway hits and a number of films, including *The Player* and *A Few Good Men*. And he has published several best-selling books and is currently working on a book about the era of the 1930s.

David Brown was born in New York City in 1916. His parents were divorced soon after he was born, and Brown and his mother moved to Long Island. Brown was interested in journalism before he could even read. He loved to listen to radio broadcasters like Lowell Thomas, and from the age of five he pored over newspapers. "I looked at the advertising and the drawing and the pictures," he says. "I was interested in the world outside and I was interested in how it would impact on me."

As a high school student on Long Island, Brown was a science fiction buff who built his own radio station. He intended to major in science but found that higher mathematics and applied physics—both prerequisites for the degree—held little interest for him. Instead he concentrated on social science and psychology, graduating from Stanford and receiving a Master of Science degree from Columbia University.

After graduation Brown went through a succession of magazine jobs. His first was at Fairchild Publications for $25 a week. Over the next few years he worked for *Women's Wear Daily* as a drama critic and copy editor, wrote horoscopes ("It paid well," he says), and did some free-lance writing. In 1940, newly married, he decided he had to get a "real" job.

His father hired him to do public relations for the milk industry but fired him in short order. "I couldn't keep regular hours," Brown says. He next became the nightclub editor of one of the burgeoning picture magazines, *PIC*. "I covered nightclubs, cabaret, and theater. I got up at noon and then went to work. That's how I got interested in show business," he recalled.

A stint of writing comedy skits for the comedian Eddie Cantor led to a job with *Liberty* magazine and eventually to a position as managing editor of *Cosmopolitan*. Later on, in the 1960s, Brown would encourage his new wife, Helen Gurley Brown, to buy *Cosmopolitan* and transform it into a single-women's guide to life. He stayed at *Cosmo* until 1951, when Hollywood beckoned in the person of Darryl F. Zanuck, who offered him a job with Twentieth Century–Fox. Fascinated by the motion picture industry, Brown accepted.

At Fox, Brown rose from story editor to producer to head of the scenario department. The studio went bankrupt in 1963, so Brown returned to New York and fell into yet another occupation: book publishing. He founded a company called New American Library, which published, among other things, Ian Fleming's James Bond books. But he wasn't satisfied in the publishing industry for very long.

In 1964, Brown purchased the film rights to a popular play, *The Sound of Music,* and the following year went back to Fox to help supervise its production. The film put Twentieth

Century–Fox back on the map. During the next six years, Brown rose to be executive vice president of creative operations. In 1970 Brown was fired, along with his friend Richard Zanuck, in a political coup against Darryl Zanuck. Brown says he learned something from this experience: "In my fifties, I was out of work twice, sending résumés around. I had had it with that. Getting fired convinced me that I was never going to let a company control my destiny again—except my own company, which controls my destiny on a daily basis."

Brown and the younger Zanuck did form their own company—on July 28, 1972, Brown's birthday. They were extraordinarily successful. One of their blockbusters was *Cocoon,* a landmark film examining attitudes about aging. In the film, residents of a retirement home are rejuvenated by contact with space travelers. Some refuse to become younger because they believe it is morally wrong to reverse the aging process. Others joyfully welcome their renewed vitality and join the spacemen for the voyage to their home planet. Brown recounted that after shooting began and he saw the first rushes, he and his staff realized that the performances of Tandy, Cronyn, and the other older actors did not convey the sense of age because they did not move, gesture, nor talk like "old people," even though all of them were well over sixty-five at the time the movie was filmed. As a result, all the older actors had to be trained to act elderly for their work on the film. They were taught to change the way they walked, held their heads, sat, gestured, and talked so they would be convincing in their roles.

Brown also served as executive producer for the Academy Award–winning *Driving Miss Daisy,* starring eighty-one-year-old Jessica Tandy, which, like *Cocoon,* proved that a story about the experiences of an older person could be the subject of a highly successful and critically acclaimed movie.

After a long and fruitful partnership, Brown left to start his own development and production company, the Manhattan Project. In 1991, Brown's producing efforts were recognized by the Academy of Motion Picture Arts and Sciences, which presented him and Zanuck with the Irving G. Thalberg Award, the highest honor for a film producer.

Today, at the age of seventy-six, Brown attributes his physical, mental, and emotional well-being to the fact that he has never stopped working. "I'm healthy and energetic because I work. I take pleasure in my work. I still work seven days a week, and I enjoy it. As Tennessee Williams said, 'Make voyages. Attempt them.' That's all there is."

Dr. Lewis Thomas

Dr. Lewis Thomas, the celebrated president of Memorial Sloan Kettering Cancer Center in New York, became known worldwide for his brilliant meditative essays on biology: *The Lives of a Cell*, *The Medusa and the Snail*, and *Late Night Thoughts on Listening to Mahler's Night Music*. He developed his career as a writer well after the age of fifty.

A slender, reflective man with a wry sense of humor, Thomas had considered becoming a writer in his childhood. But his strongest desire, as far back as he can remember, was to be a doctor like his father. As was true for many other study participants, Thomas skipped several grades in school and entered college young, at fifteen. Following Harvard Medical School and an internship at Boston City Hospital, he launched a type-B Explorer-style career that took him to a half dozen cities over a period of thirty years, doing viral and bacteriological research, teaching and heading several departments, ultimately becoming president of Memorial Sloan Kettering. ("I never could hold a job," Thomas joked about the string of distinguished appointments he had held.)

Thomas's career as a physician, researcher, and administrator was an extremely fine one. It had not made him world famous, but that wasn't really something that he sought. Then in 1970, something unpredictable happened, a tiny pulse within the framework of his life that ultimately led to a totally new direction in his work and a tremendous flowering of a talent he had chosen to leave behind in childhood.

In his mid-fifties, Thomas began keeping a journal, writing down ideas and observations as they occurred to him at various moments during the day. He did this strictly for himself; no one else, he said, even knew about it. Then he received a chance invitation.

"I was asked to give an after-dinner talk at an immunology meeting in Brooklodge, outside of Kalamazoo," he said. "It was laid on by one of the pharmaceutical companies. I gave a light talk about inflammatory reactions. I didn't realize it, but it was recorded. The company, whichever it was, printed it up in a little folder and sent it around to a lot of people. It fell into the hands of Franz Inglefinger, who was then the editor of the *New England Journal of Medicine*. He wrote me a letter and said he'd like essays like that for the journal once a month. . . [no] longer than one page, which would have been about eleven hundred words. In return for that, there would of course be no payment, but he would guarantee that nobody would ever be allowed to edit whatever I wrote. That was irresistible, so I started writing essays for the *New England Journal of Medicine*."

After about three years, Thomas got a "very nice letter from Joyce Carol Oates, who said that her doctor up in Windsor, Ontario, had been collecting these things and giving copies to her. She thought they'd make a good book." Roughly at the same time, Thomas received a letter from an editor at the Oxford University Press who had been given the essays by his doctor; he wanted to make them into a book, provided that Thomas would do a lot of rewriting and link them together with "threading pieces." This offer Thomas rejected, saying that he was really busy as he was about to become the dean of a medical school and didn't have time for that.

Then, Thomas recalls, he got a nice telephone call from Elizabeth Sifton, than an editor at Viking, who had also seen the essays through her doctor. She told him that Viking would like to publish the essays as they stood—no changes. So Thomas agreed. The first printing was about five thousand copies. No one expected the book to be the best-selling classic that *Lives of a Cell* became.

"I must say I was surprised by the public reaction to the book," Thomas reflected. "Astonished. So was everybody, including my editor. She told me once they'd had an argument at Viking and had decided to publish *Lives of a Cell* because they had so many books they were making a lot of money on. She said they thought [they would feel] better if they had a loser."

Thomas was fifty-seven when he began writing essays and sixty-one at the publication of *Lives of a Cell* in 1974. Almost eighty at this writing, he has retired from active work at Sloan Kettering, where he has been given the title of Scholar in Residence, and devotes much of his time to his writing. His current projects include a collection of poetry and more essays, which he intends to put together in another book.

Like a number of other participants, Thomas had a youthful ambition that he put aside for years while pursuing a different career. Then a combination of circumstance, talent, and desire allowed him to realize that ambition later in life.

LATE BLOOMERS

In the past there have been well-known examples of people who have had late-life careers that have been considered lucky accidents. Given the new perspective provided by the Long Careers Study, we can now regard these as part of a larger pattern. One famous late-bloomer is the American primitive artist Grandma Moses, who lived on a farm in upstate New York and began painting at the age of seventy-five because, as she said, she was "too old to work on the farm and too young to sit on the porch." Her late start made her a curiosity rather than a threat to male artists, and her advanced age ensured polite, if occasionally patronizing, treatment. She remained active until her death at 101, in 1961.

Grandma Moses was a remarkable late bloomer. She chose a field—art—that harbored few women at the time. Because she was a primitive painter, however, a style that studio artists thought inferior, she became a celebrity without encountering much opposition from the art establishment, which had little interest in primitive art.

The idea of beginning a career, or developing a new aspect of a career, at fifty or sixty or seventy, may initially seem strange. But if you adopt the view that adult life is a continuous process of growth and development, and that the potential for new learning and new activity exists at all ages, then a late-life career is no longer an idiosyncrasy but a part of that process of growth.

LATE STARTERS

The careers of the late bloomers, especially those who didn't start their careers until after fifty, were difficult to rationalize. "Getting a late start" is an uncomplimentary phrase; it suggests something that is off schedule when it shouldn't be. In a career, it implies lost time that needs to be made up, a work life that will trail behind those of the on-time starters around you. Although we are taught that people achieve at their own rate, we also learn early on that it is a disadvantage to be behind the crowd. It is almost a reflex to assume that a late career start would mean fewer opportunities for achievement and success.

In practice, at least for some people, it does not work out that way. Just as psychologist Dean Keith Simonton observed[2] in the late achievers he studied, the late-blooming Long Careers Study participants were not handicapped in the degree of success they were able to achieve. Their late starts had two discernible effects on their accomplishments. First, the late starts undoubtedly changed the nature of what these participants did; at twenty-one, they would have chosen a different type of work than at fifty. And second, it meant that their careers were shorter and perhaps fewer in number than those of the earlier starters; someone who started "on time" might have had two or three careers by the age of seventy, whereas someone who started "late" may have had only one.

LATE ACHIEVERS

Among the late achievers, whose career peak came after fifty or sixty-five, there was a great deal of variety: some achieved first or second career peaks in new late-life careers, others hit first or second peaks in the same field in which they had been working for years. Career peaks after fifty were considered late peaks, but some of these participaants had career peaks after sixty-five as well: two participants had their first career peaks after sixty-five, and seven had second peaks after that age.

One historic example of this pattern was Col. Harlan Sanders, the founder of the enormously successful chain of Kentucky Fried Chicken fast-food restaurants. Before the age of forty, Sanders was assumed to be one of his Kentucky hometown's failures. Up to that point he had not been able to stay with any single career. In something of a desperate move, he opened a service station and added a restaurant to it, serving his own concoction: a well-seasoned, crisply fried chicken. To everyone's astonishment, including his own, the restaurant earned a statewide reputation and flourished.

When Sanders was sixty-four, a new highway was built that bypassed his restaurant. No longer on the beaten track, the restaurant's business declined and its value decreased. Sanders decided to franchise the name and the method of making the chicken, and he traveled around the United States selling the franchises. By the time he was seventy, he had 400 franchises; by age seventy-four, they numbered 638.

Sanders is an example of someone who had a long growth curve with two career peaks: one before age sixty-four, when the restaurant became popular; and a much larger one after that, when he began franchising the Colonel Sanders chain. In an appearance before the U.S. Congressional Committee on Aging in 1977, Sanders concluded his statement against forced retirement by saying, "We're wasting a lot of brain power and energy making people retire. I'd like to see it stopped. And one other thing— letting people work past age sixty-five might help keep the Social Security system from going broke!"

Another example of the late bloomer was offered by broadcaster Hugh Downs, who related how he interviewed Dr. Walter Alvarez, age ninety-five, for his PBS show "Over Easy." "All of his fame and scientific achievement occurred in the last thirty years of his life," Downs said. "If he had been forced to retire at sixty-five, none of that would have come about. He was an obscure doctor at sixty-five. And from sixty-five to ninety-five he just made tremendous contributions to medicine and other philosophic areas. Those thirty years were really golden years for him."

CAREER PEAKS AFTER FIFTY

Five of the participants did not really begin their careers until fifty years of age or later. All of them were women. Three are profiled here: Shirley Brussell, Toy Lasker, and Frances Lear. (The other two, Helen Breed and Janet Sainer, are discussed in chapters 7 and 13, respectively.) These participants raised a family first, and only when the nest was empty did they have the freedom to think about what to do with their own lives.

SHIRLEY BRUSSELL

Chicagoan Shirley Brussell had an early, successful career, but it was not something in which her whole heart was invested. She falls within the Transformer group because she moved from one field to another, with a twenty-year-plus gap in between. Brussell graduated from college during World War II and was sent immediately to Detroit as a civilian personnel officer for professionals who were converting military vehicles for desert use in the invasion of North Africa. As a result of her training, she is extremely knowledgeable about outfitting tanks—an expertise that she has not used very much in her subsequent life.

Next she was transferred to the War Labor Board. After the war she returned to Chicago and went into private industry, becoming the employment manager of a large food and restaurant chain.

At the age of thirty she married Judge Abraham Brussell, a man slightly older than she, who did not want her to work. They both wanted to have a family and felt that an active home life was important to them. Moreover, his career limited the amount of time he could contribute to that goal himself. It was possible for her to do volunteer work, however—as it was for most women at the time. So in addition to raising the children and managing the home, Shirley Brussell ran a staggering list of volunteer projects.

Twenty-four years later, Brussell went back to school and completed a master's degree in community organization. While studying and doing volunteer work at the university she became involved in creating employment programs for older people, and that led her to design the first temporary agency for older people, Re-Entry. She then received a grant to develop a program called Life Options, which the Chicago Community Trust asked her to direct. That was the start of Operation Able.

"There was nothing at Able when I started," Brussell says. "There were some by-laws. The Metropolitan Welfare Council had given it some space. There were three of us: I had an assistant who was a gerontologist ex-nun with a Ph.D., who had left the church a few years before, and I had a secretary. That was it. And a lot of good advice from the trust; and a very supportive and involved board." Their initial funding was about $47,000.

Since the June 1977 beginnings of the agency, Brussell has built Operation Able into an organization with a staff of 345 people, including 70 permanent staff, 125 temps, and 100 independent career counselors; a yearly budget of over $4 million; and offshoots in seven American cities with four additional communities slated for "baby Ables." Operation Able offers a variety of services to older adults, including career counseling and job placements.

"I didn't retire at sixty-five, because I thought I was only getting started," says Brussell. "I don't think of retirement; I think of what other areas I would like to help in or grow in. It's corny, but if you can feel growth and development, you don't feel old. It's when you feel you can't learn anything or do anything new that it's the end of the road."

TOY LASKER

Toy Lasker, creator of the widely popular Flashmaps, pocket-size books of subject-matter maps for large cities, began her career after opening an old box of paints she kept hidden away until she was nearly fifty years old.

Lasker, the descendant of a family of Swedish settlers, was raised a Mormon in Utah. At twenty-one, Lasker married a young lawyer, Morris Lasker, whom she met when he passed through her hometown on the way to a military assignment during World War II. They decided to get married while the war was still in progress and began a family immediately; for the next twenty-five years, Toy Lasker raised children.

When the last of their five children was grown enough to be reasonably self-sufficient, Lasker knew she could begin a new phase of her life. For years she had longed to be an artist. "I walked upstairs that first Monday morning, to a room on the third floor where I kept various projects that I had worked on. I picked up a box of paints I had bought for myself years ago, but had never had time to use, and I said to myself: Now! And I started to paint."

Lasker became a good artist, but eventually she realized she would never be an outstandingly original painter. In addition, art was too isolating for her gregarious nature. It was fine as a hobby or for a short period of time, but it did not provide enough human contact for the long run. Lasker was extremely proficient technically, however—good enough to make passable copies of both old and new masters. She filled her house with copies of paintings she loved, doing such a good job that visitors invariably ask her in hushed tones about "the Renoir in the dining room."

One day she had to drive into Manhattan for a social function. It was raining, and she got abysmally lost. She found herself asking no one in particular why there weren't maps that were a convenient size to put in a pocket or handbag and guide people around the city. The idea stuck in her head. She checked the newsstands and bookstores; nothing of the kind was available. She began sketching and making notes; there could be a map for museums, a map for the theater district, a map for restaurants, and so on. "I had always drawn maps for the kids when they went into New York," she said, "so it was just something that came naturally." Although they are commonplace today, Lasker says, no one had ever prepared subject-matter maps for the general public at that time.

The idea seemed good enough to her to try to find a publisher. Through an acquaintance who worked at Time-Life she got an appointment with the company's top executives, who seemed very interested in the project. But one of them let slip a comment during their meeting that indicated to her that the Time-Life staff didn't understand the concept at all. By that time, Lasker had a very clear idea of how the project ought to look. She said thanks but no thanks and decided to try to publish the maps herself. "This is when I started learning," she says. "Sometimes I think I know more about the book industry than anyone else, because I had to handle every stage of a book from concept to the final product, even the store display."

Lasker found a cartographer to draw the maps and spent hours doing the research: visiting restaurants, finding addresses and phone numbers to include, jotting down the hours when museums and other cultural attractions were open. A family friend loaned her enough money to get the project off the ground. The first Flashmaps volume came out in 1971; within a few years she had published volumes for all the major cities in the United States and was working on Flashmaps for London and Paris. The little books were a huge success. They are clearly drawn, in bright colors on white, easy to read in a dark car interior or a telephone booth, and just the right size to fit into men's jacket pockets or most women's handbags. In addition, Lasker was brilliant at marketing her product, constantly thinking up new ways to make Flashmaps accessible to more people.

Lasker was both apprehensive and excited about her new-found career. "When Flashmaps was first published, I was fifty, and that's when I really got started. I didn't realize what I had gotten into. Then it opened up, and it brought out a whole different me." Lasker soon found that updating the books was almost a full-time occupation. "Nobody has any idea of the work that went into it," she says.

By the late 1980s, when Random House unexpectedly offered to buy Flashmaps from her, Lasker had been running the company for twenty years and was ready to move on to other pursuits. She explains, "I think people enjoy different stages in life.

There is a time when your children are going to leave your house, there are times when you're in business, times when you're going to retire." But instead of retiring, Lasker spent a year writing a monograph on New York City's problems, as a pro bono activity. Now she has started another commercial project, "one too hot to tell anybody about just now," she said. And when this one is wrapped up, she says, "I want to get back and do some painting. I want to do lots of things."

Frances Lear

The participant whose career got off to the latest start was Frances Lear, who began her real career at sixty-two. When she and her husband, celebrated TV producer Norman Lear, decided to get a divorce, Lear moved from Los Angeles to New York and set to work realizing her lifelong dream of being a journalist. In New York, she started her own magazine for women who, like herself, were past the relatively young age normally addressed by women's magazines at the time.

Born in a home for unwed mothers, Frances Lear was adopted at the age of fourteen months by Herb and Aline Loeb, a well-to-do suburban couple. Herb had a company that manufactured uniforms for nurses and maids, and he earned a good living until the depression. When his fortunes began to disintegrate as the country slid into economic chaos, he committed suicide. His death was a tragedy for young Frances, who was far closer to him than to her distant and capricious mother.

Lear's mother remarried quickly, in part for economic reasons, to a man who shortly afterward began to sexually abuse his new stepdaughter. When she was sixteen, Frances ran away from home and got a job in New York.

Lear's ambition had always been to be a journalist. In her high school class prophecy, she was slated to be the first woman editor of the *New York Times*. But women couldn't get jobs in journalism fifty years ago. "I wanted to be a journalist, but I did not have the education or the experience, and it was a rare woman who was paid to be a reporter in the 1940s," she says. So she had a succession of jobs that led nowhere, like selling blouses at B. Altman's. I had "fifteen different careers," Lear says, "because I was forever hating what I was doing, and wanting to be something better, and use my head more." She was ambitious and extremely smart, and that combination in a woman was not always welcomed in post–World War II America.

After two short marriages ended in divorce, she married Norman Lear and moved to Los Angeles. In her years in Hollywood, Lear frequently collaborated on her husband's projects, in the process learning a great deal about the television industry. But Hollywood is essentially a company town, where spouses don't necessarily count. She found the experience of being a "nonperson" galling. She compensated by becoming involved in the women's movement and by opening her own executive search firm in the 1960s, specializing in jobs for women executives.

Lear grew increasingly frustrated in Los Angeles. When her marriage disintegrated, she decided to move back to New York with the idea of starting her own magazine for "women like me." In 1988, she founded *Lear's* magazine, "an early road map to much of the second half of life," as she describes it. The adventure of starting the magazine was bittersweet, however. Many people in the magazine industry did not believe that there was enough of a market to make the project successful, even though women in the over-fifty age bracket outnumber men almost two to one and form a very large group in the population. The work it took to shape the magazine and get it established was arduous, but it paid off. The magazine has been such a success that recently Lear was able to hire someone else to serve as editor in chief; Lear continues to act as publisher. This will free some of her time to work on new projects, like a television show and writing a second volume of her autobiography. The first volume, *The Second Seduction,* was published by Knopf in the spring of 1992 to universally favorable reviews.

On her career, Lear says: "I'm the latest bloomer. . . . I *started* my career at sixty-two! I think that, although I hate to chart anything by chronology,. . . I've had more growth from fifty-five on than during all the rest of my life put together."

CAREER PEAKS AFTER SIXTY-FIVE

DR. W. EDWARDS DEMING

The longest growth curve and the latest career peak of all belong to Dr. W. Edwards Deming, the management consultant who more than any other single individual provided the conceptual base for the economic resurgence of Japan after World War II.

A type-A Explorer, Deming is the son of a small-town Wyoming lawyer. He was educated there as a mathematician and engineer. He held several positions as an instructor in engineering, a professor of physics; later a business consultant. At the age of thirty, he became interested in statistics, then a new science. At this time, he had worked at the Fixed Nitrogen Research Laboratory of the U.S. Department of Agriculture as a mathematical physicist. He was happy in his job but when he received an offer from the Bureau of the Census in Washington, he jumped at the opportunity. "I could not resist the offer. Also it was a promotion," he said.

Once at the bureau, Deming became deeply engaged in learning how statistical methods could be used for a variety of functions, ranging from monitoring intercity motor freight to consumer research. In 1947, he was invited by Japan's census bureau to advise the Japanese on how to use statistical science to restructure their agency. Deming went, and he enjoyed the experience thoroughly. He became fascinated by the question of how to rebuild the Japanese economy after the war and thought that theory of a system would be extremely useful.

Deming was right. His ideas found an eager audience in Japanese industrialists, and they began to devise ways to integrate these concepts into their work. Deming's method enabled the Japanese to construct the most stunning economic recovery in the world, eventually wresting the superiority from the United States as a manufacturer and exporter. It is a system based on collaboration rather than competition.

"I didn't have to teach the Japanese about cooperation," Deming remarked. "They already understood it; it was part of their culture." So successful were his concepts in their application that the Japanese in 1951 established an annual prize in his name, the W. Edwards Deming Prize. Over the next decade he would return to Japan every few years to meet with leaders of industry to conduct seminars. In 1960 the emperor of Japan decorated him with the Second Order Medal of the Sacred Treasure, one of the country's highest honors.

Despite the brilliant success of Deming's method in Japan, he was almost completely ignored in the United States for decades. Only when the Japanese economy began to pull ahead of the U.S. economy in the 1970s and 1980s did American business begin to pay attention to Deming's concepts.

Deming—ninety-two at the writing of this book—feels that this latest phase of his career has been the most productive period. "I would say that the best part of my life has come from the last twenty years," Deming explained. "I work because I like it. I do it because I wish to do it. And I'm responsible only to myself." Deming believes that his career reached its peak during this period. In describing exactly what has made his recent years so fruitful, Deming went on to say, "I can see things in perspective. Time brings vision. I see where to put emphasis. What I've learned becomes clearer—week by week, day by day." Deming is a master at observing a process and understanding exactly how it is constructed and why it succeeds or fails. He feels now a sense of mission in teaching personnel at U.S. companies how to introduce the theory of a system and other cooperative practices into their work. His deepest regret is that so many industries were slow to recognize their need for the different theory of a system.

Deming has made an extraordinary contribution to the careers of many young people through his practice of mentoring. The way he has nurtured this practice is typically ingenious. A bout of phlebitis at the age of twenty-six left him with a permanent tendency toward this illness, which, when active, affects his legs and makes him less agile than his travel schedule demands. With his characteristic genius for working with daily experience, however difficult it might be, he adopted the custom of permitting companies that he consults for to appoint one or more of their promising younger employees as Deming interns. An intern travels with Dr. Deming periodically during the year, taking care of practical arrangements for him carrying bags and at the same time learning intensely from listening and observing during that time.

Busier than ever, Deming travels every week to two or three different cities where he consults for major corporations, helping them revamp their style of management to be more productive. He spends half his time on public seminars, the other half with clients. His four-day seminars have reached more than ten thousand people per year for more than a decade; they become more popular every year, which delights Deming. "Many people are interested," he says. "My seminars are overbooked months ahead!"

MILLICENT FENWICK

Millicent Fenwick's most important career peak began shortly before her sixty-fifth birthday, when she was elected to the U.S. House of Representatives.

Born and raised in New Jersey, Fenwick married in 1929 at the age of nineteen and began a family immediately. She undoubtedly thought her life would be spent comfortably as a housewife, much as her mother's had been. But the marriage did not work out. Divorced in her early thirties, she found herself with no professional or career training (she had not even finished high school), two young children, and a huge burden of debt run up by her former husband. She could not even get a job at Bonwit Teller's as a sales clerk, she recalled ruefully, since jobs of that kind required a college degree in those days.

Spurred on by desperation and her sense of responsibility, she spoke with another friend, who put her in touch with someone at *Vogue* magazine, and she found a position at last on their staff. There she wrote *The Vogue Book of Etiquette,* which became quite popular and widely used. Meanwhile, she was gradually repaying the financial obligations left over from her marriage and putting her children through school.

During the years when she was at *Vogue,* Fenwick gradually became active in public service. When she moved back to New Jersey after her children had left home, she was asked to join a local recreation commission, which became highly successful under her chairmanship. It was then suggested that she run for local council. At first she was doubtful. "They had never had a woman elected," she says. But to her surprise she won. This initial success encouraged her to run for higher office, and it led eventually to a seat in the House of Representatives in 1974. Fenwick served four terms in the House, with distinction, before launching a bid for a Senate seat in 1982. Although this campaign proved unsuccessful, she was appointed the following year as U.S. ambassador to the UN Food and Agricultural Commission in Rome.

When I asked Fenwick if she had thought of retiring at age sixty-five, and why she did not retire at that point, she drew herself up instinctively and looked at me with surprise bordering on indignation. "I was first elected to Congress when I was sixty-four," she responded, "and it didn't even occur to me that I should be thinking about retirement at that point. I was much too busy getting ready to take my first seat in the House of Representatives!"

In March 1987 Fenwick returned to the United States from her service in Rome. After that, she lived in New Jersey and remained active in public affairs until her death from heart disease in September 1992.

Fenwick was very blunt in giving advice on how to deal with one's older years, displaying the candor and face-the-facts attitude that made her so successful in politics. "I don't think you can prepare for old age," she said emphatically. "Nobody has any idea what it's like. Each person's old age is a little different. Aging is highly individual. So is growing up. The main thing is: are you interested in something beside yourself? You can't be a sissy and you can't have self-pity."

DR. LAWRENCE WEED

At age sixty-nine, Lawrence Weed, M.D., appears to be moving into the upswing of another period of intense creativity in his work. Weed is a physician and biochemist, a type-B Explorer whose original qualities of mind have generated two major innovations in medical practice. The second of these is still in its developmental stage.

Born in 1923, Weed grew up in Middletown, New York. Like Dr. Linus Pauling he spent a great deal of time outside in his childhood, living in a world of his own imagining and inventing projects mostly related to science. He attended Hamilton College, a small, extremely fine liberal arts school, where each student received a great deal of personal attention.

His move to a larger institution, Columbia University Medical School, was traumatic. Weed's intelligence had been allowed to range freely until then, and he was incensed at the rigid, hierarchical atmosphere of medical school in the 1940s. Until then he had taken his mental liberty for granted, but being forced to memorize large quantities of facts without having time to evaluate or think about them left Weed constantly frustrated. He persisted, nevertheless, and went on to do postgraduate work in medicine and biochemistry at several other major universities.

In the 1950s, while on the faculty at Yale University, Weed realized one day during rounds that the traditional way of organizing medical records actually made diagnosis and treatment harder instead of easier. Until then, information about each patient was organized on the basis of its source—laboratory data on orange sheets, X-ray reports on grey sheets, narrative data from doctors in one place, nurses' notes in another. This unassembled mosaic was the patient's record. The pieces had to be put together in the mind of the person reading the record; if that person missed seeing an essential connection, then their conclusion might be wrong.

In a moment of insight, Weed reshuffled the file folder in his hand so that it focused on a list of the patient's problems. Later, as director of medical education at the Eastern Maine General Hospital in Bangor, Maine, Weed worked out a detailed implementation of this new record-keeping system, which he called the problem-oriented record. Articles about the system, especially one solicited for the *New England Journal of Medicine* in 1968 by Franz Inglefinger (the editor who got Lewis Thomas to write his first article and asked Norman Cousins to set down his first account of *Anatomy of an Illness*), generated widespread interest in the idea. Weed's system, the Problem-Oriented Medical Record, is in use today in thousands of hospitals and private practices.

For Weed, however, this was just a first step. For many years he had been wrestling with contemporary physicians' struggle to keep up with the vast and growing body of medical knowledge and to use this huge quantity of new information in their practice. "The human memory has information-storage and -recall limitations," Weed said, "and it also has limitations in processing that information in terms of the unique set of problems that each patient presents. If you put an average Ph.D. scientist in a situation like the usual one in a doctor's office, and tell them there's going to be a new problem every fifteen minutes, they'd go mad. The demands made on the ordinary physician today are very close to being impossible."

The solution to Weed was obvious: use the computer to provide a supportive framework, to do what the computer does best, which is organize and access massive amounts of medical information. In the early 1980s, Weed began developing a computerized diagnostic information system that links a particular medical problem with all the existing information about that problem. It is put together in a question-and-answer format: the doctor asks the patient a series of questions that appear on the computer screen and types in the patient's responses as they are given. At the end of the sequence, the computer provides a print-out of the various conditions that match the patient's symptoms, and the degree to which they match (e.g., five out of six symptoms of a duodenal ulcer, and two out of eight symptoms of angina). It can also provide a list of treatment possibilities for each illness listed. Weed chose a name for this system that is utterly lacking in poetry but highly descriptive: Problem-Knowledge Couplers (PKCs).

The amount of information required to build PKC units is very large, and Weed has been working at it ever since he commenced the project, aided by a gradually accumulating group of interested colleagues. The PKCs are the basis of a twenty-first-century medical system, one that makes all the knowledge related to a problem available almost instantly to the physician and patient, organized in a way that bears directly on the particular patient's illness.

The PKC system is particularly important in a long-lived society because it will allow the newest research on health to be used in a physician's practice almost as soon as it is released. Since the study of aging is one of the fastest-growing medical research fields, it will benefit older people in a very direct and immediate way. Moreover, the computerized medical record will allow your medical record to be kept and updated indefinitely, even throughout a ninety or one hundred year lifespan and a variety of medical personnel.

Because the PKC system gives physician and patient a list of all illnesses with even a partial match to the patient's symptoms, less time is lost in making a diagnosis, and unnecessary tests can be avoided. The physician is less likely to miss a rare condition, so the percentage of diagnostic errors is tremendously reduced—and because of this the system may also have the potential to reduce the frequency of malpractice suits. Quality medicine can be mass-produced, and patients can assume a far greater role in their own diagnosis and treatment. Weed wants to develop a science of medical practice that can begin to match the science of disease developed over the last century.

At the writing of this book, PKC units have been developed for about thirty-five common problems and a number of less common ones, and more are in the works. The system is poised for growth into a comprehensive instrument that can incorporate hospital records, medical test reports, and any other relevant information. As its use spreads, Weed's role will broaden; and it is easy to see the possibility that, like Deming, Weed may have his greatest professional peak after the age of seventy (hopefully, like Deming, continuing into his nineties).

SUMMARY

A skeptic could look at many of these examples, and some of the others from earlier chapters, and call them too unusual to serve as role models for anyone else. Dr. Lewis Thomas, for example, already had a solid primary career when he began writing. John Gardner was well established and in a peak period in his primary career when, at the age of forty-nine, he wrote *Excellence*, launching his own delayed writing career. We might have assumed that they would be successful in their second careers, having been successful in the first, except that it doesn't necessarily follow that people are equally or more successful in a secondary career different from the primary one.

Nor is it true that these people are so unusual that everything they do is equally successful. In fact, many of them had done other things with lesser degrees of success. Gardner had gotten only rejection slips from his earlier attempt at writing. Thomas was a very good researcher, but not an extraordinary one—whereas he is a phenomenally gifted writer. Brussell, Lasker, Lear, and Fenwick, as well as late starter Julia Child, gave no particular indication in their earlier lives that they would have outstanding careers. If we had looked in on any of them at about thirty-five years of age, we probably would not have recognized them as people with outstanding potential, judged by the usual standards. All of them were housewives, in the postwar era when no one expected a woman to do anything outside the home and succeed in it. And they were absolutely unknown. Dr. W. Edwards Deming's greatest period of success began at about the age of forty-seven and has continued to expand exponentially ever since. He was famous, even revered, in Japan, during his fifties and sixties; but until he was seventy he was not widely known in the United States, except to his consulting clients. Now he routinely draws between six hundred to one thousand people for his four-day seminars and must turn down prospective participants when programs are filled up.

Is there a generalization suggested by these examples? Yes. They reinforce psychologist Dean Keith Simonton's findings that those who start late can rise to as high a level of achievement as those who start "on time," but their total production will be shortened because less time is available for it.

One can also say that, in general, some people simply need longer than others to find the field or type of work in which they are most successful. At times, a person seems to need to build up a specific combination of abilities in order to enter a particular career, or make their most important contribution in a field. It isn't just a matter of going out and applying for job X. There is an accumulation of knowledge over a period of time that ultimately provides the base for a truly original accomplishment.

It may also be true that our ideas of how a successful career develops and the age at which it starts, as well as the ages at which people have the potential to develop new careers, are distorted and inaccurate because they are based on a time when life expectancies were shorter. The individual's age at the beginning of a career is not a factor in predicting success.

The experience of these people demonstrates one thing over and over: growth and creativity are possible at any age, for all of us. What holds us back is the idea that growth stops.

11

Retirers and Returners

Most of us who are younger than sixty-five tend to think of retirement as the end of the story. But people who retire wake up the next morning, much as they've always done, and start another day of life. Everyone who retires has decisions to make, relationships to maintain, changes to manage, schedules to plan, new activity patterns to create. Retirement is another phase in life, not the end of it.

Roughly one-third (fifty-four) of the Long Careers Study participants retired at some point in their careers. However, most of these retirers quickly became returners: forty-nine went back to work either immediately or a short time after retirement. In fact, almost two-thirds returned to paid work, while the others pursued full-time or part-time nonpaying work. The three main reasons they gave for choosing to return to work were that they missed the activity, they had too much energy to stay inactive, and they wanted to contribute. Most of those who had not retired said that they were too busy to consider it or that it never even occurred to them.

Only five people who had retired were not working at the time of their interview. Of those five, two were in the process of looking for new projects.

Not all of the returners went back to the same kind of work.

Many found work in the same field as their primary career, or one very similar to it. Others found a different kind of work. Most of the returners were relatively happy with what they did. And two had post-retirement careers that were far more interesting and satisfying than their primary careers.

These post-retirement choices often depended on pure circumstance—on the chance appearance of the right elements at the right moment. There were two exceptions to this generally positive experience in finding or creating work after retirement. In both cases the person was unable to find a situation that was satisfying or appropriate, through no fault of their own. As a result, they experienced suffering and a real sense of loss.

It is important to repeat here the caveat stated at the beginning of the book: there is nothing wrong with retirement for people who want or need to retire, and there is nothing wrong with the desire to continue working. They are different choices, it is true. But it is essential in a long-lived society that both exist as options.

Also, this book should not be read as an argument for eliminating or cutting back programs for older people, or for raising the eligibility age for Social Security, because it is neither. There is such a radical polarization between the concept of retirement and the idea of continuing to work that it is very difficult to construct any argument that includes both and cannot be used as a weapon against one alternative or the other.

People who work at something that they dislike or that is physically or mentally wearing will probably wish to retire and do something different, and they should have that option, without any question. Others may experience poor health in their sixties, as did a few of the study participants, and may need to retire. Because of the tremendous individuality of the aging process, retirement should always remain a viable choice.

But I also believe that, in a long-lived society, people should not be forced to retire at ages as young as we have been accustomed to recently, if they are functioning well and want to continue working. The participants in the Long Careers Study demonstrate that there are many additional options for people who are sixty-five and older. Almost all of the participants who retired found ways to continue working in some capacity.

The reality is that extended longevity and the lengthened

midlife period of vitality have so changed the needs of many Americans that they want to stay active when they are older. This is a change that may become even more marked in the future if longevity continues to rise.

We need to discard our age-based prejudice about how age affects functioning. And, for the future, we will need a variety of roles and images for older people, to replace the narrow, one-dimensional view of them we have held until now—images that include health as well as illness, wisdom and strength as well as dependency and weakness, active lifestyles as well as sunsets on golden ponds.

HUGH DOWNS

The most famous returner in the study is one with whom millions of Americans are well acquainted: television broadcaster Hugh Downs. Not only did he retire and move to Arizona (to a town with the provocative and seemingly appropriate name of Carefree), he even took early retirement, at the age of fifty. "When I retired, left regular broadcasting," Downs said, "I felt that I had done all that I needed to do and didn't really have to work. Although I wasn't wealthy, there were a lot of other things I wanted to do."

Downs formally retired on October 11, 1971. He had plans for a few activities to help fill his time: he would teach at Arizona State University; he would write books; and he would look forward to attending to his hobbies, particularly flying gliders and doing aerobatics.

Downs learned quickly that his assumption was wrong about retirement being more leisurely than his work life. Because his energy level was high, he kept adding to his list of things to do. Essentially, Downs's drive to stay involved and to keep learning was so strong that it overwhelmed his original concept of having more time for leisure. At a deeper level, leisure appears to be the last thing in the world Hugh Downs was really interested in.

Downs started his retirement by adding commitments to several nonprofit organizations, and he became especially involved with the National Space Institute. Also, he didn't quit broadcasting altogether but worked on certain programs for educational TV. Then he was approached to host the PBS series "Over Easy," which meant constant commuting back and forth to San Francisco, where the program was shot.

"When I retired," Downs told me, "I took on such a load that Jean Ferrara, my secretary, said at one point, 'I wish you'd go back to work, you'd have more free time!' Which was true, because I had safeguarded vacations when I had contracts with the networks. So in a way, when I went back to work it was a sort of relief. I jokingly said more than once that every time I retired I got busier than before."

In 1976, Downs received a call from the producers of the pilot show for "20/20." The premiere had been a disaster, but the network thought the concept was worthwhile and decided to make an effort to get a better format and change the people involved. And as everyone knows, hiring Downs was perhaps the best move the network could have made.

Downs's return to work was surely one of the most successful comebacks in media history. His work, and the programming of "20/20," have become more innovative as the years have passed. The program tackles cultural features, investigative reports, and stories on science, space, medical issues, aging, and exploration. "We don't do the kind of feature anymore that says, 'Gee, folks, ain't this awful?'" Downs said emphatically. "Why depress people? If we deal with something," Downs said, "we try to show a reason or a remedy or a hope of redress."

A Homesteader who has spent his life in broadcasting, Downs began his career as a teenager in his hometown of Lima, Ohio, in 1939. Downs's father thought that eighteen-year-old Hugh should quit college and get a job to help the family survive the Depression, a view that at the time seemed entirely reasonable.

Downs began working for a local radio station as a staff announcer. He worked his way up from Lima to WJR in Detroit, then after a short break to serve in the infantry during World War II he went to NBC in Chicago, then to network headquarters in New York in 1954. In 1957, he was offered an opportunity that was to make his name a household word, as the sidekick to Jack Paar on "The Tonight Show." When Paar quit the show, Downs was offered the chance to move to the fledgling "Today" show, where he remained until that October day when he first retired.

Does he plan to retire again? No, not in the near, or even distant, future. "I'm going to stick where I am," he said. "Maybe down the line, twenty years from now, I will say, 'I only want to do three out of four shows. . . .'" His voice trails off as if that is a possibility so remote that he can't even focus on it. Downs learned that traditional retirement was not for him, and he relishes his long career now more than ever.

ESTHER PETERSON

Consumer advocate Esther Peterson retired a quarter of a century later in life than did Hugh Downs. In 1976, at the age of seventy-four, she left government service because Ronald Reagan had replaced her boss, Jimmy Carter, in the White House. After a long, challenging work life full of accomplishments, Peterson might have at least considered staying retired. But as she puts it, "How could I retire? I wouldn't know what to do!"

Peterson went back to work in the same field she had been in before her retirement, consumer advocacy. She accepted a volunteer job as the United Nations lobbyist for the International Organization of Consumer's Unions, where she still serves today. She has graduated from being a consumer advocate on a national level to being concerned about consumer issues affecting the world and its nations.

A slender, slightly fragile woman with a Scandinavian-style crown of white braids across her head, Peterson's appearance leaves you utterly unprepared for the strength of her views and the breakneck speed of her schedule. I had to wait three months for my first appointment with her because she was on a month-long speaking tour of Australia, with a few stopovers on the way there and back. She may have ridden horseback in the Utah of her childhood, but Esther Peterson has taken to the jet-propelled modern age like an eagle to the air.

Peterson was born in 1906 in Provo, Utah, to a Mormon family. Although she eventually rejected Mormonism, she credits her upbringing with instilling in her the sense that "you had to give of yourself, always. You didn't only work for yourself." A physical education major at Brigham Young University, she taught for two years and earned her master's degree at Columbia University, where she met her future husband, Oliver Peterson, a sociology student and a socialist.

Her relationship with Oliver led her to an interest in the labor movement. From the early 1930s until 1961 she held a series of jobs in various unions and labor organizations; at the same time, she also raised four children and spent nine years overseas when her husband was named a foreign service labor attaché.

While working as a union lobbyist in Washington, Peterson

became friends with then–Sen. John F. Kennedy. When Kennedy went to the White House, he asked her to join his administration as director of the Women's Bureau of the Labor Department, where she organized the first Presidential Commission on the Status of Women. Later she became assistant secretary of labor.

Kennedy had begun carving out a position for Peterson, that of special assistant for consumer affairs, and Johnson made that appointment after he took office. Peterson thus became the first woman to serve as special assistant to a president. She was too outspoken for Johnson's taste, however, so in 1967 she resigned to return full-time to the Labor Department.

Her activism gave her a wonderfully pragmatic approach to her work. "I didn't just wait for someone to tell me what was going on at an agency," she confided with a mischievous smile. "I'd put on a babushka and some old clothes and go stand in line at their benefits office, and see first hand. It's amazing what you can learn when you do that." Officials were universally disconcerted to discover that the somewhat shabby-looking little old lady standing in line was their boss, and that she had a list of suggested improvements in service all ready to slap into their IN boxes.

After Nixon's election, Peterson took on the corporate sector. On a dare from the president of Giant Food Corporation, she went to work for the large supermarket chain in Washington, D.C. It was a very successful move: she established many reforms, including open dating, unit pricing, nutritional and ingredient labeling, and certain safety programs. She described her reforms in the *Harvard Business Review,* and her techniques remain classroom examples of "consumerism as a marketing tool."

In 1976 President Carter asked Peterson to resume her previous office as special assistant for consumer affairs. She agreed, and kept it until Reagan took office in 1980, when she retired.

It took Peterson several years to find her next project. Meanwhile, she hosted television and radio shows on consumer issues. When she received the offer to work for the Consumer's Unions as a lobbyist at the UN, she knew immediately that this was the next logical step in her work: to be concerned about consumers on a global scale rather than in just one country. "The international consumer movement is going to be a big new force, just like the labor movement has been and the women's movement," she remarked.

In 1992, Esther Peterson turned eighty-six. She had one birth-day party in Washington and then flew to Utah for another party her friends there insisted on giving. When asked why she never truly retired, Peterson laughed and said, "It never occurred to me. I need to be active, doing something, feeling that I can make a dif-ference, even as little at it might be."

Peterson's career has followed a pattern found in many other careers. She made a number of shifts in scale as she matured in her work, going from small to large; from the grass-roots level of local and individual concerns, she changed focus to the larger scope of regional organizations and wider issues, then progressed to the national level; now finally she is working with international concerns. Not until the age when many people now retire, sev-enty, did she have her first job in a corporation, another enriching change for someone who had always taken the cause of the unions and their workers. A type-B Explorer, she has remained firmly rooted in labor and consumer issues during her entire work life, serving that commitment in a variety of settings.

ALAN PIFER

Carnegie Corporation president Alan Pifer also retired by choice, but for a different reason than did Hugh Downs: to start a new career for himself before he reached the age of sixty-five.

Pifer, who was John Gardner's successor at Carnegie, had had a distinguished career and had been at the corporation for thirty-five years. He described how the idea first came to him:

By the time I was sixty-one, I had been president of the Foundation sixteen years. I was getting bored with it, frankly. I was walking through Grand Central Station on my way to the office one morning. I said to myself, "Gosh, I really don't feel like going to the office today," the first time I'd ever had that experience. So when I got there, I thought about it a little and I called up the chairman of the board and said, "I think the time has come for me to figure out how I'm going to get out of this." Just like that.

Pifer was able to stay on at Carnegie for four more years, until he was sixty-five, and pursue projects of his own interest—a great opportunity, to be sure, but also one demonstrating excep-tional courage and resourcefulness. He created and chaired two projects, one on population aging (the Aging Society project) and a second on the reform of federal policy (the Federal Social Role project). As sixty-five approached for him, he formed his own nonprofit organization, the Southport Institute for Policy Analysis, near his home in Connecticut. The institute has thrived and now has a Washington office in addition to its Southport headquarters, and its agenda has been broadened to include projects on adult illiteracy.

Like Downs, Pifer notes that in some respects he had more leisure time while he was working full-time than he does in "retirement." "I have worked much harder since I left the corporation presidency," he said. "There were periods when I had to work terribly hard there, of course, but day in and day out I did protect most of my weekends. And now I can't." For the moment, however, he is enjoying his activities enormously, so working weekends seems to be a minor inconvenience.

OLLIE THOMPSON

Sausalito, California, resident Ollie Thompson started his life as a farmer and was a motel maintenance man in his last full-time job. He retired thinking he would enjoy having more leisure. But Thompson, who has always been very active and interested in the world around him, very quickly made an amazing discovery: he was bored beyond anything he would ever have imagined.

Thompson grew up the youngest of nine children on an Alabama farm in the 1930s and thought he would remain there all his life. Circumstances worked against that, however. His father died when he was fifteen, and Thompson took over the farm. Earning a living there became difficult, and eventually he sold the farm and headed for the nearest city, in search of urban employment, as many blacks did during that period. He got a job in a pipe-fitting shop, and when the war began he enlisted. Unfortunately, the war helped break up his marriage: he came home on leave to find his wife had had a child by another man, and she refused to go back to Thompson, who was devastated. But a year later he married again, this time very happily. When he was discharged from the service, Thompson decided to go to California, settling in the San Francisco area.

California was a great place for entrepreneurs. Thompson started several businesses: in house-cleaning, in landscape gardening, and in catering, as well as a small cab company. When one business became established he would sell it and go on to the next. From time to time he would also work on passenger trains, making the run from Oakland to Salt Lake City and back. In addition, for some years he managed staffs for several wealthy clients. Finally he took the job at the motel because it seemed easy, and at that point he wanted some free time for himself.

By the time he was sixty-eight, Thompson had worked very hard for a long time, and he thought he was really tired of it. He decided to retire and take his well-earned rest. Boredom was the last thing he expected to feel; he thought retirement would be heaven on earth. Thompson's retirement lasted about three months. "I sat at home and ate," he recalls, "and gained thirty pounds, and drove my wife crazy. I've always worked, and I was lost without something to do. Finally I said to myself, 'To hell with this! I'm going to go out and go back to work!' And I did. And I've been much happier ever since. And so has my wife!"

Thompson started his own chauffeur service, a smaller, one-man version of his earlier cab company. His interest now is not in building up a company but in having his own personalized clientele. He derives a great deal of pleasure from driving his clients around the San Francisco Bay area where he lives. He works mostly because he enjoys the activity, the human contact, the sense that he is being useful. He is in good health and has too much energy, he says, to sit around. And, of course, the money he earns provides a welcome addition to his Social Security income.

Thompson is a type-A Explorer. His career demonstrates that the pattern holds true regardless of a person's type of work or socioeconomic level. Thompson outgrew farming; enlisted in the army and moved away from Alabama to start over in response to external factors; and fueled by his internal drive worked his way up through a series of business ventures in California, finally going back to working for other people just before his retirement. He loves the independence his current work provides, and he plans to keep going as long as he can.

JUDGE MORRIS LASKER

Judge Morris Lasker, a New York federal district judge since 1968, has found that a judgeship provides tremendous variety and flexibility. Because judges are appointed for life, the judicial system does not have a traditional retirement policy for them; instead, special options have been devised. At sixty-five or seventy, depending on how long they have served, they may choose to retain a full caseload; or to retire almost completely, with a minimal caseload; or to take "senior status," as Lasker has, which means they have a reduced but still active caseload.

Lasker worked tirelessly as an active judge for over twenty years. Taking senior status is a compromise that works well for Lasker. "It means I don't work under pressure," he explained. "Whereas when I was an active judge I used to have to work over weekends and nights and so forth in order to keep up with things. Now I'm finished at the end of a workday." Lasker still goes to his chambers almost every day, but he now takes longer vacations and days off. Meanwhile, a younger judge can be appointed and begin to gain experience. This unusual arrangement, which emphasizes the value of experience and wisdom, provides a much needed example for other professions; it is possible for senior people to cut down their schedule, while continuing to be engaged in their work. Especially in an era when "increased productivity" has become a buzzword (meaning "too little time to do the amount of work that has to be done"), a form of senior status could be useful in many occupations.

Lasker was born in Hartsdale, New York, in 1917. After his father died when he was barely three years old, his mother remarried a successful lawyer who was a member of a well-known law firm by the name of Battle, Levy, Fowler and Neimann. "I suppose I must have been influenced to some extent to go into the law as a result of his being a good lawyer, but it was never through any effort on his part to influence me in that direction, or my mother's," Lasker commented. In fact, Lasker says he did not make the decision to become a lawyer until the very end of his college career.

After graduating from Yale Law School, Lasker worked in Washington as a staff attorney for the Truman Committee. He longed to make a career in public service, but on returning to civilian life after serving in the army air force, he chose to join his stepfather's law firm so he could support his young family adequately.

In 1968, Lasker finally left his private practice when he was appointed a district judge, at age fifty-one. His new position did not disappoint him. Becoming a judge has vastly widened the scope of Lasker's professional life. He appreciates deeply the opportunity to combine and apply all the wisdom learned through his prior experiences as a lawyer. "The remarkable thing about this job," Lasker said, "is its infinite variety. . . . I feel that the total corpus of my work has contributed something to the development of the law."

At the time of his interview, Lasker had written over fifteen hundred opinions, which fill twenty volumes. He strongly believes that he becomes a better judge every year. "I can tell you without any question or doubt that I am a remarkably more capable judge today than when I'd been on the bench even five years, because I know what it's all about," Lasker said. "My decisions are more informed and they are made with consciousness of much more of the body of law behind them." His own experience as a judge has convinced him that our youth-oriented culture, which so often wants to throw experience "on the trash heap," must begin to value the achievement of wisdom in older people.

DR. KENNETH CLARK

Dr. Kenneth Clark has had a brilliant career as a teacher and social psychologist. With his wife, Mamie, he was responsible for ground-breaking research on the damaging effects of discrimination on children. His research was cited in the Supreme Court opinion in *Brown* v. *Board of Education* and was a key factor in the court's decision.

In 1975 Clark voluntarily retired from teaching at City College of New York, to the surprise and protest of his students and colleagues. But Clark didn't believe he was in fact "retiring." "I believe that people should go on with what they are doing as long as they want to," he explained. "I never thought about retirement; I thought about changing focus. I wanted to spend less time teaching, and more time on my research."

Clark was born on the Canal Zone, Panama, in 1914. His parents, Jamaican immigrants to Panama, separated when he was a child, and his mother and sister moved to the United States, leaving Kenneth behind in the care of his grandmother. Two years later, he joined his mother and sister in New York. He still remembers coming through Ellis Island with his grandmother.

Clark's mother taught her children to persevere and strive for achievement, not allowing social and racial restraints to discourage them. "The process of being afraid of what people would say was not part of my socialization," he added. Clark's career has always stayed true to that lesson. He received his B.A. from Columbia University and an M.S. from Howard University, returning to Columbia for his Ph.D. in social psychology, which he received in 1940.

"I didn't think of my studies in terms of using an understanding of psychology to improve racial understanding," Clark said. "I thought at that point that I was using psychology to understand *human beings.*"

Clark was the first black academician invited to join the faculty of City College of New York. During World War II, he was assigned to the Office of War Information, where he worked with a group studying the morale of civilian blacks to find out whether racism and prejudice had a persistent negative affect among blacks in the war. Ironically, he himself left the office after a year because of prejudice: he wasn't getting enough support and his efforts were being undermined by the FBI. "I never stayed in a situation where I had to adjust to racism or interference," he adds.

Clark often had to deal with discrimination in his career. For example, he was not accepted at Cornell's graduate school because the admissions committee felt "he wouldn't be happy there." When he was studying at Howard University, he was shocked by the degree of segregation and racism in Washington D.C. As a teacher at Hampton Institute, Clark was scolded by the president for "frustrating my students by talking to them about race." But Clark also had many mentors who supported and encouraged his work throughout his career; these mentors, aware of discriminatory practices, were consciously trying to advance bright minority students and employees. Thus, Clark believes his minority experience had both positive and negative aspects.

When Clark left the Office of War Information, he returned to City College. His wife was conducting a study on self-image in children for her master's degree and wanted him to participate. Together they received a fellowship to pursue that research. Mrs. Clark then became pregnant with their first child, so Clark conducted the field studies alone, traveling around the country and using pairs of white and black dolls to test children's self-image. Their research was published in 1940 and generated great interest. It was the first clear, objective evidence gleaned from research that black children were being conditioned into negative self-images by gender and racial prejudice.

A colleague, Otto Kleinberg, asked Clark to write a summary report on his findings. Thurgood Marshall, then a practicing attorney, saw the report and recruited Clark to work on the *Brown* v. *Board of Education* case. He became part of the team that put together a social science brief used as expert testimony during the trial, and Clark's research was cited in the final decision. When the decision came down, Clark says, "I was jumping for joy. . . . We certainly didn't anticipate that our research was going to have any revolutionary impact."

Clark was next commissioned to do a similar report on adolescents in Harlem, and he participated in the creation of Harlem Youth Opportunities. This research led to his prize-winning book *Dark Ghetto* (1965), in which he examined the plight of youths in Harlem. He has been awarded many national honors, including the Presidential Medal of Liberty (1986), and is the author of several books and numerous articles.

After thirty-one years, Clark left his teaching position at City College because he felt strongly that it was time to move on to other things. "I never gave retirement a thought. I just wanted something different from teaching," Clark explains. "My definition of retirement was retirement from thirty-one years of teaching. I wanted an easier approach to looking at the world rather than the curriculum approach. I just wanted greater freedom in that area."

Since his university retirement, Clark has started the Metropolitan Applied Research Center and is currently president of Kenneth B. Clark and Associates, Inc., a firm that provides professional consultation to educational institutions, private corporations, and government agencies on personnel matters, emphasizing race relations and affirmative action programs. He has advised organizations such as the NAACP Legal Defense and Education Fund, the United States Department of State, AT&T, Chemical Bank, Con Edison, IBM, and NASA. Clark has also served as president of the American Psychological Association and sits on several important boards. At this point, Clark says, "I plan to go on being active as long as I can."

Clark is surprisingly severe in his assessment of his own achievements. He believes that his life "has been a series of glorious defeats" because he dedicated his life to the improvement of conditions for young people and, he says, "I do not see that that has been accomplished." Nevertheless, he will admit, when pressed, that *Brown* v. *Board of Education* has changed the course of American history and was a major victory in combating racial discrimination and injustice.

Clark has never felt confined to society's expectations, either by his race, his profession, or his age. He refused to accept the idea that he was "retiring" in the traditional sense, just as he has always refused to submit to racial discrimination. That independent approach to his career has allowed it to grow constantly in new and valuable directions.

MARGARET FOX

Another returner was Margaret Fox, who sold catalogs and managed the window at the William Doyle Auction Gallery in Manhattan from the age of sixty-two until shortly before her death at the age of eighty, in 1989. Slender, fragile-looking, and sweet, with a distinctive fluff of white hair, Fox's angelic smile belied her inner strength and determination.

Fox was born in New York City and grew up in a townhouse in Chelsea, the oldest of five children born to Irish parents. After graduating from St. Vincent's College, she taught school and then went to work on Wall Street as a secretary for $37.50 a week—a great improvement over her $15-a-week teaching salary.

After stints of secretarial work at a linen importing firm and a rubber company, Fox was hired by the U.S. Customs Agency. She remained there until she reached retirement age, at sixty-two. Then she went to work at the William Doyle Gallery, a job she got simply by walking in off the street—because she thought it looked like a nice place to work.

Before World War II, Fox had been engaged to be married. However, her fiancé died of strep throat just before he was to leave for the army. Fox never found anyone else she cared as much about, and she then centered her personal life about her parents, brothers, and sisters. An Explorer, Fox was a highly people-oriented individual. She liked some of her previous jobs, she said, but she loved her job in the gallery best of all because it involved being around beautiful things and being in touch with a lot of wonderful people. She considered this job to be the high point of her career, and she worked steadily and happily there until about three months before her death.

MAGGIE KUHN AND SAMUEL SADIN: POST-RETIREMENT
CAREERS THAT OUTSHONE THE "REAL" CAREERS

Two participants created post-retirement careers that were actually more satisfying and interesting to them, and in many respects more successful, than their primary careers. Both Maggie Kuhn and Samuel Sadin had relatively unexceptional jobs beginning in their twenties all the way to retirement. In other words, they had what we would think of as normal work lives, culminating in retirement at age sixty-five. Then, without intending to do so, each developed a career far more brilliant and meaningful than their primary career had been. Both were cases of pure serendipity; neither Kuhn nor Sadin had anticipated having a second career after retirement, and they would certainly not have predicted the degree of success that lay ahead of them at that point.

MAGGIE KUHN

Maggie Kuhn, founder of the Gray Panthers, was born August 3, 1905, in Buffalo, New York. She grew up in a succession of cities where her father worked as a manager for Dun and Bradstreet. Ultimately the family settled in Cleveland, where Maggie attended Western Reserve University. She wanted to be a teacher, but her supervisor decided she couldn't maintain discipline, so her teaching career ended abruptly before it even began.

After graduating, Maggie was offered a job with the Young Women's Christian Association, working with young women in industry. She was a natural organizer, good at her work, and she loved it. She earned the equivalent of a master's degree at Columbia University's Teachers College in a joint program with Union Theological Seminary. And when her father was transferred to Philadelphia, Kuhn moved too, taking a job in the YWCA in Germantown.

Kuhn's work in Philadelphia was with businesswomen, but it quickly developed a wider scope, supervising WPA workers and maintaining liaison with forty other agencies in the greater Philadelphia area that also had WPA workers assigned. She also worked with the federal Job Corps and the Youth Conservation Corps, which was geared toward the environment as well as toward the training of young people.

During World War II she moved to New York to work for the USO. After the war, Kuhn was sent to Boston to help reorganize the Unitarian general alliance. (Kuhn's father called this "missionary work among the Unitarians.") But after several years Kuhn returned to Philadelphia to help care for her ailing mother and took a job with the Presbyterian church, where she remained for twenty-two years, until she reached sixty-five. During the last several years of her tenure she was posted to the Interchurch Center in New York, near Riverside Church, and commuted from her home in Philadelphia.

So far, so good. Kuhn had had a perfectly respectable career, but she was hardly a household name. What happened next could never have been predicted; it was as if a cocoon that had been lying dormant for many years suddenly began to crack open, and an astonishing butterfly began to emerge.

"They told me that I would be retired," Kuhn recalls, "that this was mandatory—on my sixty-fifth birthday. There were six of us women in the New York area who were confronted with the same difficulty. A real interesting group of women, and all of them having to retire." If they had been men, Kuhn reflects, they would have been given consulting contracts until they reached seventy. But they were women, so they were just "thrown out."

"So we got together and discussed it," Kuhn continued, "and we said, The question is, what do we do with the rest of our lives? And we said, We can't answer that alone. We've got to deliberate it, and get some kind of a collective answer. So we wrote that in a very simple manifesto, and called a meeting at the International House of Columbia University. A hundred people showed! It was in June 1970; it was a [historic] moment."

Kuhn and her friends had chosen to discuss the war in Vietnam. They decided to demonstrate, to "stand with the kids," and concocted a name for themselves, the Consultation of Older and Younger Adults for Social Change. They got an engagement on a talk show at WBAI radio in New York. While they were there the producer, hearing their name, winced and said, "That name will get you nowhere. You're the Gray Panthers!" The semantic link to the Black Panthers delighted them, and they adopted the name on the spot.

But it wasn't until two years later that the nation learned about the Gray Panthers. In May 1972, Kuhn attended the annual meeting of the General Assembly of the Presbyterian church in Denver, Colorado. On that particular morning, someone in the Presbyterian organization had called a press conference in the

hotel, featuring, Kuhn said, "some VIP who didn't show." There
was a huge turnout for the conference—all the wire services, the
Denver Post, the *Washington Post,* the *New York Times.* In desperation, the press officer called Kuhn and asked her to talk
about "those old people you're working with." Wanting to help a
friend out of a tight spot, she obliged. "A month later," she says,
"I was on the 'Johnny Carson Show.'"

Like the account of how Julia Child's TV show originated,
Kuhn's retelling of her rise to fame through that impromptu press
conference has a flavor of how things really happen. Sometimes,
when last-minute snafus threaten disaster, people who can
improvise and think creatively discover an entirely new path for
themselves. Occasionally, they create new organizations at the
same time.

The serendipity was genuine. Like so many other study participants, Kuhn had a goal in mind, but she did not expect her life to
develop as it has. "I didn't set out to start a movement," she said.
"In many ways it was to answer this very odd question: what do
you *do* with the rest of your life, when you've been so involved
with your work? You see, people who have a certain amount of
privilege have work that they love. And the work and their personal lives—their personal and their professional lives—are
blended."

But it isn't just those who are privileged to have work that
they love who must worry about what to do after retirement.
Kuhn saw very clearly that it is a universal problem. "Those who
do not have work they love, who hate what they do and aren't
affirmed by their jobs and are glad to leave them, *then* what do
they do? They're miserable, too."

A Transformer, Kuhn sees a continuity linking her first career
with her work for the Gray Panthers over the past twenty years.
"I'm building today on all the things that I learned when I was
younger," she says. "For instance, when I worked with the Pres-
byterians, I did seminars on international affairs and foreign policy and things like that. So it's not new to me to have some
agenda items that are forward looking and progressive."

"But my feeling is that in late life we are free to transcend our
own history, and to be progressive," she added. "To take a new
view of ourselves and the world. And we are concerned about the
tribe's survival, not our own. And to get *that* across to people."

Like Esther Peterson, Kuhn has moved from the grass roots to the mountaintops during her work life. She started out organizing working women, went on to work with church agencies on a regional and then national level, then created an organization embracing several age groups and issues of universal importance. She sees this last stage of her career as a potential model: older people have the time, the perspective, and the resources to be concerned about the whole of society rather than just one little part of it. And Kuhn firmly believes that that is what they ought to do.

SAMUEL SADIN

Another Transformer, New York businessman Samuel Sadin, also found his post-retirement career more passionately engaging than his pre-retirement work. Sadin was born in 1918 and raised in Brooklyn, the third of three sons. His father worked in a corrugated box factory, and his mother ran a small retail candy store to bring in extra money. Sadin's childhood was marked by a vivid awareness of the impact of money. His family was poor, but they knew there were many families who were even poorer, in truly desperate straits. The poverty he saw around him lit in his heart a deep concern for justice.

After completing a business degree at City College, he became a CPA and went to work for an accounting firm. Later he started his own business in New York City, a lumber supply company, which he ran successfully for twenty-five years.

Eventually he began to outgrow his interest in the company. "I got impatient and bored with doing the same thing every day and selling the same product," Sadin says. Looking around for other outlets close at hand, he took a creative writing course; became executive secretary of the *New York Quarterly,* a poetry magazine; and took college classes in the Bible and in literature. "That was, I think," he says, "the sign that it was time to go. That there were all these other things waiting to be done." Ready to move on to new endeavors, Sadin sold his lumber business in 1975.

During this period, Sadin's wife had been working in the Department of Senior Citizens of Nassau County. Frequently she told Sadin about clients who had problems with Social Security and didn't know where to get help. That struck a chord in Sadin's mind. You can't go to the agency itself if you're having problems with it. But where could you go?

Soon afterward, Sadin accepted a volunteer assignment for the American Jewish Committee, where he organized a project that involved informing people about their legal rights in various areas. When he met Dr. Rose Dobrof, founder of the Brookdale Center on Aging at Hunter College, he asked her whether Brookdale would be interested in sponsoring an institute to train social workers and senior center staff to advise older people about their legal rights and entitlements. That was the germ of the Institute on Law and Rights of Older Adults at the Brookdale Center, a major program affecting the well-being of thousands of people throughout New York City. Sadin created the institute and served as executive director of the program from 1977 to 1989.

Sadin believes that the law institute is his greatest professional achievement. "This is the best life work I've ever had, in terms of all-around satisfaction," he said. "I think it fulfills the need I had to accomplish something for other people." Like Kuhn, Sadin was able to advance from being a volunteer to being a paid member of the staff when the fledgling organization had enough money to support a salary. That was important, he said, in terms of respect for his work within the organization, which was made up entirely of paid personnel, and also for the continuation of the institute as a fully integrated part of the Brookdale Center.

Sadin also found that much of his business experience was transferable to his career at the institute. His background in accounting turned out to be especially useful in counseling older people, enabling him to interpret figures and read statutes. "If there is anything you should put in your book," he added, "it's that people ought to look at the possibility of either new or related careers—they don't have to be completely new—that draw on some aspects of their life, or the life of their family, or their culture." As a volunteer he learned how a nonprofit organization functioned and was able to apply this knowledge later when he had to run such an organization. In 1989 Sadin stepped down from his administrative position and became a deputy director at the Brookdale Center on a part-time basis. He was also appointed to the National Committee on Social Security Administration. He continues to work for the rights and interests of older people, while spending more time with friends and family. As he puts it, "If my aging career has to come to an end for one reason or another, I'll go find something to do with children or alcoholics or, it really doesn't matter. There are disadvantaged people wherever one looks."

RETIRERS

What about the five people in the study who retired in the classic sense, without replacing their regular work with some other consistent pursuit? Their stories are somewhat less positive. A number of people in the study got caught at some point by mandatory retirement rules, but most wanted to continue working and found an alternative way of doing so. Several took up volunteer work; others found consulting positions or advisory work where their age was not a factor.

Of those who were forcibly retired and not working at the time of their interview, Richard "Buzz" Gummere was happy and Dr. Lawrence Wylie was still unhappy and looking for alternatives. Of those who retired voluntarily, Dr. Alan Cott retired for medical reasons, Sam Cross was looking for new projects, and Sam Goody deeply regretted his choice later on.

RICHARD "BUZZ" GUMMERE

Richard " Buzz" Gummere, for many years associate director of career services at Columbia University, was forcibly retired but later said he was happy in his new situation. Gummere compared his adapted mandatory retirement (at age seventy) to being pushed out of a nest—expecting to fall and flying instead. "It's just marvelous," he said. "You can set your own timetable. I enjoyed my work at Columbia; but I had already enjoyed as much as you can possibly enjoy in a nine-to-five job. There's one thing I had always wanted to do and that's write, and write and write and write."

Gummere had harbored this aspiration since 1952, when he wrote his master's thesis. When he was forced to retire, he immediately set about applying his need for professional activity to writing. He brought me copies of several articles published in *Columbia* magazine, including one entitled "Life Begins at Seventy."

Gummere gives the impression that he has made the best of his involuntary retirement partly because he deliberately turned his attention to other interests and partly because he felt he had no other choice. If the stakes had been higher, however, or if he had been engaged in work that had gotten cut short, the outcome might have been less positive, as it was for one other participant with roots in the academic world.

DR. LAWRENCE WYLIE

Dr. Lawrence Wylie, an internationally famous teacher and researcher in French language and civilization, had his career cut short by administrative rules and departmental politics just at a point when his work had entered a new peak period—one that was as important and inventive as any of his prior work. Wylie was not able to find another work situation with the right elements to allow his work to continue, and his research was in effect terminated.

It is useful to explore this example. Because so many of the other people in the study found alternatives and made successful transfers, it might seem as if it is always possible to do so. In fact, it is not always possible for the person to find a new situation that provides an adequate replacement for the old one, however much the individual might want to do so, especially in fields where the accumulation of expertise takes place over a lifetime and where the particular combination of knowledge in one person's mind becomes a unique creative or professional instrument.

Wylie's first career peak came in teaching French language and civilization; his second was as an anthropologist of modern French life. His book, *Village in Vaucluse,* describing life in a southern French mountain village named Roussillon, is a seminal work in contemporary sociology and anthropology.

By 1970, Wylie had begun to move into a third area: the study of how body language differs between language groups and how foreign language teaching can be adapted to include nonverbal as well as verbal language. In the mid-1970s, Wylie received a major foundation grant to make an experimental teaching videotape on nonverbal French. His work was generating increasing interest and gave promise of helping students achieve much greater skill and fluency in a foreign language than had been possible before. Wylie had years of research and observation of nonverbal communication behind him; he was, and probably still is, one of the two or three most knowledgeable people in the world on that subject.

One day Wylie's department chairman took him to lunch and informed him summarily that the department was removing Wylie from his endowed chair because he was about to turn seventy and they thought that the chair should go to a younger person. Wylie did not expect this turn of events, because the university quite commonly made exceptions to the retirement rules for certain people. He assumed that extensions were given on the basis of merit, and because he was so successful in his field he assumed that the value of his new line of research would be factored into any system based on merit. He now concludes that these exceptions were more political than he realized—favors granted to particular people who were useful to the administration. In addition, his immersion in his research had kept him from thinking about the university's retirement system, much as many other Long Careers Study participants had told me that "it never occurred to them" to consider retiring at sixty-five because they were busy and enjoying what they were doing. In short, he was caught by surprise.

Wylie then decided to continue his research with outside funding and was told that the university wouldn't approve his grant application because of his age. This was the final blow. Even though he was angry and dismayed by this turn of events, he did what he could: he accepted guest teaching stints at Stanford University and at Hampshire College; he continued writing; he taught a few courses for the extension division. But lack of access to students and to funding made it impossible for him to continue his research at a professional level. Moreover, he found himself treated like a doddering old man because he wouldn't play the docile role the college staff obviously expected from someone his age.

"I was talking about this with one of the assistant deans, the one in charge of finances, at the faculty club one day," Wylie said. "He said, 'You know, you're getting older, and we have to protect you from yourself. You mustn't overdo.' And I had just come back from a two-week canoe trip down the Allegash River, on white water; it rained for nine or ten days. And he tells me I should be careful! It's the kind of thing that makes me furious."

Wylie at seventy was too young and full of energy to retire; he was at the peak of his teaching and research abilities. At eighty, his current age, Wylie said his research would undoubtedly have been completed and he might well have been ready to retire. But that option did not exist for him, and the work he might have done is lost. And although he and his wife, Joan, have a very happy life together in Cambridge, Wylie will always regret not being able to complete his research.

Often the societal response to someone who is forced to retire and cannot either "adjust" or continue his or her work under new circumstances is to blame the victim. We seem to assume that the person didn't try hard enough, or simply didn't want to make it work. This assumption can be both untrue and unfair. A person whose work requires an organizational or institutional setting may be genuinely unable to find another satisfactory home for that work. Sometimes the right working conditions can be duplicated, and sometimes they can't. Simonton's research indicates that scholarship is one of the types of work in which people have the longest and latest productive periods. But scholarship in a field like Wylie's, on the expanding edge of research breakthroughs requiring a particular setting in order to continue, may not be transplantable. It is hoped that in the future more universities will explore ways of providing continued affiliation for faculty members who are still active at older ages. A lifetime of experience in a given field is an asset for the entire society and should be treated with respect.

SAM GOODY

The most poignant retirer was one who voluntarily retired from his business but was never able to find a substitute for the work he loved and gave up. Sam Goody built a record business that was nationally famous and which still bears his name. It was the joy of his life. The walls of his home in Woodmere, Long Island, are lined with photographs of celebrities who visited his store: Ava Gardner, Angela Lansbury, Harry Belafonte, Benny Goodman, Shelley Winters, Mohammed Ali—the list seems endless. Hanging beside them are seven framed apostolic blessings that Goody, a Jew, received from different popes. "He enjoyed his business so much, his business was his vacation," remarked Goody's son, Barry.

"When I reached the age of seventy-five in 1979, I said, enough is enough. I want to retire," Goody remembered. So I sold my business to the American Can people for a very small sum. And two years later I suffered a heart attack."

Goody's contract with American Can prevented him from using his own name to start another business for some years after the sale. He consulted for the company for several years, but after his heart attack he could no longer do so because he needed time to recover. He took up oil painting, became proficient at it, produced several hundred canvases, and gave most of them away. But painting did not replace the store nor satisfy his longing for it.

Goody acknowledged that to a great extent his decision to retire was influenced by social pressure. He heard other people talking about looking forward to retirement, as if, he said, it was a kind of nirvana. "I thought it was like heaven, you know—to be able to do what you want to do, go where you want to go, that kind of stuff. Well, I found out it isn't like they say, [that] on the other side of the street the grass looks greener. It's not so. I'm eighty-six, and I would love to get involved in something which would make me get up at 7:30 or whatever time I'd have to get going; be there; come back." If he had it to do over again, he said, he would not have made the sale. "I would have stayed there until I died."

Goody filled his time with family activities, which he loved—the children and grandchildren who lived nearby were constantly in and out of the house—and with advising friends informally. But he always missed the business and regretted bitterly having walked out of it at the time that he did.

Goody's regrets seemed even sadder after his stores (resold by American Can to Musicland) expanded to a nationwide chain of 250 locations. Ironically, when I was originally trying to locate him, I had called the Musicland general offices in Minneapolis and asked the operator how I could find Sam Goody. "There isn't any Sam Goody," she said. "He's just a fictitious figure. They had to have some kind of name for the chain."

Sam Goody died a year after I interviewed him. Throughout the Long Careers Study, I had heard many anecdotes from the participants about people who had retired in good health and then became ill soon after their retirement. Goody was the only example of this phenomenon that I actually encountered, since almost all of the other study participants were involved in some form of work at the time of the interview, including those who had officially retired.

But other participants made observations about their friends' lives. "I've known guys who retired and then just died," said Hugh Downs. From all accounts, Sam Goody was in good health when he retired; it seems plausible that his frustration at no longer having his beloved stores could have contributed to his developing ill health. In any case, he was unable to replace the satisfactions of his business with another activity that might have provided similar satisfaction and engagement.

Goody's story is also a useful lesson. Goody's was another work environment that simply could not be replaced after retirement; finding alternative projects that provided as much stimulation was difficult or impossible. Gregarious and highly motivated, Goody thrived on the crowds of customers who came to his store, on the contacts with celebrities, on the creativity of his marketing ideas. He was a marketing genius, and his success was highly nourishing to him. When he retired, these pleasures vanished along with the stores. They could not be reconstituted.

SAM CROSS

Making radical career changes has been Sam Cross's trademark. A type-A Explorer, so far he has had five distinct careers, beginning as a metallurgical engineer at Bethlehem Steel, then spending four years as a ballistics officer in the navy. After leaving the navy, he decided to go to the Harvard School of Business, but through a fluke in the timing of the application process he ended up going to law school instead. After law school, he worked first as a patent and trademark attorney and next as a corporate officer in a high-tech manufacturing company, the Perkin-Elmer Corporation. In 1964, he decided to open his own practice in Connecticut; it grew into a large and distinguished firm that was later acquired by the New York firm Kelley Drye and Warren and now serves as its Connecticut office.

In January 1989, at the age of seventy, Cross took of-counsel status in accordance with the firm's policy. Because he has always enjoyed changing careers, Cross was not unhappy to retire from the firm. "I wanted to do something else with my life," he explained. Although he has yet to return to work, Cross is actively looking around for a new career path. "My broad objective is to start a business from scratch," he added. He has taken time to analyze his personal affairs, participate in various organizations, and examine business possibilities in Europe. Meanwhile, he is still active as a lawyer for friends and former clients.

Cross's retirement is not very different from the rest of his career; in fact, he clearly regards it as just another change bringing new opportunities and challenges. Because he is financially secure, he is taking his time in choosing his next pursuit, but there is no doubt that when he finds the right project, he will be off and running on his sixth career.

SUMMARY

The message underlying the varied experiences of the people in this chapter is that finding a successful match after retirement involves several different factors. Because of this, it is essential to think ahead. If you are going to be caught by an organization's retirement rules, thinking about it in advance is a definite advantage, since it allows you to consider alternatives. Although these few examples are not enough to generalize, it seems reasonable that people who are taken by surprise, as Dr. Lawrence Wylie was, fare less well, partly because they have less time to think about and plan a strategy and partly because of the psychological burden of losing their job. Such a situation can be particularly destructive for a person who is still at the height of his or her creativity.

The people who made the transfer most successfully usually took two to three years in the process, thinking about what they would like to do, networking with organizations and people they knew, "putting their name in the hat" when they came across something they found interesting. In general, as Douglas Dillon said, it was better to have several things lined up instead of just one, since that provided more options if one didn't work out.

The majority of the retirers in the study found new roles and new work very successfully. Since the group as a whole consisted of motivated individuals who had always pursued active work lives, it makes sense that their experience of so-called retirement would not conform to the traditional definition of the word. Retirement options can be as varied and as individual as career choices.

It is important to remember that the nature of the Long Careers Study in examining people over sixty-five who have continued working made it unlikely that any of the participants would be happy in an inactive and leisurely retirement. But their experiences with retirement are not as atypical as we might assume; they are not simply workaholics. Like millions of older Americans, they are people who want to remain engaged in the world around them.

12

Reinventing History

WOMEN AND WORK IN THE TWENTIETH CENTURY

In a book that explores career patterns of twentieth-century lives, it is vital to examine the development of women's careers apart from those of men. The careers of the women in the Long Careers Study were often shaped by the fact that they were women. Society's expectations of their role in the work force have shifted many times throughout the century, and as a result, women have been pushed and pulled in several different directions. Each woman in our study dealt with those shifts differently, according to her personality, interests, and circumstances. All contributed in one way or another to the development of the women's movement, whether they did so intentionally or not. Their careers have opened up new opportunities for women across the country. They have shown that a combination of flexibility and determination is important in a successful career and that many barriers, even formidable ones, can be overcome with persistence.

Until very recently, the twentieth-century women's movement and the drive for equal opportunities for women had been presented as if they had begun in the early 1960s. Certainly Betty Friedan's 1963 book, *The Feminine Mystique,* unleashed a cascade of social upheaval, which has yet to settle into a stable, identifiable social pattern. But the life histories of the women in the study clearly indicate that the struggle for equal rights for women has had a much longer history.

This movement actually began in the nineteenth century. It has been a fight shaped by periods of great advances and strong leadership as well as by defeats and episodes of "backlash."[1] The two world wars had a major impact on the role of women in the workforce, as women were recruited for the jobs left behind by men who had gone to war.

The Long Careers Study women are divided into three groups on the basis of age. The oldest group, born at the end of the nineteenth century or the beginning of the twentieth, includes the daughters or granddaughters of suffragists, who remembered a time of ferment, agitation, and victory on behalf of women's rights. They grew up assuming that women were entitled to equality with men, and these assumptions were reflected in their careers. The middle group, women who had come into adulthood before the outbreak of World War II, were less political and more practical in their involvement with the women's rights movement. They were recruited to fill factory jobs vacated by men, and they flooded the work force during the war—only to be sent packing when the men came home.

The youngest group, the mothers of the baby boom generation, were still in high school and college at the end of World War II. After years of being admonished to finish their educations so they could be of service to their country, they found upon graduation that society's expectations for them had suddenly made a 180-degree turn. They were now expected to be the quintessential happy homemakers and to manufacture babies, just as during the war they had manufactured weapons. They embraced this goal wholeheartedly at first; then over time they became deeply disillusioned by the narrowness of the role they had been thrust into.

The most recent phase of the women's movement, which began in the early 1960s, affected all three groups of women to some degree. It particularly influenced the youngest, many of whom were profoundly ready for a change from their constricting domestic life-styles.

DAUGHTERS OF THE SUFFRAGISTS: THE FIRST GENERATION

The oldest women in the study—those who were 85 to 102 at the time of their interviews—were born between 1890 and 1905. They were children around the turn of the century and into the 1910s, and their mothers, aunts, cousins, and grandmothers had been suffragists. They were born into a nation that did not regard them as citizens, because they were female. As young women, they witnessed the success of the women's campaign for the right to vote. The passage of the Nineteenth Amendment seemed to validate their aspirations to equality: it said to them that women had finally come into their own, that they had been recognized as the political equals of men, and that therefore the questions of equality were settled.

What was most surprising about this oldest generation of women was their confidence in making choices and in standing up against discrimination. Their sense of entitlement made them impervious to guilt for "stepping out of line." On the contrary, they delighted in retelling stories of how they got jobs for women, overcame inequities, steered their careers around attacks of prejudice, and, in general, how they, their mothers, sisters, aunts, cousins, grandmothers, and friends triumphed.

In terms of their careers, most of these participants felt that women should be given exactly the same rights and prerogatives as men. For example, in the 1920s and 1930s several of them filed complaints that their job contracts were shorter or more temporary than those of male colleagues; they asked for salaries equivalent to those of the men who had held their jobs before them; they crusaded for what they thought was right even if their husbands happened to be less than enthusiastic about their views. One participant told me about a women's network that channeled names of women into the appointment process for high-level government positions during the Roosevelt administration, and saw to it that a percentage of all the appointments made went to women.

This group also suffered defeats. Women who took men's jobs during World War I were forced to leave them at the end of the war—not in the same numbers as would later work during World War II, but the retreat was discouraging nevertheless. Many of these women entered a network of women's institutions in which they could work freely without encountering prejudice: foremost among these was the YWCA (Young Women's Christian Association) with settlement houses a close second.

With the onset of the depression, women's jobs were often sacrificed first to give men preference. But throughout these experiences, these women seemed to have maintained an unquestioning commitment to the equal position of women. Some in fact were pushed into their careers by the Depression, but once they began working they never left.

Perhaps most remarkable from the perspective of a contemporary woman is that not one person in this oldest group believed that being a wife, mother, and housewife was enough to fill a normal adult woman's life. All of them simply took it as a given that, while raising a family was important and part of a woman's life, it certainly didn't use up all her time and energy, and it didn't take the place of some kind of outside activity or work.

This attitude cut across social, economic, racial, and geographic lines. Mother Clara Hale, who grew up in a poor black neighborhood in Philadelphia, and Judge Lucy Somerville Howorth, who grew up in a middle-class household in a tiny rural Mississippi town, were as liberated as Elisabeth Luce Moore, who grew up in China the daughter of missionary parents, and painter Theresa Bernstein Meyerowitz, who moved from Philadelphia to New York City to study art.

Judge Lucy Somerville Howorth

Judge Lucy Somerville Howorth, a type-B Explorer, was ninety-three when I interviewed her in her home in Cleveland, Mississippi. Born July 1, 1895, in Greenville, Mississippi, she was the youngest of four children. Her father was a civil engineer; her mother worked for women's suffrage and later became the first woman member of the Mississippi state legislature.

Howorth attended Randolph Macon College, and, in 1918, when she had completed her B.A. in political science and enough work for an M.A., her mother decided she should take a year off "to be a lady." She was sent to New York, where she attended classes at Columbia University taught by the famous sociologist, Talcott Parsons.

World War I was still in progress; Howorth, like many women, was eager to take part in the war effort and to show her value as a worker. She found work in a metal machining factory in New York as a machine screw gauge inspector, a job vacated by a man who had gone to Europe to fight. She enjoyed the work and quit only because her mother decided she should have a more professional job. Mrs. Somerville used her connections with other suffragist women to get Lucy a position at the YWCA. Meanwhile, the war ended, and Howorth saw the famous Armistice Day parade in November of 1918.

Howorth recalled vividly the passage of the Nineteenth Amendment, which gave women the right to vote. It was finally approved in 1920 (it had to be ratified state by state), and Howorth cast her first vote in New York. She thus voted before her Mississippi friends were able to, since Mississippi had not yet ratified the amendment. Howorth was jubilant that women were able at last to exercise this precious right of citizenship.

She attended law school in Mississippi, where she was one of two women in her class. Her sister's husband offered to take her into his own law practice and served as her mentor, taking her to court, allowing her to question witnesses, and otherwise teaching her the ropes. Howorth had to learn to sublimate aspects of her personality to avoid censure from the men with whom she worked. She told how she wore a bright print suit to court one day and got snide remarks from her colleagues at the bar. "I never made that mistake again," she said firmly. "After that I always wore something plain, like navy-blue serge."

In 1927, partly as a result of her work with the Red Cross in helping Mississippi recover from the great flood, Howorth was made the first woman federal judge in the Mississippi district. In 1928, she married a law school classmate, Joseph Howorth. She had delayed their marriage until she was established professionally, reasoning that otherwise she would not have any credibility as a professional. The couple moved to Jackson, Mississippi, and set up practice together.

In 1934, Howorth was offered a six-month appointment by President Roosevelt's office to the National Board of Veterans' Appeals. The Howorths moved to Washington so she could accept, and Joseph Howorth set up a practice there.

Howorth was one of three women appointed to the board. The other two were not lawyers, so she organized the three of them and began educating the other two about the legal aspects of their duties. Then a man was appointed, a Mr. P. D. Gold, from North Carolina. One day Gold happened to be bragging about his appointment and pulled out his letter of appointment to flaunt it. Howorth saw that Gold's letter had no mention of the six-month limitation that the women had been given. She asked if she could copy his letter and did so on a manual typewriter, sending the copy to the chairman of the appeals board, telling him that they were happy to welcome Mr. Gold but that they were unhappy to note the discrepancies in their letters regarding the time limitations. Howorth suggested that a new letter be written to the three women members, without any time limitation. To the women's surprise, the chairman wrote back saying that the discrepancy had not been called to his attention before. The three women received new letters of appointment with no time limitation, as they had requested.

Howorth was amazed to find that there were a lot of women in high-level civil service positions during the Roosevelt administration. She discovered that this had come about because Roosevelt, running scared at the beginning of his campaign, had decided to go after this large new group of voters and had organized a Women for Roosevelt group. It was extremely successful, and because of this its chairperson, Mary W. Dusen, was appointed cochair of the Democratic National Committee after Roosevelt's election. The Democratic National Committee cochairs had to approve all political appointments, which meant that Dusen had a great deal of leverage. She saw to it that a reasonable number of women were always included among potential appointees; and, said Howorth, when Dusen was given trouble about an appointment, she would call up Eleanor Roosevelt, and the appointment would go through.

Howorth and her husband stayed in Washington until they were sixty, and then decided to move back to Mississippi. They set up a law practice in Cleveland and continued it until his death in 1975; since then, Judge Howorth has carried it on alone.

Theresa Bernstein Meyerowitz

A gifted painter who began selling her work by 1914 and continues to sell today, Theresa Bernstein Meyerowitz has had a career lasting almost eighty years. Like the lives of Dr. Michael Heidelberger and Edward Bernays, her life has encompassed all the drastic changes of the twentieth century.

As a young artist in Manhattan in the early 1920s, she had a small studio above a horse stable on Fifty-fifth Street (today a crowded, busy midtown street). "When I grew up in Philadelphia, the form of transportation was the horse and buggy," Meyerowitz recalled in a newspaper interview. "Everything was done by cranking in those days. Even if you took a cup of coffee, you had to crank the beans. If you wanted to hear great music, you had to turn the handle."

Born in 1890, she began to paint seriously in high school and won a scholarship to art school. Attending both schools became too difficult, so Meyerowitz left high school to study art full-time for four years. She insists that she didn't know she was going to be an artist. "I had no idea about it. I just worked."

One of her most powerful traits has been her determination to succeed in spite of the many obstacles placed in her way. For example, for an art school scholarship competition, Meyerowitz painted a canvas of Adam and Eve being expelled from the Garden of Eden by the angel of the Lord. Three days before the judging, someone stole her painting. She was desperate, offering a reward for its return even though she had no money. Finally she realized that someone had taken the painting so that she wouldn't win the scholarship. In a fury, she locked herself in a studio and painted another painting from memory of the original. This second painting won the scholarship.

She graduated from art school in 1911 and studied at the Pennsylvania Academy of Fine Arts before moving to New York, where, despite her eagerness to do her own work without further instruction, she enrolled in the Art Students League. "I was very determined to express myself and I only needed [the league] because I wanted to work from models, and I didn't have any money to pay a model."

Meyerowitz's paintings of street life in New York are full of her own vivacity and energy, with brash colors and bold strokes. In spirit and technique, her work exemplifies the famous Ashcan school of realism, but this style was seen as masculine because of its boldness and strength and because its founder would not allow women to belong to the school. Thus, Meyerowitz has often been ignored by critics and historians.

Throughout her career, Meyerowitz suffered from the discrimination of galleries, museums, and critics who were not predisposed to appreciate women artists. When she began showing her pieces at the National Academy in 1913, she signed her work just "Bernstein" because "a woman had no chance whatsoever. They threw them out like cupcakes. No matter how good you were, you couldn't get a picture on the wall." Reviews of her work contained comments like, "This man has a very interesting viewpoint." She was able to maintain her anonymity for only two years before word finally leaked out. "After that," she says, "it was much harder!" Often her work was accepted but not hung, with no explanation.

During this time, she met her husband, William Meyerowitz, a painter from the Ukraine who was helping to provide art education for children in settlement houses. In 1919, they were married, and she had her first one-woman show in New York. The money she made from painting portraits supported them as well as her husband's many siblings from the Ukraine, even through the Depression. To date, she has painted more than one hundred portraits on commission.

Meyerowitz also was involved with the suffragist movement in New York, and she painted several canvases of women marching for voting rights, the only painter to have captured this historic movement. And she became an integral part of the New York art scene, with friends such as Edward Hopper, Georgia O'Keefe, and Alfred Stieglitz.

Although she received some critical acclaim in her early career, Meyerowitz had difficulty sustaining her popularity, as stylistic tastes shifted toward abstract expressionism and discounted the contributions of American realist painters like herself. Meyerowitz increasingly turned to promoting her husband's career, often at the expense of her own, and became known as part of an artistic couple, a situation that undermined the impact of her own work. Nevertheless, she is now receiving the praise she deserves: in the last five years, major retrospectives of her work have been shown at museums around the country, and art historians and critics are acknowledging her place among the most accomplished painters of the century. Thanks to her longevity, Meyerowitz luckily is around to receive that long-denied applause.

About ten years ago, Meyerowitz began work on her husband's biography after his death in 1981. She sent four chapters to an editor she had met at a party. He told her that she wrote with enthusiasm and that her style was gripping, but, he added, "I don't think at your age you will ever write a book." Taking that statement as yet another challenge, Meyerowitz went on to write not one but six books, including two books of poetry and a children's book (in order to entertain young children who sat for her, she made up elaborate stories, which evolved into a collection called *Rabbitville*).

Through all the changes in her life and world, Meyerowitz has retained a commitment to her art that brought her successfully through many obstacles. "In my life span, all my negatives were roads to my achievements because I never let them stop me," she explained. "That's the whole secret of my being alive."

JOAN ERIKSON

A dancer, artist, jewelry designer, and therapist, Joan Erikson has had an enormously varied career, fitting it around her role as a wife and mother, raising four children, encouraging and helping her husband in his career, and still managing to create an identity of her own. It was, she emphasizes, a process that took place over time—often difficult, often bumpy. But the result is a work of art in itself.

Erikson is one of the subjects of Mary Catherine Bateson's book, *Composing a Life*. Her work life experience as a type-A Explorer is a model for both women and men in the uncertain society of the 1990s. American careers have increasingly become a crazy quilt of different jobs, instead of one smooth, connected climb within the same company. Joan Erikson's experience is a priceless guide on how to manage and adapt to change.

Born in 1903 in a tiny community in Canada where her father was the local Episcopal minister, Erikson had what she called a "chaotic and disorganized" childhood. Her mother left her and her siblings in the care of their grandmother, later returning to take them on a four-year tour of Europe. Soon after, her father died of cancer, and Erikson was sent to boarding school. Her difficult childhood fueled her desire to have a strong and healthy family of her own one day.

After two years of college without a clear career objective, Erikson, who loved studying dance, decided instead to become a teacher and enrolled in Columbia Teacher's College. A wonderful dance teacher who was tall (like Erikson) convinced her to consider dance again. "She was as big as me and she danced beautifully and I thought, 'To hell with it. I'm going to be a dancer.' Erikson recounted. "So that's what I became. Suddenly I knew who I was, and what I was doing, and why I was doing it. It was grand. Of course, that brings success! You can't help it if you're that enthusiastic."

In 1928 she went to Europe to work on her dissertation in modern dance for a year and ended up staying for two, to marry a young psychologist she met there named Erik Erikson. The

Eriksons returned to the United States and spent time at several universities—from Philadelphia to Cambridge to Yale, finally settling at Berkeley, where Joan became deeply involved with the schools. After World War II, when the McCarthy period began, Erik Erikson was so profoundly offended by the university's practice of requiring loyalty oaths, and its strikingly preferential treatment of senior professors versus younger faculty members, that ultimately he resigned. Buoyed by the favorable reception of *Childhood and Society,* which had just been published, the Eriksons returned to the East Coast, where Erikson accepted a position at Austen Riggs Hospital in Stockbridge, Massachusetts. In Stockbridge, Joan Erikson finally came into her own.

When I had been in Stockbridge for no more than five or six months, I began to be very unhappy about what they were doing about the patients. They were doing the most up-to-date kind of psychiatry; but what they did when they weren't in psychiatry was just stupid. Here were these young people, kids out of college, and they just jumbled along, not getting up in the morning and having nothing to do. They had one room that was devoted to reading. Then they had very organized things that they taught them to do in woodwork, and that was it. It was take it or leave it.

Erikson went to the head of the program and got permission to see what she could do to organize things differently. First she mobilized the young patients to set up a kitchen for themselves, so they could make their own tea in the afternoons. She developed a studio, a drama group, and classes in leather work, pottery, and fiber work; young artists were brought in from the community to give the woodwork classes a different flavor. The drama group held performances and invited the townspeople, beginning the process of improving relationships between the patients and the local residents. Finally, they created a nursery school. For five years, Erikson generated programs and health-giving relationships among the patients and staff at Austen Riggs.

When her husband took a sabbatical to write *Young Man Luther,* Erikson gave up her position so she could take the year off with him. For many years she had edited her husband's work—his English was still craggy enough that he needed editorial help setting things down and in polishing his written work. They went first to California and then to Mexico, where the book was finished.

Meanwhile, Erikson had become interested in beads and, through them, in jewelry making. It was an interest that was to continue for many years; eventually she acquired a high degree of skill and won prizes for her work.

On returning to Stockbridge, she set to work to organize a halfway house for Riggs patients, so that they could "stretch out into the community when they got past Riggs." By that time, she had also begun a book, which was published several years later, launching her career as a writer.

A tall, graceful woman who at eighty-nine is still strikingly beautiful, Erikson was a childhood rebel. "I got educated in dance, an area where what I was doing was not in competition with men," she said. "I haven't fought the patterns particularly, because the things that I did were outside the pattern. It didn't run me up straight against the judges."

Erikson also found an outlet for her defiance by playing an apparently traditional role that was actually a genuine act of rebellion: helping her husband in his career. Erik Erikson had psychological insights that challenged traditional Freudian psychotherapy and met with resistance among traditional-minded psychoanalysts of the time. By working with her husband as an invisible partner—as many wives of gifted husbands did until very recently—she helped reshape and greatly expand psychological theory and practice.

OTHER EXAMPLES IN THE FIRST GENERATION

The outspoken desire for equality and the vigorous networking of the first generation that Howorth describes were present in the accounts of other participants. Esther Peterson, some ten years younger than Howorth, was determined to work despite her Mormon childhood and married a man who encouraged that desire. Another study participant, Nell Eurich, described how, early in her career, she discovered that she was being paid less for one job than the previous incumbent, who was male, and straightforwardly requested an equivalent salary, which she got.

Even the mothers of some of the male participants were unusually liberated, by today's standards. William Greenough recalled that his mother was a "tremendous influence" and adds:

Mother was what we would now call a women's libber. She had finished college at a time when not that many young women were attending college.

She was in the initial Phi Beta Kappa group at Indiana University. Immediately after graduation she helped to establish the Women's Franchise League in Indiana, to secure voting rights for women.

After women got the right to vote, she was asked to be the first president of the new League of Women Voters, and was for many, many years. Mother wrote the first voter magazine describing the candidates.

[My father] was active in the legislature on behalf of banking legislation. I remember him occasionally saying to my mother: "Kate, you know that I support everything you're doing and I'm glad you're interested in good government instead of the spoils system, and all of the other things you're doing. Could you hold off this month, while I'm trying to get some banking legislation through?"

Dr. Rose Dobrof, a social worker and founder of the Brookdale Center on Aging, reminisced about her mother, Lydia, who "was one of the first three women in Colorado who had a Ph.D., having earned it in 1914, in history, at the University of Denver. Daddy was an immigrant and married this lady who was a college professor and had all this education. He was very proud of her."

There is an unexpectedly moving quality to these accounts. In the most recent phase of the women's movement, we have come to associate ambivalence and deep guilt with questions related to women's participation in work outside the home, and with women's desire for status and respect equal to those accorded men. The accounts of these women—who are so much older than women now in their thirties and forties, yet so totally guilt-free, so much more certain of their value as workers and as human beings—suggest that *the sense of guilt is itself a product of prejudice:* a conflict created by the society to slow down or stop the drive for change. These oldest participants raise the possibility that there are solutions that we have not yet rediscovered, which would offer equal citizenship to everyone, male or female, without condemnation.

WOMEN OF WORLD WAR II: THE SECOND GENERATION

The next oldest group of women, who ranged in age from seventy-five to eighty-five, were born between 1906 and 1916 and were children during the 1910s and 1920s, the era of World War I and the Roaring Twenties. In the Depression-ridden 1930s they were young women. They resembled the older women in many respects, and they had a highly pragmatic approach to their mar-

riages and their work. Many of them retained some kind of outside work while raising a family, aware that marriage and a family were not enough to keep them fully occupied. But there were
also some who chose not to have careers outside the home, either
because they wanted to stay home or because they wanted to
please their husbands.

In general, feminists of this generation were lonelier in their
egalitarianism than were the first-generation women. They witnessed a rising resentment of women's freedom at the end of the
depression and biting attacks from "Mom-ism," depicting women
as greedy, self-indulgent tyrants who dominated their husbands
and emasculated their sons. And they saw most of the gains won
during the first forty-five years of the century wiped out after
World War II. The prejudice that had been at times concealed by
other more urgent issues surged back in full force almost as soon
as the war was over.

Two women in this age group never married because their
fiancés were killed in the war. Explorer Margaret Fox experienced
two such losses: her first sweetheart was killed early in the war,
and she then met and fell in love with another young soldier, who
was also killed. She simply did not have the emotional energy to
try again. And then, there were fewer available at the war's end,
since so many young men had been killed.

ELINOR GUGGENHEIMER

Elinor Guggenheimer describes her career choices in the manner
of a true type-A Explorer: "I think I am one of those people who
wherever she saw an open door rambled through." Guggenheimer
has been involved in an impressive variety of fields: theater, television, film, city government, women's rights, philanthropy, writing, publishing, consumer affairs, child care, senior citizens rights.
In all of these areas, her career has always been motivated by a
deep concern for social issues.

Guggenheimer, born in 1912, was the daughter of a commercial banker. Her father died when she was twelve, and her mother
and grandmother were key figures in her childhood. She attended
the Horace Mann School in New York City, which, she remarked
with satisfaction, taught girls that they could *do* things. "They
didn't just bring us up to be little ladies." However, none of the
rather well-to-do girls she grew up with were expected to have a
paying job. Even in Guggenheimer's long, varied, and extremely

active career, 50 percent of her work has been on a volunteer basis.

During Guggenheimer's junior year in college, she married Randall Guggenheimer, and several years later she and her husband began their family. At about the same time, she became involved in volunteer work and philanthropy and began her life-long involvement with child care.

During the 1930s Guggenheimer started making documentary films. During World War II, she volunteered for civilian defense and became involved in the development and distribution of films made to train civilians to fill jobs vacated by men who had gone to war. She also worked on a film that focused on what happened to children when thousands of women were recruited into the work force.

Immediately after the war, government funding for child care was withdrawn because of the assumption that women would now stop working and go back to homemaking. Guggenheimer was incensed. She wrote articles, testified before committees, organized marches with other activists, and became founder of two organizations—one local and one national—to support day care. In 1992, federal funding for day care still has not been restored.

In 1960, Guggenheimer was asked to fill a vacancy on the New York City Planning Commission. She noted in her statement to the press: "I think city planning in some ways is an extension of homemaking. It's housekeeping on a larger scale." The statement created a miniature scandal. Her male colleagues on the council were offended and dismayed; they saw city planning as a complicated engineering process. The contrast between the male and female perspectives was striking:

I remember the first meeting I had with my colleagues on the planning commission and this weird little scene in which we were discussing the location of a housing project. The commercial area was going to be at the bottom of a hill and I said, "Oh, dear, all those women are going to have to carry their groceries uphill!" It was such a strange concept to those men that the meeting stopped dead. I remember all of them looking at me. I thought: None of these men who are planning these neighborhoods have ever lived in them.

After working in government, television, and civic affairs for several years, Guggenheimer returned to child care, founding and serving as executive director of the Child Care Action Program. "Every time I get irritated about something," Guggenheimer told me, "I end up founding an organization. That's how I founded the New York Day Care Council, the National Day Care Council, the New York Association of Senior Centers, the New York Women's Forum, and the National Women's Forum. Now I'm trying to pull all the women's organizations in New York City together into one interracial and intercultural council called the New York Alliance of Women's Associations."

Volunteer work was for many years considered a "proper" activity for women, one that supplemented a woman's role as wife and mother without conflicting with the husband's status as breadwinner. One of the interesting aspects of Elinor Guggenheimer's career is that she used this proper role to fight for rights and services that supported the cause of equality: women's right to work in paying jobs, their need for child care while working, and the inclusion of women's perspective in areas previously dominated by men, like urban planning.

Another original element is that she has combined her role as a crusader with a traditionally feminine love of entertaining. Guggenheimer and her husband are famous for their grace and ingenuity as hosts; Guggenheimer has even written several books on how to give successful dinner parties. As part of my interviewing process with her, she included me in one of their evenings; it was superbly planned and at the same time wonderful, spontaneous fun. Her life is convincing proof that no role is inherently either masculine or feminine, and anything can work if it is what you really want to do.

Louise Brown

Louise Brown (a pseudonym), an eighty-year-old secretary in a prestigious New York City organization and a type-A Explorer, made time to talk to me at the end of a workday because her boss was a friend of mine. She agreed reluctantly to let me interview her—on the condition of strict anonymity. When she was in her fifties, she unexpectedly lost one job because her employer died of a heart attack; she went out to find another job, going to employment agency after employment agency, and was turned down repeatedly because of her age.

Brown is a fighter. She decided that if age was a handicap, she would overcome it. She dyed her graying hair, bought some new office clothes at Bloomingdale's, removed all references to age from her résumé, and went back to the same agencies she had originally gone to. She was hired immediately. The experience made its impression. Although Brown is extremely happy in the office where she works now, and is highly valued by her employer (who knows her age and brags about it), Brown does not want any unnecessary publicity. "I work because I enjoy it," she says, "but also because I need the money. I can't afford to put myself in a position where if I had to find another job, I'd be thought of as too old."

Born in 1912, Brown left high school in her senior year and devoted herself to intensive training in singing, dancing, and dramatics to prepare for a professional career which was halted because of an injury incurred doing back flips. When the war broke out, she joined the Red Cross blood donor service for one year before enlisting in the WACs. She was impressed by the rigors of training for her role. She learned such skills as judo and how to combat gas attacks. She served overseas in Italy, and she still stays in touch with many of the women with whom she served, who were and still are a surrogate family.

After the war, she decided to teach voice instead of pursuing her own singing career. She attended the Juilliard School of Music under the G.I. Bill and after her graduation in 1950 taught singing until 1968. Since then she has worked full time as a secretary for a number of prominent organizations.

Brown never married nor had children yet feels very lucky that things turned out the way they did. "It's a lucky man that didn't get me because I had always planned to have a dozen children, not all my own," she said. "I planned to adopt some." Despite this ambition of hers as a young woman, she appreciates her independence and feels no loss that her life took a different course.

Brown works regularly and is outraged by the idea that she should retire. She has always worked and enjoyed it. She likes the feeling of making extra money. She sees no reason that because "one day you're sixty-four and the next you're sixty-five, you suddenly aren't able." She thinks this is also a good lesson in how to treat children, saying, "You shouldn't push a child either just because he's a certain age."

FRANCES ETTER

Memphian Frances Etter has filled many roles during her eighty years. In addition to raising children, caring for and spending time with her husband, keeping a well-loved home, and doing volunteer work for charitable organizations, she has also had three very distinct careers: in journalism, fashion, and real estate.

The spacing and timing of these careers were influenced by the demands of her life as a wife and mother and by the ethic that was widely held in her community that women did not work while their children were young and needed their care. In addition, Etter and her husband both felt that her husband's active professional life required her participation as a housewife. She obligingly tabled her work ambitions, apparently without any sense of frustration or resentment. Once her obligations had been fulfilled, she went back to work, ultimately with her husband's approval, and has had an immensely successful career.

Born in 1911 in rural Tennessee and raised in Nashville, Frances Etter attended Southwestern College in Memphis. While in school she wrote articles for a local newspaper, the *Memphis Press-Scimitar,* and after graduation she landed a job in the society department of its rival, the *Memphis Commercial Appeal.* In 1934, she became the *Commercial*'s society editor.

When Etter married Dr. Charles Barton Etter in 1934, she quit her job in journalism at his request. He did not want her to work, but she also felt strongly, as she says many women did at that time, that for her to have a career would "reflect upon my husband's professional ability." She added, "I didn't think it was proper for a woman to work if her husband was working." She settled down to life as a housewife and mother of three children.

During World War II, her husband spent two and a half years overseas. Largely out of financial need, Etter and a friend developed a business: they created and manufactured a changeable sweater collar, called "Tucker by Fran and Lou." The tuckers—so named because they tucked into the round neck of a pullover sweater to give it a dressier look—were wildly successful with young girls. They became a national fad and spread to older girls as well; as late as the early 1960s they were still a kind of uniform for high school and college students. But, like many women who held jobs during the war, Etter simply walked away from the Tucker business when her husband returned home in 1946, giving her share to her partner.

Etter's talent for business surfaced again in 1951 when she joined forces with a friend to start a real estate business, Coleman-Etter Realtors. By this point, her children were grown and her husband's career was well established. She had been in the real estate business for a couple of years when she said to her husband, "Barton, you made me get out of the Tucker business, and that's the best business I could ever have. Why don't you make me get out of real estate?" And he said, "Frannie, I'll tell you why. Because I'm afraid of what you might do next!"

Dr. Etter was undoubtedly right; if she had not stayed in real estate, Etter would probably have ended up running for Congress. As it is, she has been in real estate now for over forty years and is a charter life member of the Million Dollar Sales Club. "I love real estate," she said. " It's the most wonderful people business I can think of. There is nothing in the world more important than helping a family find the right home; it makes everything in life so much easier. You've got to give it your full time and interest."

Etter still works as a saleswoman, but she has turned over all the major responsibilities for administration to her other partners. Her feelings about retirement are answered with an emphatic, "And do what?! Go into recluse boredom?" In addition to sales, she maintains a busy schedule of church activities and fund-raising for her alma mater, Southwestern.

Etter's role as a housewife and mother took precedence over her career pursuits. What is remarkable about Frances Etter, however, is that in addition to this very traditional role—and despite it—she has had an extremely successful career anyway. She was able to apply her natural business talents first when the need arose and again after her family commitments had diminished.

Other Examples:

Like Etter, writer "Lucy" Scott discovered that being a housewife greatly influenced her pursuit of other careers. She candidly admits that the periods of her life when she was single have been the most enjoyable: "I think the process of being a housewife and a mother is interesting over the long pull. It was a job to me and I wasn't a frustrated housewife. I used to think every little while that there must be more out there than I am getting, but it wasn't a serious objection. I don't think most of my contemporaries did either.

"The happiest time of my life was the two years that I was

divorced and since I have been a widow. Now that sounds like a terrible thing to say because I had what, I think, was a very good marriage. Certainly when my husband died the loneliness was brutal at first, but there is a great deal to be said for being a single woman."

MOTHERS OF THE BABY BOOM: THE THIRD GENERATION

Members of the youngest group of women in the Long Careers Study were born between 1917 and 1927, making them sixty-five to seventy-five at the time of their interviews. They were children during the Roaring Twenties and the Great Depression. The oldest members of this group who went to college finished school just as World War II was beginning; the youngest were in college or high school during the war. Some of them married during the war; many of them did not get married until after the war, either because they were too young or because the men they might have wed were in the armed services. And a few never married.

What these women had in common was their assumption during the war that they, too, had to pitch in to do whatever was necessary to help in the war effort. They also shared the sudden reversal of their role and their world after the war, when society's message to them changed to, "Go back home and have babies."

Joan Erikson recalled that "there was new emphasis after the war on children and their development. Spock's book [1946] would have been the beginning of it. In the late forties, I think there was a lot of talk about mothers, 'Mom' being so overriding, and pushing particularly their sons around. Then in the fifties, there was a conference on the healthy child, the White House Conference on Children. That is when I date the change in attitude about women staying at home."

"At that point everybody was saying, 'What makes for a healthy child?'" Erikson continued. "At the conference it was decided that a healthy child has a happy home, a doting mother. It didn't leave the fathers out, but the emphasis was certainly on the women. I associate it with that period."

While some of these women were lucky in having good female role models and families who supported careers for women, others had a harder time in getting an education and making a career for themselves.

JULIA WALSH

Stockbroker Julia Walsh has had a Homesteader career that was shaped by external influences as well as her own interest in her work, including her father's prejudice and later her role as a wife and mother. Walsh, who became famous after building her own successful brokerage firm in Washington, D.C., recounted how she won a scholarship to Smith College. "They offered me quite a lot," she remembered, "but my father, who thought education for women was a complete waste of money, beyond high school, wouldn't even lend me the money to [travel] from Ohio to North Hampton, [Massachusetts]." It didn't occur to her until years later that she could have written the college to ask for transportation money. Walsh ended up going to nearby Kent State University.

Walsh was very straightforward about this disappointment of not being able to attend Smith, but she felt equally strongly that Kent State was a good university for her and that she gained a great deal from going there. "Because all the men were away," she continued, "I ended up being president of the student body. I got more opportunities than I would have otherwise. I was always looking for opportunities to move ahead."

Walsh began her career as a stockbroker in the 1950s to make a little extra money as the young wife of a career army officer, with two young children. She had just made her first thousand dollars when her husband was transferred to Kansas, and she went with him. Two years later, in 1957, her husband was killed in a tank explosion during battle exercises and she became a single parent overnight. To support her family, she moved back to Washington and returned to the same brokerage firm, Ferris and Company, where she discovered that she had a real gift for investment. She stayed at the firm for over twenty years, serving as senior vice president and then vice chairman. In 1977 Walsh decided to leave Ferris and open her own firm, Julia Walsh and Sons, in Washington, D.C. The event made newspapers all over the country.

There were no women in the investment business when Walsh started out. She was candid about the biases she has faced in her career because she is female. But despite the gender handicap, Walsh generally did well. However, twice she suffered major losses, partly because her conditioning as a woman made her a vulnerable target. In the first case, the senior partner at her first firm decided to change the partnership structure. The change meant that her taxes for that year doubled, and she was almost wiped out. In the second case, when she left Ferris and Company, she was told that although she had been there twenty-two years, it was not long enough for her to become properly vested in the pension fund. As a result, she left without a pension. Subsequently, she regretted not having protested more vigorously.

"I wasn't as sophisticated as I might have been, as a man," she explained. "Both times I should have fought harder. I should have had them make an adjustment on my taxes the first time; I certainly should have sued them for the [pension] money—I was a major holder. Life's been very good to me, but I figure [those incidents cost me] about a quarter of a million dollars out of my pocket." If her experience at Julia Walsh and Sons hadn't been so good, Walsh says, she might have been bitter. As it is, she is at a point in life where she recognizes very clearly that the money, particularly the pension, would have been important, and wishes she had known how to do things differently.

Walsh's career is interesting because it was generated largely by negative external circumstances: her father's choice of school for her and her husband's early death. Her innate talent for finance was called into use in response to her family's financial needs, and because she was widowed and trying to raise her children, her being a woman was tolerated more than it would have been had she been single. Even so, it did not protect her from being subtly disadvantaged at times by male partners who guessed that she would not know fully how to protect herself.

As she began to use her skills she found that she enjoyed the work a great deal and that she had a unique talent for it. Walsh was perhaps the first woman to become nationally known in the field of finance and to start her own firm, major accomplishments in a field that even in the early 1990s is largely dominated by men. If her husband had not died so young, it is possible that Walsh might never have returned to her career as a stockbroker, heeding the expectations of the day to stay home with her family.

Evelyn Cunningham

Evelyn Cunningham, founder of the New York Coalition of One Hundred Black Women, changed her distinguished journalism career at midlife to work in public service and government for the rights of women. Although she experienced both racial and gender discrimination, Cunningham was determined and committed to pursuing her interests and convictions. And though she has been married several times, she feels she was fortunate in always having husbands who encouraged and supported her professional life.

When asked about her marital life, Cunningham informed me that she was currently married to her fourth husband. She explained her husbands' lack of negative influence on her career choices as a racial phenomenon: until fairly recently, "it was much easier for a black woman than a black man to find a good, high-paying job," she said. "So black men welcomed a woman who had a good job, and they weren't threatened by that." Black women, she further explained, were less threatening to society than were black men, and they advanced more quickly in what she considers nonthreatening fields like education, social work, and nursing. Cunningham said that, in her mother's day, it wasn't uncommon for a black train station porter to be married to a black woman who was a high school principal.

Born in Elizabeth City, North Carolina, in 1918, Cunningham moved with her family to New York City when she was only four years old. Cunningham feels that the move was prompted by a response she gave to that age-old question, "What do you want to do when you grow up?" Cunningham recalls, "I said I wanted to pick cotton, and I shook them up quite a bit." Her parents, who encouraged Cunningham in creative areas and fostered a very supportive family environment, certainly did not want their daughter picking cotton.

Cunningham soon adjusted to life in New York City, attending Hunter High School and later Long Island University. While at college a guidance counselor discouraged her from pursuing a career in journalism; she had wanted to become a writer once her interest in cotton-picking waned. Cunningham explains: "I really wanted newspaper writing. [But] he said that if you're colored you'll never get a job. And the papers don't take women." Although Cunningham didn't get to study journalism at the university, she feels that her background in sociology was just as valuable and that impression was borne out of experience; years later when she enrolled in Columbia University's School of Journalism, she attended only two semesters because, she said, "I knew it all."

After graduating, Cunningham got her first job as a reporter in the New York bureau of the *Pittsburgh Courier* in 1940. She soon became editor of the New York and Philadelphia editions of the *Courier*, and within the next ten years she became city editor for the New York edition; in doing so, she became the nation's first woman city editor, black or white. She remained in that position until 1962.

In the early 1960s Cunningham became increasingly aware of the violent civil rights battles being waged in the Southern states. Eager to report on the changes taking place, she convinced the paper to let her go; they agreed. While covering a story in Montgomery, Alabama, she found herself involved with Martin Luther King and the city's legendary bus boycott. She was the first journalist to publish an in-depth article about Dr. King, and her decision to travel with him through the South saw her attacked by dogs and hoses and jailed three times during the ongoing struggles.

After leaving the *Courier*, Cunningham hosted her own radio program, "At Home with Evelyn Cunningham," on WLIB in New York, during which time she interviewed many important political figures and celebrities. But it was while working at the *Courier* that Cunningham had her first experience with male chauvinism and became interested in the women's movement. Being the only female editor among many men, this was not surprising. Though she does admit that there were times when she found it difficult to handle, she remained positive about the experience: "I was the boss and I had to go through all that. It was a wonderful experience in learning."

In 1969, Cunningham became special assistant to Gov. Nelson A. Rockefeller and served as director of the Women's Unit Office of the Governor. She found her earlier experiences of discrimination invaluable. "When I got deeply involved in the women's movement, I was way ahead. I really knew when things had happened and how they happened." Throughout the 1970s Cunningham played a leading role in women's issues, accompanying Vice President Rockefeller to Latin America for a six-month study of women's problems in 1975, and later working with HEW on a ground-breaking report on federal programs and single mothers.

Cunningham continues to be actively involved with a number of organizations, including the World Service Council, the Alvin Ailey American Dance Theater, and Resources for Midlife and Older Women, and she remains committed to advancing the rights of women and minorities.

Cunningham's many accomplishments continued throughout her long career, which she has no intention of halting. "I didn't retire at sixty-five because I've got a lot of energy and I'm not senile," she said bluntly. "I think the social pressure to have to retire is ridiculous. I didn't let it affect me at all."

ELIZABETH McCORMACK

Elizabeth McCormack, the former president of Manhattanville College in New York (originally a Catholic women's college), is a dramatic Midlife Transformer. For many years she was a Catholic nun involved in education. But in 1974, at the age of fifty-two, she left her order and the presidency of Manhattanville to do philanthropic work with the Rockefeller family—and to get married.

Born in 1922, McCormack went to a convent school in the Bronx before entering Manhattanville College. During her senior year in college, she decided to become a nun because "I believed it was the right thing for me to do, though it wasn't something I particularly felt like doing." But she was very committed to a career as a teacher and chose an educational order, the Religious Order of the Sacred Heart.

"What made it easy for me to have a career," McCormack explained, "was that I was a nun and all nuns had careers." She went on to add that most of her college friends had become engaged by graduation and that for them "it was absolutely understood that you didn't have a career. What you did was you married soon after college and you had a lot of children and your career was to be a wife and mother. I wonder if not wanting that as my whole life had anything to do with the motivation that caused me to enter the convent." She insists that it was not a conscious motivation that guided her, but in retrospect it seems clear to her that it was a crucial impulse.

Because nuns live in a separate type of world, there was no competing with men, no discrimination. "You simply had to appear to be somebody who could do the job, and you had to be chosen." McCormack was grateful for the opportunity the order provided for establishing her career in an egalitarian setting.

After graduating in 1944 and joining the order, McCormack returned to her convent school, the Academy of the Sacred Heart, to teach for several years; she said that those early years of teaching were the most enjoyable for her because she had the closest contact with the students. In 1954 she became headmistress of the school for four years, then received an offer from Manhattanville to assist their president. McCormack accepted the offer and earned her Ph.D. from Fordham University while in the position.

In 1966 she became president of Manhattanville and soon faced a barrage of divisive issues as students led aggressive protests against church and national policies. Because more top secular colleges were admitting women, McCormack decided that the college should become coeducational and sectarian in order to attract more bright students. Both decisions were strongly opposed by many on the board of trustees. Reflecting on the situations, she preferred dealing with the protesting students to battling with the board.

McCormack began to feel it was time for a change after eight years as a college president. She accepted a new position as the assistant to the president of the Rockefeller Brothers' Fund. Two years later she moved into the Rockefeller Family and Associates office as their philanthropic adviser, a position she continues to hold today, with no plans of retiring.

McCormack believes that change is central to maintaining a healthy and productive life. "I think very few people should have one career," she remarked. "I think people should change what they do. Changing at about fifty or fifty-five is a very healthy thing to do because you have to learn a whole new world." McCormack's observations about the value of stimulation to older people are quite perceptive. In her order, older nuns lived alongside much younger nuns and maintained many important roles in the community through their nineties. In this living situation it was rare to find senility among the older nuns. Now that the order has become smaller, the older nuns are segregated and there has been a corresponding rise in senility. In brief, McCormack believes that to have a purpose in life is more helpful as far as health is concerned, "more important than oat bran and all the other things you're hearing about all the time," she remarked. "Much more important."

By choosing to become a nun, McCormack removed herself from the societal pressures on women her age to get married, have children, and stay at home. Then she made another unusual choice by leaving the order and marrying in her early fifties.

FELICE SCHWARTZ

Felice Schwartz, another type-B Explorer, was born in 1925. She has had a career focused on starting new social service organizations. While attending Smith College, she first developed what she calls a "very strong sense of mission." It centered on the plight of blacks in society, particularly their access to college education. When she was a college junior, Schwartz created the idea for the National Scholarship Service and Fund for Negro Students (NSSFNSS), an organization dedicated to getting scholarships for qualified black students to the best colleges. She started the organization immediately after graduating, at first under the auspices of the NAACP. Independent in its second year, the organization placed 750 students and went on to become a major success. It marked the first time substantial numbers of black students had applied to and attended previously all-white colleges.

Schwartz had been in college during the war years and, as many other women did, accelerated through college to graduate in three years instead of four, so she could join the war effort. However, the war ended and the message suddenly changed. "My generation was the quintessentially sexually polarized generation," she said, "because after World War II, the message was, 'We haven't produced goods or babies for five years, so women, you go home and produce babies, and men, you go back and produce goods.'"

Schwartz says many women welcomed this new message; after a long war, they were eager to see loved ones and settle down to happily married lives. Schwartz herself was eager:

Irv and I knew we were going to get married before he went overseas. His coming back was certainly something I loved the idea of and found very exciting. Now if that meshed in with the message that society wanted to beam out to you, then you were also excited about that. On one level or another this was happening everywhere: you were dreaming about your guy who was going to come home, and you were going to get married, and you were going to run up curtains out of nothing, and always look wonderful, and be ready there to support your husband, and have the children bathed, and the martini ready, and dinner hot. This is the generation that did that. They did not go sobbing to the suburbs.

But still, Schwartz acknowledges, "we were being programmed; there was a very unified voice in the country. If you didn't marry, there was something wrong with you. You were an old maid. It was all very pat."

Schwartz did get married, but she and her husband chose not

to have children right away. She continued to direct the scholarship fund (NSSFNS) for several years, and then spent three years
running her father's metal embossing plant following his sudden
death, so that it could be sold. She was successful, the plant flourished, and her family was able to sell it at a profit. (Her résumé
lists this as three years as vice president in charge of production for
a heavy manufacturing firm, a credential few women can claim.)

When the plant was sold, Schwartz and her husband moved to
the suburbs and started their family. There for the first time
Schwartz encountered her peers: the women who had gotten married right after World War II and were already raising 3.7 children
in suburban homes, "these women who'd done what society told
them to do." It was her generation of women, Schwartz says, who
started to realize that just having babies wasn't enough, "because
they were the women who were so tremendously pressured into
that." Not only were they pressured, they were also told how to
feel about it. "It was expected of them," she said, "not only that
they would be home full-time, but that they would love it. And
that they would love every minute of it."

But the dream did not match the reality; many women were
finding the experience extremely confining and restrictive, feeling
terrible conflict because they believed that there was something
wrong with them because they were not enjoying every minute.

Schwartz stayed at home for eight years, and when her
youngest child started nursery school, she began to put into action
her idea for creating a women's career resource organization,
which she ultimately named Catalyst. The agency was founded,
Schwartz says, "to bring to our country's needs the unused
capacities of educated women who want to combine family and
work." This mission statement was very carefully crafted so that,
between the lines, it communicated to men that it was not
intended to act in competition with them but to tap into
the unused abilities of women ("not just to pursue *careers*,
God forbid, at that time," Schwartz said, "but to *combine* family
and work").

Schwartz didn't think the organization could sell private businesses on the idea of part-time women workers, so she started
with the public sector. Catalyst's board of directors wanted to
establish a library on women and work, build a network of career
counseling centers for women around the country, and create
informational material on work that was directed at women.

They accomplished all three goals. Moreover, they created several experimental projects that showed that women could function extremely well in part-time jobs, with little absenteeism, a very low turnover rate, and good relationships with their clients. Over the years, Catalyst has evolved as the progress of women has changed; now it concentrates on working with companies interested in taking initiatives to develop and retain women.

In January 1989, Schwartz gained notoriety by publishing an article in the *Harvard Business Review* that gave rise to the idea of the "mommy track," that women who want to raise families should not be forced by companies to compete on the same career track as women who do not want children. The furor raised by this article led her to write a book, *Breaking with Tradition*. "It is about my view of where women are in this country, and where I think we have to go," she explained. "My generation started the feminist movement because we wanted to do something else with our lives. We got nowhere for ages, because we were viewed by employers as superfluous. . . . It's really only in the last four or five years that it's begun to swing. Women are no longer superfluous. They've finally arrived."

Stimulated by the discussion her article raised and by the experience of writing her book, Schwartz is planning her own career change: she will step down from the presidency of Catalyst and spend more time reading, lecturing, and writing. "Every year in my professional life has been more exciting than the last," she said. "The wonderful thing for me is that I have for the first time legitimized some thinking time for myself. You have to think to be a social activist, of course, but life is so frenetic, and so much of your time goes into fighting to survive! For twenty-nine years I've loved every year—and now I really want just to think, and to communicate with other people who think. I can hardly wait."

CHANGES IN DOMESTIC LIFE

The question that naturally arises here is: what happened? Given that many of the women born around 1900 were so sure of their equality and their entitlement to the same human rights as men, why didn't the generations following them inherit the same attitudes?

Although the possible answers to this question are too complex to address here, one contributing factor that became apparent through the study interviews was the difference between the domestic lives of the older and younger women. Many of the older participants, both men and women, describe growing up in families with at least one servant and often several, even if they came from middle-class or lower-middle-class families. In the early part of the twentieth century the wide availability of domestic help enabled middle-class as well as upper-class women to delegate part of the work of housework and child-rearing to servants.

Most households early in the twentieth century included other adults in addition to the mother and father: aunts, cousins, grandparents, and servants. In families that did not have servants, there was often a female relative living with the family who helped with the housework, and the children would be required to do a certain number of chores on a daily basis. It has only been since the end of World War II that the "nuclear family" has come to mean just a couple and their children.

Few labor-saving devices existed at that time, so it was physically impossible for one person—the wife and mother of the family—to do all the work necessary for a family of four or five people (which was a small family at the time; many families were much larger). Clothes had to be washed and ironed by hand; meals were cooked from scratch, including making some kind of bread for every meal and preparing desserts, most of which had to be baked. House cleaning similarly had to be done by hand—even such heavy tasks as cleaning carpets, which before the invention of the carpet sweeper meant pulling up every carpet in the house and hauling it outside to the clothesline to beat it to remove the dust. Many families made part or all of their own clothes, as time-consuming a task as the other domestic chores performed by women.

Despite all the labor involved in housework, if a household was well organized and had the right amount of help, the woman of the house would be able to take time for some outside activities. In fact, according to the social habits of the period, she was *supposed* to have time for outside activities, such as volunteer or church work. And she could take on outside activities without sacrificing the organization of her household.

The Great Depression had an enormous impact on the structure of domestic lives. Many families lost all they had. Social historian William H. Whyte dates the change in women's domestic roles from this period. In the town where he grew up, every middle-class family, "even the ones who were considered the wrong side of the tracks," had cooks. "I don't remember a single woman before the depression who did her own cooking," he said. After the depression and the war, the servants vanished. The days of large households with many servants were over for most Americans, and women had to adapt to taking on more time-consuming domestic chores and raising their children alone. Under these circumstances it may have seemed important to keep women's outside activities limited so that they could fulfill their obligations in the home. But the change is too sharp and too distinctive to be based on pragmatic consideration alone.

SUMMARY

The women in the Long Careers Study have been the foot soldiers of the women's movement in this century; all established strong, independent careers at various points in their lives, whether they were married and had children or not. Many of them have pursued their careers out of the limelight of the women's movement, and yet their achievements have undoubtedly advanced the movement's progress. Frances Etter's multimillion-dollar real estate business is as significant in this regard as Frances Lear's highly visible and important magazine (discussed in chapter 10).

The careers of the women in the study confirm that the women's movement has been with us since the very beginning of the century; it has come through many victories and defeats since then. Their experiences serve as instructive testimony on the history of the movement. As Lucy Scott, a journalist in the study, remarked, "Younger people forget what women my age and the ones who actually got the vote went through. . . . It is very interesting to me to tell younger people about that."

The experiences of the so-called mothers of the baby boom in contrast to that of the oldest women in the study supports the argument that it was not the start of the 1963 women's movement that interrupted an unbroken dedication to traditional roles; rather, the return-to-the-kitchen movement following World War II broke a long continuous tradition in the recognition of women's equality and the drive for women's rights.

All but seven of the women in the study married at some

point in their lives. It was surprising that twenty-two of those who had married were able to develop successful ongoing careers while maintaining their marriages and, for some, raising a family. Others participated in nonpaying volunteer work while raising a family and developed careers when their children were grown. Eight waited until their fifties to actually start their careers.

The women with long-standing careers had chosen fields in which they were self-employed or that provided flexible work schedules. Many of these women had careers in the creative arts—painters, writers, actors, designers. Other fields included psychiatry, law, politics, and scientific research, all of which have the potential for flexibility.

Several women had careers that were initially shaped by their husbands' interests; their careers grew to be completely equal to or independent from their husbands' later on. For example, Liz Carpenter ran a news bureau with her husband, Sayra Lebenthal and her husband ran an investment firm, Evelyn Nef became interested in the Arctic through her second husband, and Margaret Chase Smith filled her husband's congressional seat when he died prematurely of a heart attack. Eileen Ford did the reverse; she planted the seed of the Ford model agency, then her husband joined her in the agency after their first child was born. Julia Child's husband retired and then went back to work producing her TV show.

There were also a group of women who developed careers after a divorce or the death of their spouse. Some, like financial adviser Julia Walsh, started careers out of financial necessity. Others, like actress Helen Breed, found themselves free to pursue new directions or lifelong dreams of their own.

The varied designs of these women's lives provide excellent models for today's women who are grappling with often conflicting desires for a successful career and family life. One of the most important qualities that the women in the study seemed to possess was the ability to adapt productively to changing circumstances and to take on new roles and purposes. It is not surprising that many of them followed the Explorer career pattern in order to accommodate their many priorities and interests. The adaptability, flexibility, and energy required to develop a career that incorporates several successive stages, which may or may not include parenthood, are exactly the qualities that men and women alike need to sustain successful careers in the modern world.

PART IV

GROWING AND GROWING OLDER

13

The Responsibilities of Aging

PHILANTHROPY AND VOLUNTARISM

The longevity factor has not only extended the abilities and opportunities of people over sixty-five; the gift of long life carries with it new responsibilities as well. In the traditional image of aging as withdrawal and disengagement, people over sixty-five increasingly relinquish their adult responsibilities and expect to be taken care of by others. But that image no longer conforms to what most people over sixty-five want. Certainly most older people don't want to be dependent. Older Americans who are enjoying the gift of healthy longevity have much to offer younger generations, as we have seen in accounts of the many outstanding people profiled in this book. All older persons can use their experience and enduring energy to make significant contributions to the world in which they live.

Dr. James Birren, founder of UCLA's Borun Center on Aging, addresses the responsibilities of older Americans through precepts that he calls "My Responsibilities for My Old Age." These nine so-called commandments are focused on dispensing with negative attitudes and encouraging mental, emotional, and spiritual growth. Birren emphasizes again and again the importance of older people's engagement in the world, not just for themselves but for younger people who need their guidance and support.[1]

I have included these nine precepts because I believe they address directly the traditional problem areas of individual aging:

- I should honor my children and all children and foster their growth. May I remain close to my children but not hover over them and stunt their maturity.

- I should avoid becoming bitter if overlooked by the passing young and by events. May my spirit not be eroded by the acids of life. I should not blame or rage against others for their inability to control the impossible.

- I should continue to seek information and learning and avoid dogmatic positions and postures. May I be a source of experience for solving or moderating the problems of life.

- I should use the experience of my years for attaining fairness and justice for others.

- I should foster my physical and mental health. Should I have poor health, I should cushion its impact so that it does not weigh unduly upon others, and I should refrain from seeking an unreasonable share of resources and placing a disproportionate load upon others.

- I should manage prudently and with affection my relationships with others and initiate the expression of caring and love for others. May I manage the passing along of my possessions with fairness and avoid manipulating them to gain attention or to cause others to vie for material gain.

- I should continue to weed the garden of my life, remove yesterday's flowers and dead branches, and foster new growth.

- I should prepare myself and others for my death. May I promote my passing with poise, dignity, and peace. I should consider making provisions for the use of my body parts by others.

- I should leave the land and its people better than I found them. May I plant seeds that will bloom for others in springs I will not see.

The study participants confirmed the importance of a continuing and renewed sense of responsibility in the lives of older people. Many of them relished the fact that their personal responsibilities had diminished, whereas their more global responsibilities were expanding. They finally had the time and the financial security to direct their energies to making broader contributions; in addition, they now had the experience and wisdom that make their contributions most valuable. Moreover, although most of them did not say so explicitly, it was suggested that the older decades had brought them a sense of increasing altruism. They were genuinely concerned about the needs of their communities. They sought out certain activities, not to satisfy their egos or to prove that they could still "cut the mustard," but because they wanted to see the quality of human life improve. Robert McNamara, in a discussion on research, wondered aloud why there isn't a research institute where talented older people could come to try to devise solutions to society's most insoluble problems.

Advertising genius David Ogilvy sees John D. Rockefeller as an example of someone whose philanthropic career gave him a whole new life along with a new identity. "If John D. Rockefeller had retired at the normal age of sixty-five, no one would ever have heard of him," Ogilvey said. "But he had a second career for another thirty years in philanthropy. And he became the most famous philanthropist in the history of the world. The same thing happened with Andrew Carnegie."

The philanthropic careers of the study participants have often been, like Rockefeller's, more outstanding and productive than the individual's previous career. In every case, the participant found the move into philanthropy extremely rewarding.

PHILANTHROPY

JOHN L. LOEB

John L. Loeb, founder of Loeb Rhoades, one of the most successful investment firms of the twentieth century, has become an active and generous philanthropist, particularly in the fields of art and design.

Loeb began his career following in his father's footsteps but later changed fields, only to be joined by his father in his new pursuit. Born in 1902, he was the son of a brilliant and talented businessman, Carl M. Loeb, chairman of the American Metals Corporation. Loeb and his father were very close; young John always knew that his father wanted him to join him at American Metals, and their mutual affection made it a foregone conclusion.

John Loeb, like J. Peter Grace, was the son of a chief executive officer at a time when it was believed that everyone—even the heir apparent—should start at the bottom of the company. Loeb first spent six months in Pennsylvania unloading zinc ore cars with a team of Polish immigrants. He was next transferred to cost accounting and then became a combination of office boy and salesman. Eventually, he says, he "graduated" to New York in the mid-1920s, remaining in that office for two years.

In the meantime, Loeb had gotten quite interested in the stock market. His father had asked him to handle some of the family accounts; the market was strong and investing was very productive. After a good deal of reflection, Loeb went to his father and told him that he thought he would like to go to work for a financial firm. His father was disappointed, but gave his approval.

Loeb by this time had married a beautiful young woman he had met in college, Frances Lehman. Her father steered Loeb to the firm of a family friend, Wertheim and Company. Again, Loeb started at the bottom, first as a "runner," or messenger boy. After a month, however, he tactfully suggested that he might be better used in some other way, and he got a different assignment.

About a year later, Loeb's father unexpectedly had a falling out with the board of directors of American Metals and left the firm with a handsome golden parachute, six months before the 1929 stock market crash. But the senior Loeb was energetic and vigorous, and he felt lost without something to do. This encouraged John Loeb to venture an idea: the two of them could start their own office, simply to look after their own investments if for no other reason. Loeb's father agreed, and they opened a modest office on Wall Street in January 1930. A later merger added "Rhoades" to the corporate name.

Father and son built one of the great investment firms of this century, Carl M. Loeb, Rhoades and Company. Loeb senior had a large network of contacts both in the United States and in Europe, and he was widely respected. From the beginning, opportunities came to the firm in a very natural fashion, and the two Loebs were masterful administrators. The kind of intuition that guided John Loeb to choose finance over American Metals is a crucial skill for an investor. Although Carl Loeb died in the mid-1950s, the firm thrived.

When he was in his thirties, John Loeb had an experience that caused him to think a great deal about his life and ultimately drew him to become more involved in philanthropy. In 1936 he had an operation and needed about a year to recuperate fully. "It really changed my philosophy of life," he said. "I suddenly realized that the amount of time I had in this world might be limited. It occurred to me that whatever good turn I could do, I should do it because I wouldn't be coming back too soon. Or maybe never. I think that's what developed my interest in education, in hospitals, and in philanthropy generally, in which I have been very active and so has my wife."

A few years later, when he tried to enlist in the war effort, he was turned down and discovered that the "illness" he had had was cancer. He was not told about his condition by doctors because at that time doctors often thought it was unwise to tell the patient about such maladies.

Loeb's exceptional concern for the well-being of the larger community is nowhere more clearly demonstrated than in an incident related by his nephew, Thomas Kempner. Apparently, Loeb had personally influenced the stock market at great risk to his own company. During the Bay of Pigs crisis in April 1961, the stock market was falling quickly because of the threat of war. Loeb was convinced, however, that the situation would not develop into war, but he was very worried about the financial stability of the market. Early in the afternoon on "Black Friday," he came out of his private office and walked into the bull pen (the area of the office where traders normally sit) and, choosing an empty desk, sat down and began buying stocks. Everyone else in the office saw him and began to buzz that "Mr. Loeb was buying." Soon the word spread to other companies. The stock market decline ground to a halt, and on the following Monday, the market was on the rise. While there is no way of knowing to what extent Loeb influenced the rally, it was a very powerful display of concern and undoubtedly contributed to the financial turnaround.

When John Loeb reached the age of seventy, he felt he should think about stepping down. "I thought I was getting old," he said with a chuckle. "Of course from where I stand now at eighty-nine I was a teenager then!" But in the decade of the 1970s a wave of seismic shocks hit the financial industry: an oil shortage caused a painful minor recession, the laws were changed on how profits were made, and the first merger storms appeared, heralding a typhoon of such ventures that would strike in the 1980s. Moreover, no single person at Loeb Rhoades had John Loeb's combination of intuitive perception and keen intellectual judgment. The firm made a wrong choice in direction and ultimately was swallowed up by Shearson and American Express, along with several other distinguished financial houses.

Loeb has been a very active and loyal trustee and patron for many nonprofit institutions, including the New York University

Institute of the Fine Arts, New York Hospital, the Museum of Modern Art, and the Pierpont Morgan Library. He has been a dedicated alumnus of Harvard University, giving funds to the Harvard School of Design and, with his family, establishing the Loeb Drama Center at Harvard. He was also on Harvard's board of overseers for many years.

THOMAS CABOT

Highly successful businessman and philanthropist Thomas Cabot spent more than twenty years as CEO of his own company, before retiring in 1962. He then decided to pursue philanthropic causes, doing so with the same vigor that had shaped his earlier career. Over the next twenty-five years he would raise large sums of money for many institutions. He was elected an overseer of Harvard for two terms (an unprecedented record), during which time he raised millions of dollars for the university. These efforts, he said, earned him the title "The Biggest Beggar in Boston." He also undertook a major consolidation of the Harvard Medical School's health care programs throughout the city, merging four hospitals into one corporate ownership.

This work continues to keep Cabot busy. "I've given big money and raised big money, and I'm still doing it," he said recently, after spending a weekend on a fund-raising drive. Cabot sums up the principle that has sustained his career: "I believe very strongly that a person is happier if he keeps busy." This philosophy also prompted him in 1979 to write a book about his life, *Beggar on Horseback*. "I wrote my book to prove that a busy life is a happy one."

Cabot was born in Cambridge, Massachusetts, in 1897. His father, guided by puritanical tenets passed down from his ancestors, instilled the importance of duty in his young son. "Despite their austerity," Cabot says, "my parents did encourage an interest in science." His father had a strong interest in chemistry and in 1892 had set up a small chemical company to produce carbon black (a substance used to color rubber tires black).

Growing up in the shadow of several great universities only increased Cabot's interest in science, and by sixteen he had passed all the college entrance exams. However, he was deemed too immature for college life and was sent to Arizona to "grow up." There, says Cabot, "I developed a love of the out-of-doors." This experience marked the beginning of Cabot's love affair with the wilderness. In later years his zest for exploration and adventure would take him to all corners of the globe.

At eighteen he went to Harvard, where he met his future wife, Virginia. The outbreak of World War I disrupted their romance along with Cabot's college study; he enlisted as a flight instructor. Like his father, who was a pilot in the navy, he loved flying, and by the end of the war he was a veteran. But his aviation career would be short-lived. Upon his return he was persuaded by his girlfriend to give it up because she "wanted a husband, not a daredevil." He agreed. They married in 1920, and seventy-two years later they are still together.

On completion of his A.B. at Harvard, he went to work for his father's carbon black manufacturing company, Godfrey L. Cabot (renamed the Cabot Corporation in 1960). Once there, he discovered that things were in a "dreadful mess." Cabot seemed a natural in both business and technical areas of the company, and he soon convinced his father that he could manage the company. Shortly thereafter he found himself running it.

The price of carbon black rose considerably after World War I, and the company prospered. Plants were soon established in Texas (nine would be built between 1925 and 1930). This prosperity was abruptly halted by the Great Depression, during which the price of carbon black plummeted. In 1930, Cabot fell ill with a severe bout of scarlet fever, which left him in such poor health that his physicians declared he would "never go back into business."

He proved his doctors wrong, but it was five more years before he returned full-time. This period of convalescence was important for Cabot. He spent many hours hiking and camping with his family to help regain his strength. "The change in life-style enhanced my happiness and improved my effectiveness as a business leader," he said.

By 1940, he was back running the company, in time to see business boom once more with the outbreak of World War II. This time Cabot supervised the company's expansion overseas, first establishing a plant in England before eventually branching out worldwide. In 1951, Cabot was appointed director of International Security Affairs and would serve one year with the State Department before returning to his business, from which he retired in 1962.

Cabot continues to pursue the physical activities that he loves, such as horseback riding and sailing. Still passionate about traveling, in early 1992 he and his wife, both in their nineties, took a three-week tour to Antarctica. They plan to continue traveling and do "all kinds of things together" in the near future. Summing up his own philosophy of life, Cabot said, "A life without dedication can never be a happy one."

VOLUNTARISM

As longevity expands and good health is extended, millions of older people are willing and able to be involved in their communities, either through paid work or through volunteer activities. In fact, the number of people already engaged in these activities is surprisingly large. The Commonwealth Fund's study (discussed in chapter 14) found that more than 80 percent of those fifty-five and older who were working (whether it was paying or nonpaying work) were also involved in volunteer activities, either through organizations or by providing direct care to families and neighbors. The equivalent value of their voluntary contribution is 8.2 million full-time workers. The study also found that millions more older Americans were willing and able to work and/or volunteer, and that half of the total population over the age of seventy-five was involved in volunteer work, either through organizations or on a direct-care basis.

The responses of the Long Careers Study participants resembled these findings: almost 90 percent say they have done volunteer work during their careers, and more than half did most of their volunteer work after age forty-five. Almost two-thirds of the participants feel that older people are obligated to do some kind of volunteer work. Clearly they felt the sense of responsibility toward their community and the world that Birren has addressed.

The types of volunteer work the participants have done varies as widely as their careers do. Many volunteered their time and energy throughout their careers for causes and organizations they believed in. Others had to wait until their careers shifted sufficiently before finding time to do volunteer work. But at some point almost all of them found the time to contribute, living up to their belief that they as older Americans also have a responsibility to the larger community.

The amount of volunteer activity participants could take on

was usually based on their financial security. Many participants were able to do volunteer work only after they had achieved a stable income level, which for many came in their fifties and sixties. There was also a clear pattern in volunteer work and philanthropy along gender lines: the "career volunteers" were married women whose husbands were able to provide enough security for them to devote their energies to nonpaying work, while the philanthropists who contributed the largest monetary amounts were men who were able to generate incomes during their careers substantial enough to support major philanthropic interests. As traditional roles change and women continue to make strides in their earning power, this pattern may alter so that both men and women can be equally active in volunteer work and philanthropy.

MOLLY KIMBALL TODD

One of the two participants who made a career out of volunteer work is Molly Kimball Todd. Named in *Newsweek*'s July 1987 issue on "American Heroes" as the hero from the state of Tennessee (she was captioned "a quintessential doer"), Todd is known for her determination and her bluntness, which have earned her the nickname "Redoubtable Molly Todd" in her adopted hometown of Nashville, Tennessee. She explained, "I have a way of speaking out the way I feel, not always very tactfully, but sometimes it would encourage others who agreed with me to push for changes that I thought were important."

Throughout Todd's long career, she has championed the causes of women's rights and civil rights; she was in part responsible for the 1953 Tennessee convention to redraft the state constitution, in which the poll tax was abolished and other major reforms were implemented. The most interesting factor about her career is that it has been almost entirely nonpaying; she is essentially a professional volunteer, using her time and energy to exert leverage on social and political causes.

Born in Utica, New York, in 1904, Molly Kimball Todd grew up in a comfortable middle-class family, in which her father ran a garment business and her mother ran the household and played the piano. As an undergraduate at Vassar College, Todd got involved with a social services center in a slum area of Poughkeepsie; it was at that center that she "started being interested in doing things for other people."

This experience inspired Todd to become a social worker.

After attending the School of Social Work in New York City, she returned to Utica and worked for a local organization called the Associated Charities of Women. Through a friend, she met a young woman from Lexington, Kentucky, who was living in Utica. The next summer, the three young women decided to drive to Kentucky for a visit. It was highly unusual for young ladies to take "road trips," and her parents were, to put it mildly, not thrilled.

At a Lexington party given for the three women, Todd met both her future husbands. When she returned home from Kentucky, one of the young men, Robert Massie, went to visit her. They were married a few months later in 1928 and moved back to Lexington, where he started a private boys' school. In 1930, after the school closed because of the depression, Massie died of cancer. Todd was alone with one small child, and she was eight months pregnant with another.

Todd decided to go home to her parents, who had moved to Summit, New Jersey. There she began doing volunteer work for local charity agencies, bringing people money for groceries and rent. Later, she got a job in a welfare agency doing social work. She returned to Lexington several times to visit her in-laws, and during these visits she came to know the best man from her wedding, James Todd, whom she first met at the party long before. They were married in 1935, and she moved back to Lexington with her two sons.

In Lexington, Todd started an effort to create a birth control clinic at the local hospital, a cause that was strongly opposed by many in the community. She found a woman doctor willing to run the clinic, and the hospital agreed. "It was really quite radical at the time," she added.

A few years later, Todd's husband was transferred to Nashville. There she soon got interested in local politics, particularly in the state constitution, which she believed was in desperate need of reform. During this time, she had two more sons. In 1941, with a few other women, she started a branch of the League of Women Voters; the group studied the local council and legislature, worked for police reform, and targeted their efforts to reform the constitution. Their lobbying efforts finally proved successful: in 1953 Tennessee held a state constitutional convention. Todd ran and was elected as a delegate, and the convention achieved the goals Todd had set out to reach.

Todd's next cause became civil rights. She had been disturbed by racism since she was a child. In 1954, with the *Brown* v. *Board of Education* decision, she was mobilized into action, organizing the mayor and leaders of the black and white communities to promote desegregation. Todd took part in lunch counter struggles, joining black women at a previously all-white drugstore counter. After lunch counters, Todd and her friends took the battle to restaurants and movie theaters. Later she ran for the state legislature and the city council from her conservative district, but she lost those elections. She had spearheaded so many state and local reforms that some opponents branded her a communist. But that never dimmed her passion for political activism, and, she said, it meant "that I could go on doing the things I was doing."

In the 1970s Todd became involved in the growing environmental movement, as a member of the Tennessee Environmental Council and the nuclear freeze movement and, more recently, in soliciting aid for the homeless. Her neighbors always knew which Chevrolet Chevette was hers—the one with all the bumper stickers on it. In 1986, she traveled with a church group to Israel and the Middle East to better understand the religious and political difficulties of that region. And when she cracked a hip a few months later, doctors and nurses who came to her hospital room would find her registering any eligible voters she could find.

To this day, Todd continues her involvement in dozens of political and activist organizations. Although she no longer drives her own car, she has one of her many friends (many of whom are at least fifty years younger than she is) drive her to meetings and events.

Todd insists that she has had no career to retire from, which demonstrates how deeply integrated her activities are with who she is. She has received many civic awards in the last few years, yet has a typically matter-of-fact explanation: "I guess they think I'm about to die. But I've still got some things to do and I'm going to be busy doing them."

WILLIAM GOLDEN

William T. Golden's philanthropic career not only developed in the later half of his life, but also became a full-time career. A highly paid and successful corporate director throughout the 1950s and 1960s, Golden gradually transferred his talents to numerous causes and organizations in the 1970s.

Golden was born in 1909 in New York City, in a family that valued education. Although he graduated from the University of Pennsylvania in 1930, he still did not have a clear picture of what he wanted to do. "I had read a romantic story about Wall Street and I decided that I'd try to get a job there and make some money and have the freedom to do all the things I may want to do," he recalled. So Golden enrolled at the Harvard Business School; but he did not like it and left a year later. Although it was the summer of the Depression year 1931, he got a job on Wall Street as a security analyst starting at $25 a week. He worked there for over ten years before leaving to serve in the navy's ordnance bureau during World War II.

After the war, Golden was offered a job as assistant to Lewis L. Strauss, whom he had met in the navy, in the newly created Atomic Energy Commission. After three years, he felt the need for a change and set off traveling with his wife for seven months in Europe and North Africa.

On his return, he was offered a variety of positions on boards of businesses and nonprofit organizations. Thus, during the following decades, Golden held numerous board positions with companies as diverse as U.S. Radiator Company and Crowell, Collier and Macmillan. He also helped create the Science Advisory Commission, under President Truman.

In the early 1960s Golden found that he was moving away from business to more public service and philanthropic causes. "Gradually, I increased the number of not-for-profit things and reduced the number of business activities," he says.

By the 1970s he had greatly reduced his business interests and was associating himself with many diverse causes. He became trustee of Mt. Sinai Hospital and its medical school, Columbia University Press, the New York Foundation, and over twenty other public benefit foundations, organizations and commissions.

Golden's appointments during these decades and his apparent ability to move back and forth between the fields of health, science and technology, and publishing appears to be the fulfillment of his wish as a youth: to have the freedom to explore his many interests. Such pursuits, teamed with a deep-seated belief in his responsibility to others have resulted in many people benefiting from his years of pleasurable hard work.

Elisabeth Luce Moore

Elisabeth Luce Moore, like Molly Kimball Todd, built a dynamic professional career out of volunteer work. She has been an active member of the International YWCA for many years, and headed the women's division of the United Services Organization during World War II. She then branched out into the field of education, first taking on a trusteeship at Wellesley. Later in her life she became the first woman (and as of this date, the only woman) to chair the board of trustees of the State University of New York. Moore also devoted much energy to help build the China Institute, founded in honor of her parents.

Moore, sister of *Time* magazine founder Henry Luce, grew up in China in a missionary family and returned to the United States only to go to college. After graduating from Wellesley, Moore, who as a child wanted to be a journalist, worked briefly at a textbook publishing company before joining her brother at *Time* to help him get his then-fledgling magazine off the ground.

Moore then decided that she wanted to get magazine publishing experience from beyond her family. She landed the plum position of assistant editor at *Junior League* magazine, with a promise of the editorship within a few years. She was eager to begin work on the magazine, but her beau, lawyer Tex Moore, had been offered a long-term job with an Italian law firm; he asked Moore to go with him to Italy—in those days, an invitation that was understood to be a proposal of marriage. Initially, Moore refused; but almost immediately she realized that her new job was not going to work out as easily as she had expected. After a disagreement with her boss, she resigned, married Tex, and sailed for Italy.

Moore settled into married life, and eventually motherhood, which she enjoyed, but a few years later, when a friend asked her to help out at the International YWCA because they desperately needed volunteers, she was eager to try something new. Moore liked the work and was so impressed by the organization she decided to get more involved. "I met these fantastic women who were doing such a good job in countries where it was even harder to fight for women's rights," she explains.

Over the next ten years Moore built herself a new career in voluntarism with extraordinary energy and ability. She also discovered that her work enabled her to carry on without conflict the family role she had chosen. "In a way," she reflected, "I think it was a positive factor rather than a negative one; when my husband came home from a trip I had something interesting to talk about, in addition to the household things."

During this time, Moore developed a keen understanding of the role of a volunteer. "The volunteers," she explains, "bring a down-to-earth, fresh outlook and make a contribution that is far beyond the time they spend in actual hours doing their work because they represent the community and the many differences between one community and another, whereas the professional in most instances comes from outside the community."

Moore found her work to be both challenging and fun. "When we had to raise money," she recalled, "we'd have an event, and then you'd have a speaker that had an opportunity to talk not just about money, but the status of women and make people realize this was something pretty important to be working for. It was a lot of fun!"

Moore's efforts came to the attention of several high-ranking officials, and during World War II she was asked to head the women's division of the USO. She recalls with delight the day she was offered the job. "I'll never forget these two handsome men sitting down rather stiffly in our very old-fashioned reception room. Both rather tall and good looking, beautifully tailored, and the YWCA was such a funny Victorian shabby old place."

Her new job was even more demanding than her previous position and meant traveling around the country attending the numerous local USO meetings to give pep talks. "It was a matter of giving them some inspiration," Moore says. "I literally spent the whole war years on trains and buses. My poor husband!"

Moore worked tirelessly throughout the war. "It was an amazing time. We had a very patriotic verve. It seemed to us that this was the one thing we could do," she says. After the war Moore returned to the International YWCA to help with the rebuilding urgently required after the disruption of wartime. Over the following five years she performed various activities, including helping to organize the World Emergency Fund for the YMCA.

Moore's success with the YWCA and the USO was followed by an invitation to be a trustee at her alma mater, Wellesley. Her efforts there brought her to the attention of Nelson Rockefeller, who asked her to chair the board of the State University of New York. Moore was the first woman to hold the position, and she rose to the challenge, once more spending countless hours traveling to conduct council meetings at local colleges and university centers.

Always a tireless worker, after twelve years on the State University board she left to begin work at the China Institute. Headquartered on Sixty-fifth Street in a building donated by her brother Henry, the organization was still in its infancy, and Moore knew it needed work. "I was certainly going to see that anything that was headquartered in a building named for [my parents] was going to be good," Moore says.

Today Moore has lessened her workload, spending more of her time advising and mentoring and doing less hands-on work. She still works at the China Institute and attends International YWCA meetings. "I'm still very involved with the international work," she says, "but mostly in an advisory capacity. But I like to get in there and see that things happen."

MAXWELL DANE

Maxwell Dane, one of the founders of the legendary advertising agency Doyle, Dane and Bernbach, created a highly satisfying post-retirement career for himself. At the age of eighty-five, Dane is still deeply engaged in his volunteer work, which he began when he stepped down from his position at what was then mandatory retirement age, sixty-five Dane and his partners had established the retirement policy themselves, and Dane felt he should abide by it to make room for the younger members of the firm. But although he retired, he did not stop working; he simply shifted his focus to activities outside the firm.

A Homesteader, Dane spent his entire work life in the field of advertising. He started out as secretary to the advertising manager of Stern Brothers in Manhattan, soon moving up to become assistant advertising manager. After many years of experience in the advertising business—magazines, retail, radio broadcasting—he opened his own agency in 1948 and called it Maxwell Dane, Inc. In 1949 Dane merged the company with two friends, Ned Doyle and Bill Bernbach, who had recently left the Grey Advertising, Inc. Doyle, Dane and Bernbach became one of the largest advertising agencies in the world, handling multimillion-dollar accounts, including Volkswagen, Avis, and American Airlines. Dane was responsible for the internal administration of this rapidly growing firm, which went public in 1964.

Doyle and Dane both took advantage of the mandatory retirement policy they had instituted. Dane retired from his administrative position in 1971 but maintained his position as a board member until the company's merger in 1986 with two other large agencies (Batten, Barton, Durston, and Osborne and Needham Harper). He still has an office in the agency's quarters on Madison Avenue, as well as a part-time secretary; he uses the office as a base of operations for his own work. After his retirement, Dane began concentrating on his own writing and became more actively involved with the many boards of which he was a member. He has also been involved with the efforts of the United Jewish Appeal and other Jewish organizations. In addition, he still manages to find time for other volunteer work. His post-retirement volunteer activities keep him as busy as his successful advertising career did.

Dane has remarked, "When people ask me, 'Are you retired?' I don't know how to answer. I'm not being paid for what I do. But if I work, it means devoting efforts and talents to something I enjoy, and the economists don't understand that."

Not everyone wants to take on responsibilities after retirement as large as the ones they handled during their working lives. Instead, some choose to assemble several smaller volunteer activities in areas that interest them.

JANE GOULD

Jane Gould built her career around an organization that she helped create; then she retired to work on the same issues on a volunteer basis so that she would have greater freedom.

Born in 1918, Gould grew up in New York and, at her father's insistence, attended Barnard College. After graduating, Gould worked for two years as a secretary before marrying her husband, Bernard, and following him to army bases around the country. She raised two children and, in 1954, decided that she wanted to go back to work, at least part-time.

Gould contacted the placement office at Barnard, only to discover that no placement services existed for women who wanted to return to work. Undaunted, Gould eventually got a part-time job as an assistant at the Alumni Advisory Center, a nonprofit membership organization that offered counseling and placement for college-aged women in New York City.

Over time, Gould spoke with "a trickle of Barnard alumni who were coming back saying, 'Hey, is this all there is to life? I can do more.'" She became known as "the person to see if you wanted to return to work." Through the center, Gould organized informal workshops and seminars for women who wanted to go back to work. Barnard's president, Millicent McIntosh, was very supportive of the initiative and, in 1959, successfully solicited a grant from the Carnegie Corporation to continue the center's activities on a larger scale.

By 1965, Gould was ready for a change, so she accepted the position of director of the Office of Placement and Career Planning, again at Barnard. Through individual and group counseling and varied career programs, she helped students and alumni of all ages develop and implement satisfying careers. Seven years later, she became president of the Women's Center.

Although she has technically retired from her administrative career, Jane Gould has continued to pursue her interests in women's issues just as aggressively on a volunteer basis. Gould explains: "I have found that working [gives women] an identity. It seems men always seemed to know that they were people. Without a job, women tend to feel lost in this society."

JANET SAINER

Janet Sainer, commissioner of the New York Department of Aging for twelve years, is legendary among senior citizens for her tireless dedication to the needs of the elderly. Referred to as the "hands-on" commissioner, never "timid at taking a stand," she began her career at age fifty, after having raised a family and having worked only part-time since her marriage in 1941.

Born in Brooklyn in 1918, Sainer was raised by her mother, a teacher, after her father died when she was five years old. She developed a keen interest in group and community work during summers at camp. Sainer obtained her bachelor's degree in social work from Hunter College in 1938. She attended graduate school (where she would meet her future husband) but decided that group work was of more interest to her than individual therapy. After graduating, Sainer worked for a short time before moving to New Jersey and settling into family life.

While raising her children, she worked part-time in volunteer community organizations, primarily with children. It was not until 1956 that she was introduced to the field of aging. Asked to head the Golden Age Club, a community program run by elderly volunteers to offer services to the community at large, Sainer jumped at the challenge and spent ten years creating what would prove to be a highly successful project. Even after this success she still did not look on it as a "professional career." "It was something I was doing because I liked to do it," she explains.

Sainer's volunteer work at the club nevertheless required a full-time schedule, and she soon decided that she might as well get a salary and benefits if she was to continue to work full-time. She first applied for social work positions in her local area but then realized that she was more suited to organizational work than to dealing on a one-to-one basis with the institutionalized elderly. She applied for a position with the Department of Public Affairs in New York and landed a job in the Community Service Society (CSS). This job was a challenge from the beginning. "It would open up a whole new area," she remarked.

Her first task was to assess a recently completed research study of elderly people's interest in employment. When told to "see what she could come up with," she "was floored. I didn't know what I was going to come up with!" Sainer took to tackling such "nonconcrete" requests with great initiative and intelligence. Soon she would launch her first program to bring elderly volunteers into community work. During this time, Sainer adopted a principle that she would maintain throughout her career: "I decided that if we were to do this, our primary goal had to be the older person and meeting his [or her] needs." This volunteer program, the first of its kind, called Serve (later to be known as RSVP [Retired Senior Volunteer Program]), now operates in seven hundred communities across the country.

After fourteen successful years of work at CSS, Sainer was chosen by a special search committee and named commissioner of the New York City Department of Aging by Mayor Koch in 1978; this work proved to be as pioneering as her previous efforts at CSS. "I felt strongly that it was important to expand services, and I guess also because my own interest was in program development, I carried that same thing into the department," she explained.

During her administration she was responsible for many new department initiatives. The best known, Citymeals on Wheels, a supplemental nutrition program for the homebound elderly, supplied more than 700,000 weekend, holiday, and emergency meals in 1988 alone. Her other successes include the establishment of an Alzheimer's Resource Center, employment and job training programs, and the organization of health promotion services.

Sainer has many strong views about what she calls the "retirement mystique"—the picture of the elderly as frail and infirm, which she views as largely a media creation. "We need to demyth the current myths," she said. But she also feels that part of the blame does lie with those working in the field of aging. "We put our primary emphasis on those who are needy. . . . We don't speak about all the well aged." Instead she feels that the concept of older people as a "resource" should be promoted. And in her years as commissioner, she helped to raise public awareness of concerns of the elderly locally, as well as nationally, by leading and participating in conferences, presenting testimony before Congress and other legislative bodies, and conducting broad outreach and public relations campaigns.

After leaving the Department of Aging in 1990, Sainer planned to spend more time with her recently retired husband and felt she was "ready to do a little bit less." But she soon found herself with two major consultancy assignments. Her recognition overseas led to her being asked to perform consulting work in Israel, and she was also asked to be a consultant to the commissioner on aging in Washington in "public/private partnerships." So Sainer's remarkable work in the field of aging continues. Of her present workload, she said that although she is supposedly retired, she still has "two heads, two hats, and two cities."

SUMMARY

Although volunteer work can play an important role in planning post-retirement activities, many participants believed that it was easier, as well as more important, to be engaged in volunteer work throughout a career, instead of trying to begin after retirement.

Philanthropy and volunteer work provided new ways for the participants to continue to contribute to their communities. For many of them, volunteer work fulfilled a deep sense of responsibility they felt to the world around them. And for some, like Janet Sainer and Elinor Guggenheimer, volunteer work developed into successful paying careers, often on more than one occasion. All the volunteers have found their roles extremely rewarding and a powerful complement to their previous careers.

14

The Two Faces of American Retirement

More than fifty years after it became an American institution, the concept of retirement is going through a period of transition and realignment. Our old idea of retirement as the culmination of the American dream—a period of leisure at the end of adult life when the individual is free to do what he or she wishes, without involvement in work—has become blurred. It is evolving into another, albeit one that has not yet assumed a defined shape.

The old view of retirement was based on several assumptions: that the worker did not like his or her work; that the ability to perform inevitably deteriorated as one grew older; and that people find leisure more satisfying than work.

Those assumptions were partially true at the time they were formed. Even as recently as 1950, the majority of workers did the kind of work that was highlighted in Studs Terkel's *Working*—jobs that were unpleasant and boring and that often involved strenuous physical labor. A lifetime of work in such a job can be a crushing burden; retirement for these workers genuinely is something they look forward to for years and relish when it arrives. "There's a discontent. You see, it has to do with the nature of the assembly line," said Terkel. "The spot welder at an auto plant assembly line goes along and shoots spots all day. What is there to like? So he dreams of thirty and out. The UAW, back some time ago, won thirty—that is, after thirty years, you can get a pension, you retire. And they dream of that."

Second, a lot of work used to be so physically punishing that a man really might be too old to continue in his fifties. And working hours were longer than they are today: at the beginning of the twentieth century most people worked six days a week, ten hours a day. Because average life expectancy did not reach far beyond sixty-five, it was important for people to have time they could look forward to at the end of life that was not dominated by physically destructive labor.

The increase in longevity, the transformation of the nature of work, and the shifting economic climate have changed retirement's meaning for many Americans. Now a far higher percentage of jobs do not involve the wear and tear of physical labor. Today, many more people perform work they actually enjoy than was true at earlier periods in the twentieth century. "The teacher, or someone else, who loves the work he does and plays a role in it," said Terkel, "doesn't want to be forced to mandatorily retire. So it depends upon the person and the work."

The roller coaster ride of the economy and of corporate personnel policies from 1970 onward have steered many Americans in directions they did not anticipate: out of work at a time they did not expect, working for less money than they would have predicted, or forced into early retirement. This has happened at a time when not only the average life expectancy is longer than it has ever been in our entire history, but when the physical beginning of old age has been delayed until later and later in life.

These changes have brought to the surface a hidden contradiction in American attitudes toward aging and retirement. This conflict has been present in some form since before the passage of the Social Security Act; in fact, its existence was partly responsible for the act's passage. It is a clash in two different clusters of values that are almost diametrically opposed, both offshoots of one of the most basic and deeply felt of American values: our commitment to equal opportunity.

This contradiction surfaced repeatedly in the Long Careers Study interviews. The first part of the conflict is the belief that the institution of retirement is a good thing for the society, that older people, who have had some time in the workplace already, have an obligation to leave their jobs at a certain point so that younger people can "move up." The second part is the belief that age discrimination is wrong and that people should be able to work as long as they function well—regardless of their chronological age. Linked with these two beliefs, undergirding them in some respects and opposing them in others, is the fierce dedication Americans feel toward the Social Security program. Americans tend to believe that retirement at a certain age should be available as an option for anyone who chooses to take it.

MAKING WAY FOR YOUTH

Over and over again, participants in the Long Careers Study told me that they felt older people should get out of the workplace to make way for the young. They evoked a concept very much like the rationing of work: since there are not enough jobs for those who want to work, and since the available jobs are not equally desirable, you have an obligation after a certain amount of time in the workplace to step down and give others their chance.

This argument was summed up very neatly by historian Arthur Schlesinger, Jr., who acknowledged, with his characteristic lucidity, that he holds all the beliefs above—even though he is fully aware that they are contradictory. On the one hand, he tends to think that older people should leave to make way for younger ones. "I don't like mandatory retirement as a way to do it, particularly," he said. "But I do think that people ought to get out of the way. I see it so often in universities. . . younger historians in the 1970s couldn't find jobs, and therefore became lawyers or tax advisers or something like that. I think the case for a turnover is good; people shouldn't just stay on and stagnate. I believe in youth, giving youth a chance."

But, Schlesinger says, he also believes in letting people continue in their work "as long as they do it well, which [is] a contradiction to the other," he noted. "It's an insoluble problem, because there are arguments against mandatory retirement, and equally [strong] arguments against discriminating. That's a hard thing to work out."

"I think people are so much younger now in their seventies than they used to be," added Schlesinger. "I'm shocked every time I reflect that I'm seventy-three. Seventy-three always seemed to me aged. I never feel seventy-three. I feel forty most of the time, ninety occasionally. But I don't feel seventy-three!"

In discussing the issue of stepping back to make room for the young, the participants usually spoke of the transaction as if it were a one-to-one substitution: the older person leaves a job, which is then filled by a young person. In practice, of course, this is not really how such changes work. A sixty-year-old vice president does not retire from a position that is then filled by a twenty-three year old. The process is described as if it works that way, but it doesn't.

What probably happened originally was that when a long-term worker retired, each person who was lined up behind him on the corporate ladder got to move up one step. And at the end of the line, a new worker might be hired to fill the job vacated by the lowest person in the chain. But this is a gross oversimplification, and even if it might have applied in the early part of this century, it is questionable whether it would be valid today. The organization of most contemporary companies is so complex that trying to apply a domino theory of advancement within them is impossible, even ludicrous.

Today there are also times when someone retires and nobody moves up. Perhaps a job is simply eliminated by better technology or corporate belt-tightening. Or a candidate may be brought in from outside the system. In these cases, the true issue is the corporation's desire for a change, not a wish to give those at lower levels upward mobility.

The participants who thought older people should step down understood that they were oversimplifying the process. They also knew that age is not a measure of a person's productivity or value, and that by encouraging people to leave at a particular age, the company in fact may lose valuable talent in the departing senior staff member. Nevertheless, many of them held fast to their conviction that this was a good way for things to work because it ensured that there would be places for the young, on whose presence the future depended.

OPPOSING AGE DISCRIMINATION

During their interviews, the participants also voiced the opposite side of the conflict, as Schlesinger did: they were against age discrimination and mandatory retirement policies. They felt that people are entitled to continue holding their jobs as long as they are functioning well, without regard to chronological age. They did not feel that anyone's value as a worker or as a human being should be lower simply because they had reached a particular age.

"I think sixty-five is a phony age," said Elinor Guggenheimer. "I don't see why we should be losing the productivity of people at a certain age. There is very little reason why there should be an artificial age limitation at all—except that equally you do want to open things up for younger people moving up. But there has to be a better way of doing it."

The participants deeply resented the experiences of age discrimination they had had themselves. They did not believe that their age should have such a strong impact upon the perception of their ability. Renowned surgeon Dr. William Cahan fought a long battle with Sloan Kettering Memorial Hospital in 1984 over the hospital's efforts to retire him at age seventy. The hospital's by-laws originally fixed retirement at age sixty-five but were amended as a result of a state law raising the age to seventy. Cahan had taken stock of his physical and mental abilities, supported by a complete work-up, and found everything functioning normally. "I would quit in two seconds if I thought, technically, that I was unable to do it," he commented. Feeling that he was perfectly capable of continuing to operate, Cahan wrote a letter to the hospital administration in which he stated:

At Memorial, we are careful to deal with patients as individuals. Shouldn't the same approach apply to staff members? In which case, wouldn't it be wise to be less concerned with a particular surgeon's chronological age and more with his performance? How old I am is unimportant; how able I am is.

Although Cahan was aware of the need to promote younger surgeons, he also believed that he had acquired valuable information over his many years as a surgeon, which he wanted to pass on to younger surgeons. "It took about a year for them to come to their senses and not retire me, and then it took another six months to get them to let me do surgery," Cahan said. Cahan continued to perform surgery until 1990, fulfilling a lifelong dream of operating with his son, who had also become a surgeon. He still assists frequently at operations, mentoring and teaching younger surgeons.

Another participant, Dr. Harold Proshansky, for many years president of the graduate school and University Center of the City University of New York, was engaged in a power struggle by

CUNY's chancellor, Joseph S. Murphy, who announced that he was seeking new, "more vigorous" leadership for the six colleges in the system whose presidents were over sixty and had held their posts for more than a decade. Proshansky, a brilliant administrator and a superb psychologist, felt that age was not an appropriate criterion. During his tenure he had recruited an outstanding faculty and helped the graduate school build a national reputation; at the time of Proshansky's death, a nationwide survey found that one third of the school's doctoral programs were among the fifteen best in the nation.

Proshansky fought vigorously and ultimately was able to defeat Murphy's move to retire him immediately; he retained his post for several more years but agreed to set a date for his retirement. The struggle took its toll, however. A few months after the conclusion of the negotiations, Proshansky discovered he had contracted lymphoma. He died in December 1990.

Discrimination in less blatant ways was also a concern. Participants encountered it in many different settings, from board memberships to everyday conversations. "I am going on seventy-one," said William H. Whyte, author of the famous study on corporate America, *The Organization Man*. "I've never been busier in my life, never worked so hard or put in longer hours. I've been on the board of my old school, St. Andrew's School. [When] my term was up, one of the senior trustees said, 'I think what we should do is make you emeritus. You will be allowed to come to meetings.' I was furious. The only reason for doing it was the supposition that I am too old; everybody else got their three-year term extended. I have never been near that school since."

The conflict between the belief that everyone should have a fair turn in the job market based on age and the belief that age-based discrimination is unfair does not exist just on the microlevel of individual opinion. It is present in our society on a larger scale. Over the past fifty years we have idealized retirement as the pot of gold at the end of the rainbow, while simultaneously resenting it as an unfair system of putting out to pasture people who do not want to go.

There is widespread bitterness among older people about being shut out of mainstream society and tagged with labels they dislike; "golden ager" and "senior citizen" are expressions whose pejorative meanings are thinly veiled, if at all. Older people also resent being called "greedy geezers" (a term coined by professional journalist John Hess) because they own their own houses or have saved enough money for a comfortable retirement. They are vividly aware of how ironic it is that the nation spent decade after decade trying to reduce or eliminate poverty among older people and then, after it succeeded, suddenly began to blame the older generations for the very security that the entire society had worked so hard to create.

As recently as the 1970s, when Dr. Robert Butler wrote his Pulitzer Prize–winning book, *Why Survive?*, about the difficulties faced by the old in America, "generational equity" meant reasonable economic security for older people. In the 1980s, suddenly the concept was turned inside out, and "generational equity" became the concern that a wealthy selfish older generation was bankrupting the future of the baby boomers, for whom no Social Security benefits would be available. The framework of this conflict springs from the same decade in which Social Security was established and retirement became an American institution: the era of the Great Depression of the 1930s.

THE IMPACT OF THE GREAT DEPRESSION

The Great Depression was the most radical economic reversal that the United States had experienced in its history. Suddenly the number of job seekers outnumbered the quantity of available jobs by 40–50 percent. At one point almost half the American work force was unemployed. Families tumbled from the middle class into poverty from one month to the next; men who had taken pride in their ability to support their families were reduced within a short period of time to standing in line at soup kitchens. It is a vision that most younger Americans cannot imagine, even in view of the 1990s recession; yet it comes terribly alive in the accounts of the study participants.

Artist Will Barnet went to New York in the depths of the Depression, in 1932. He arrived at night; the bus dropped its passengers on Forty-second Street then, because there was as yet no bus station. Barnet walked up the West Side to find a place to stay in a city that had been devastated. "New York was in terrible trouble financially," Barnet recalled. "It was dark at night because the street lights had been turned down as low as possible to save electricity. Buildings were abandoned and there were thousands and thousands of places to let. Everywhere you went, it was 'To Let' or 'For Sale.' Everybody went bankrupt. There were bread lines all around the block and soup kitchens everywhere—that's just a place on the street where there's a big pot of soup. The picture is a bunch of homeless people, standing in a line that would go blocks—around the corner, down the next block—waiting patiently to get some food, because they were starving. It made a deep impression on me, and I've never recovered from it."

Older people were particularly hard hit, in a society that was fiercely ageist, with a bluntness that today seems deeply shocking. "The present recession is a Sunday School picnic compared to the Depression," remarked Dr. Norman Vincent Peale, who was the pastor of a church in Brooklyn at the time. "There was a saying in those days that nobody thirty years or older could get a job of any kind in New York City. There was just no money—and New York was the money capital of the world."

The Great Depression permanently traumatized many of the families that lived through it, scarring not just the adults but the children as well. They carried the memory of their families' suffering long after the actual events were past and conditions had improved.

Over time, the attitudes those injuries evoked blended into the texture of American values. The specter of massive unemployment helped to convince many Americans that it is better for everyone to have a boundaried work life than for some people to work as long as they can while others have no work at all. In the interests of both efficiency and compassion, age seemed to be the most logical foundation on which to base such a system.

There were two important motivations driving the passage of the Social Security Act. One was the compassionate desire to provide, not necessarily entire pensions, but extra money—supplemental or cash income—for people who retired. The other motivation was to move older people out of the job market by inducing them to retire. Both motivations are still present today.

Not everyone involved in drafting the Social Security legislation understood the extent to which this was true. Judge Simon Rifkind, who helped Sen. Robert Wagner draft part of the legislation, believed it did not have that potential. "What I visualized, and what some of the people I was working with visualized, was quite modest," he said. "Take a farmer. He's old and now he has a house to live in; he has a farm that his children are working, but he hasn't any cash income—just a little bit of cash to buy his newspaper, a suit of clothes and so on. If he could have a little supplemental income, his whole life would be transformed. And that was the Social Security concept. The idea was cash income as opposed to other kinds of income," Rifkind explains. "But Social Security appealed to so many different people for so many different reasons. That's why it's almost unmentionable to think of eliminating it," he adds.

But behind the creation of this pension program was a prickly situation: since the Industrial Revolution began to take hold in the nineteenth century, the search for ever greater productivity stimulated the invention of ever more ingenious machines. Technological advances periodically reduced the number of workers needed in various industries. Each new invention eliminated a number of jobs that had formerly been held by human beings. Many immigrants to the United States came for just that reason. Andrew Carnegie's father was a weaver who was displaced by the invention of mechanically operated weaving machines and could not find other work in his native Scotland. Unions and industry met this ongoing crisis by periodically shortening both the workday and the workweek, thus creating more human positions to go around. But the massive outflow of workers during the depression meant that much more drastic moves needed to be taken. Retiring older workers and providing a supplemental pension for them seemed to be a step in the right direction.

We need to resolve this conflict, for many reasons. As we become longer-lived, and more youthful at older ages, there will be an increasing number of people who want to remain engaged, and the pressure to create more varied opportunities for older age groups will increase. Various alternatives have been suggested as partial solutions to this impasse, but it is crucial that we find others and begin the process of implementing them on a broad scale.

FLEXIBILITY

The suggestion most often made by the study participants was that the current system is too rigid and that more flexibility would improve it substantially. Cyrus Vance, for example, said he felt a firm should have some kind of retirement age, but then he added, "I think in every plan there should be enough flexibility so those individuals that a firm or company feels a particular need to keep on, because of what that individual can contribute—there should be that kind of flexibility and they shouldn't be absolutely rigid."

J. Peter Grace was even more liberal. "I think that just as a general answer, nothing can be run by rule books anymore," he said. "I think that anytime you say that after sixty-five is the time to retire, it's crazy. Some people are old and tired at fifty-five, and some people are wild men at seventy-two." Grace defended having a general retirement age—at seventy rather than at sixty-five—because he thinks it poses too many problems to have to determine every person's retirement age individually. But like Vance, Grace believes that it ought to be possible to be flexible about those rules so that the most valuable employees could stay on longer.

Former milk company executive Robert Popper went further. "I think that there should be *no* policy on retirement," he said. "I think it's terribly important that every person be allowed to do whatever he or she wants to do. I think mandatory retirement is extremely foolish. Anybody who isn't doing his job should be kicked out; and anybody who's doing a good job should be allowed to stay on. Age is not a factor."

And although the answer to institutional mandatory retirement policies might be found in more flexible programs, flexibility is not necessarily a simple solution. Former Ford Foundation president and Kennedy administration National Security Affairs assistant McGeorge Bundy described the complexities of the flexible retirement policy that Harvard had when he was teaching there:

They had a flexible retirement age—sixty-six, sixty-eight, seventy—and nobody wanted to quit at sixty-six. The people that you invited to quit at sixty-six felt that you were telling them they weren't very good, which you were, so there wasn't any escape. You had not only to make the decision but you had to tell them. A single retirement age is much more soothing for management but it's also a terrible waste for people who are better than that. I never found a good answer to that. I knew we could dress it up and say that everybody quits at X and some people are invited to stay on for the convenience of the institution; but you don't fool anybody. People are so sensitive to that round-about approach. I think we haven't solved that problem at all. I'm not sure I know a good answer to it. When you are sixty-five and the employer of first resort doesn't want you—unless you're very good at figuring out what to do next, it's not easy.

"Figuring out what to do next" or at least going over your options is clearly an important step in dealing with retirement, mandatory or not. But for people who are very involved in their work, it can be difficult to find time to research other options thoroughly. Frank Stanton, former president of CBS and the Red Cross, is opposed to mandatory retirement but believes that even with such a policy there are ways for companies to make the transitional period—from full employment to leaving the company—easier for employees.

Stanton tried this approach on his own: on nearing the network's mandatory retirement age he sought the advice of Marvin Bower's management consulting firm, McKinsey and Company. Stanton explained: "I said to them, 'I won't have any time to worry about my own problems; you know what's out there, see if you can find some list of options that I can consider.'" Stanton was keenly aware that many other workers were facing a similar situation. "I know a lot of men who work like mad up until the time of retirement and they've never really sat down and thought it through."

Although Stanton found his next position, as head of the Red Cross, through the recommendation of its former president and not through McKinsey, he still believes that the idea of providing management consulting advice on their next careers to people approaching retirement age would be an excellent company policy. Such a system would be beneficial for everyone involved, including the management consultants. "I think this might be a whole new business for them," he said, "because a lot of guys are going to be retiring, racing against the clock the same way I was. Maybe this will be something companies can do for their retiring employees in the future."

Stanton described a similar policy CBS had several years ago. "A year before the individual retired, we took them for a weekend at a conference center with their wives. We would sit down and do financial planning: their work planning, their options to do public services and so forth. I think that taking the lid off age sixty-five as a mandatory retirement date has changed that somewhat, but you still have the problem of helping people through that rather narrow gate from inside to outside."

Noted sociologist Matilda White Riley had done a great deal of thinking about retirement policies. She spent several years as a member of a panel on college and university retirement ages. "We don't know the solution yet," she said. "We know that mandatory retirement by age is not good, because age is not a useful marker. But without that, you have to have some kind of testing. I've thought a good deal about it. I firmly believe that if you take college professors, who are a microcosm of the larger society, they ought to be tested every five years. My point is, a great many college professors get into teaching—it's considered a secure place. Many of them are bored to death after they've done it for fifteen years, but they don't know what else to do. The testing would encourage people to consider changing more often."

"The system is set up for short lifetimes," Riley continued, "and people don't have short lifetimes any longer. It's also set up for comparatively slow-moving change in society, when now we have a very rapid change process. Everybody has to keep relearning their tasks, so what's needed is to recognize this and not wait until age fifty-five; that's too late."

AGES AND STAGES IN WORK

Recent research has proposed the tantalizing possibility that people play different roles in successive stages of occupational development—roles that are frequently, but not always, age-related—and that a full range of roles is important to the healthy functioning of an organization. In other words, it is possible that we have been selling ourselves short by assuming that a workforce should be composed largely of younger people, from their twenties to their fifties. There may be both structural and psychological reasons that we have been unaware of why it is better to have an organizational age range that goes up through the sixties and seventies as well.

The existence of this research is directly related to the question of age discrimination. In 1967 Congress passed the Age Discrimination in Employment Act, making it illegal to discriminate on account of age. In 1978, the ADEA was amended so that the mandatory retirement age of sixty-five was pushed forward to seventy for most American workers. The exceptions to this were college and university faculties, airline pilots, and public safety officers (policemen and firefighters). All of the employers argued that they should be allowed to retire employees earlier than seventy for special reasons. These were disputed cases. In 1986 these exceptions were temporarily extended to 1993, and studies were ordered of the effectiveness of older people in these professions and of the economic impact on the institutions of abolishing mandatory retirement. One set of these studies has now been completed.

Frank J. Landy, a psychologist from Pennsylvania State University, was engaged to do the study on public safety officers. Landy and his twenty-one-member scientific team from the Center for Applied Behavioral Sciences reviewed over two thousand published studies on different aspects of aging. They collected data from 182 police departments, 185 fire departments, and 102 correctional facilities throughout the United States. In addition, they used national data bases showing deaths, injuries, and medical illnesses among public safety officers.

The Landy team's findings indicated that age had very little to do either with fitness or with performance. *Some public safety officers in their sixties were more physically fit than others twenty years younger.* "There is evidence for substantial variability in the physiological status of older adults," the panel concluded. "Age-associated declines in many of the principal physical abilities involved. . . are highly modifiable depending upon one's life-style."

Moreover, the researchers discovered that there was an advantage in having older public safety officers working along with younger ones. The older officers often moved into supervisory positions, where their accumulated experience was extremely useful in teaching and mentoring the younger officers.

"This isn't the only study with a result of this kind," Landy added. "There are a number of studies in various areas. For example, with typists, it's been shown that an older typist does as well as or better than a younger typist, because she takes in more at one time. Then there is the impact of stress in the workplace. If there is no stress, then experience doesn't make a difference. But if you add stress, experience counts; the experienced person will keep performing at a good level, while the inexperienced one won't be able to."

MANAGING COMPLEXITY

Another factor involved in alternatives to the current retirement system is the ability to deal effectively with great complexity. Putting together new organizations, for example, is such a skill.

Professor Eli Ginzberg, a Long Careers Study participant and the director of the Eisenhower Center for the Conservation of Human Resources, has written over one hundred books in the fields of human resources, urban studies, economics, and health policy. Ginzberg has become a master at managing a number of projects simultaneously. He explained that "one of the tricks is to know what the limits are of one's life structure. I always say to kids, 'If you don't know how to say no you're going to be in big trouble.' *No* is the most important single refrain in the English language from the point of view of careers. There are a lot of opportunities out there and if you don't know how to manage your time, you're dead. The most important single aspect is to have an idea of what you want to do and what you like to do. Make sure you handle your time, that you don't get overambitious, that you don't get seduced by all kinds of possibilities."

The flow of events in many of the life histories showed that the participants had learned how to manage large and complex activities cumulatively over a period of time. They would start out working for other people, observing and learning. Next they would take on a modest project for themselves. As they completed each project they would then move into another, which was somewhat larger or more complex.

In addition, even for the Explorers, there was at least one relatively long period when they stayed in the same organization or job, learning and expanding their managerial skills and knowledge of human behavior within a secure organizational setting. The settled Explorers reached this point when they found a position which fit their interests well enough that they could stay in it, perfect their skills, and then use it as a base to add other activities. Other Explorers, like John Gardner, found a good "learning job" relatively early. Later, this learning period became the foundation from which these Explorers would launch into new fields. Gardner started Common Cause in his late fifties and developed Independent Sector in his sixties. Elinor Guggenheimer has made a mini career out of creating organizations and is still going strong in her eighties.

COUNCILS OF ELDERS

Max Lerner told me how he published periodically a column in which he advocated the use of older people in "councils of wise men." (I think it is safe to say that Lerner would have considered this use of the term *men* generic and would not object if in my more contemporary language I rephrase it as "councils of wise men and women.") On the national level, for example, he envisioned creating an advisory organization of past presidents and cabinet officers, who could be called on to advise the government in any number of ways. An informal system of this kind already exists, based on personal communication between the president and previous presidents and some cabinet officers.

On a community level a council of elders certainly might be both practical and useful. Former World Bank chairman Robert McNamara suggested that councils of this kind, whether on a local or national level, could deal with large-scale or very difficult problems, applying the whole weight of their life experience to devise solutions. Former secretary of labor Willard Wirtz made a similar suggestion, adding, with his usual wry humor, "It isn't as if we have a shortage of major national problems on hand for people to work on."

THE VALUE OF EXPERIENCE

If we project this concept onto a larger scale, we can see that another possibility is to create an additional layer of institutional involvement in our society, which would take advantage of the special skills older people have—skills that require development over time.

Many in the Long Careers group described activities that depended on skills acquired and refined over long periods of time. Almost all of these activities (e.g., mentoring and advising individuals as well as organizations) involved human relationships and demanded a fine-tuned understanding of human personality and behavior. Elisabeth Luce Moore, who was the first woman to chair the board of the State University of New York, described eloquently the role she adopted in her work with various organizations as she grew older.

Moore is a dignified, elegant woman who has claimed as her right a frankness that would be hard for many younger people to match. "I used to spend many more hours and actually do a lot of the work myself," Moore said. "Now I'm much more in an advisory capacity. I have the courage to tell them, 'That's nonsense; quit doing that. You're wasting too much time.' Most people can't. And that's one of the great advantages of age, because I can get away with saying something is nonsense. I'm a senior citizen; they think that I've made a big contribution to these organizations, in leadership, to say nothing of money. But mostly, if I know something is going wrong, and it's stupid to go on that way, I know how to stop it. And I don't do it in a mean way. I can find a way of expressing the matter that has everybody agreeing; I really am a good diplomat."

Moore paused, and then added, smiling, "But it takes courage, and that's what old age gives you. What have you got to lose? They can just say, 'Well, that's that old battle-ax!'"

One of the most stunning examples of the value of experience was Judge Simon Rifkind's last case as an attorney, when he was eighty-eight. He had begun to taper off and "loaf a little" when he was around seventy-five; at eighty he decided he would no longer argue cases because it was a round-the-clock activity, but he still took some appeals. Pennzoil Texaco, an old client, asked him to argue an appeal of its case. Rifkind obliged. The award, at the time the largest ever won in a civil court, was $12 billion. "They settled the case for $3 billion in cash," Rifkind said with satisfaction. Believing that he was unlikely to win a larger case, he thought it was a good place to stop—he wanted to quit while he was ahead, way ahead.

"Since then, I've been a resource," he said. "By that I mean that I'm available and any partner or associate who wants to come in and talk to me about his case, can do so. I'll say to him, 'I think sometime in such and such a year I had a similar situation and I think this is what I did. Now go through the file and look and see if I'm right.' I reach into my memory bag and drag up something. Not a bad way to spend old age."

Just as judges can take senior status, so can those in other fields, those who genuinely want to continue their work and are physically able to do so. Dr. William Cahan, in effect, is functioning as a senior surgeon; Judge Rifkind and James B. Lewis are working as senior-status lawyers; Dr. Jonas Salk is functioning as a senior scientist; Marvin Bower is acting as an adviser to the younger members of McKinsey. And Nobel Prize–winning economist Wassily Leontief said that in addition to his current role as professor at New York University, "I have to play somewhat the role of the elder statesman," adding that "objective circumstances slowly turned me to [this position]." In it, he said he now has to deal with department crises, write recommendations for colleagues and students, and give consultations to visitors.

Clearly, many professions already have special but unofficial roles for their older members; these roles need to be formally sanctioned and recognized. And in professions where they don't yet exist, strategies for creating such roles should be developed.

THE VALUE OF STATURE

Some experience-oriented tasks also require stature—the kind of respect from others that is gained only through significant accomplishment over time. Former secretary of state Cyrus Vance's effectiveness as a mediator of international crises grew out of many qualities and experiences, starting with his long-standing interest in mediation, a skill he began refining in the 1960s. But in part, his ability is an extension of his personal qualities: his intelligence; his integrity and great personal courage; his understanding of other national cultures; his capacity for seeing simultaneously many different levels of a problem; his ability to be tough when toughness is required and skillful when tact is called for; his prodigious communication skills. In Vance's case, his professional history and identity—the product of three-quarters of a century of learning and experience—are among his most powerful credentials. And they are unique.

Similarly, in the late 1980s, when research on AIDS was stalled because two leading French and American researchers were embroiled in a bitter stalemate over who had first isolated the AIDS virus, it was Dr. Jonas Salk who unobtrusively stepped into the dispute and gently, patiently, invisibly, over a period of many months, negotiated a truce that allowed research to move forward again in both countries. In an exceptional gesture for the scientific community, Salk's contribution was publicly acknowledged in the text of the accords. Probably no one else could have accomplished this rapprochement, for Salk had behind him, in addition to his intellect and his many personal qualities, a monumental record of accomplishment in the field of immunology, which commanded respect on both sides, and many contacts in

France in part developed through his wife. The truce lasted for several years—long enough so that when it ultimately began to fray, the conflict was no longer an obstacle to the forward motion of AIDS research as it had previously been, and its purpose had been served.

We have grown accustomed in the industrial age to thinking of people as basically interchangeable, like the components of a machine. This is an illusion, although it is not often recognized as such. Dr. Frank Stanton, a strong believer in periodic career changes, emphasized that people are not so flexible. "If you are good at one thing, it doesn't necessarily follow that you could do the same thing in another environment and never miss a heart-beat," he said. Sometimes, experience doesn't translate directly from one business to another, and it is unrealistic to take an executive from an oil corporation and expect him to know how to run a broadcasting company, for example.

The person who first advanced this important management precept was William H. Whyte in *The Organization Man* (1956). The book was hugely popular and formative in analyzing the impact of the development of huge conglomerate corporations in the United States after World War II. These corporations, Whyte argued, were creating a new prototypical "organization man," who had lost his individual judgment in the interest of teamwork and the organization. Whyte insists that "organization has been made by man; it can be changed by man." This statement applies just as much to retirement policy today as it does to the personality tests and other corporate policies that Whyte found questionable.

Human beings are all different, and we become more individuated as we acquire experience and grow older. That uniqueness is one of our most valuable traits. In fact, in Japan, people with such a combination of knowledge derived from experience and highly developed personal traits are recognized as living national treasures.

MODEL PROGAMS

One growing trend in creating alternatives to retirement has been the development of the job bank. Such banks consist of lists of people, including many retirees, willing to work part-time during vacations or busy periods, or in some cases full-time. The Travelers Corporation of Hartford, Connecticut, was the first large company to start a job bank; the program was initiated in the 1970s and was under way by 1981. About half the names in the bank are those of retired Travelers employees who work a minimum of forty hours a month in a variety of jobs, including typists, messengers, data-entry operators, and accountants.

Managers at Travelers have praised the retirees as "reliable and conscientious," according to a 1986 *New York Times* article. "We cannot fill the requests we get from our managers for retirees," said F. Peter Libassi, a senior vice president of the company. The retirees themselves have found that working keeps them in better physical, mental, and financial states, and they are enthusiastic about the program.

Using the retirees saves Travelers about $1 million a year. Other companies that have developed alternative ways to employ retirees include IBM, Corning Glass Works, and the Grumman Corporation, where retirees function as consultants and contract temporary employees. As the demographics of older and younger Americans change, many companies are looking to retirees as a significant and valuable resource.

Dr. Eli Ginzberg described the impact of demographic change in this way: "With each passing year there will be more and more upper-age Americans interested, able, and desirous of working. Unless the country wants to pay additional taxes to support a lot of elderly people, it makes more sense to offer them the opportunity to work and earn extra income."

In Minneapolis, Donna Anderson has created a model organization, the National Retired Volunteer Center, which keeps corporate retirees active in community service. In 1989 the NRVC launched a highly successful program, Retirees in Leadership. The program was designed to empower retirees to work together along with the cooperation of the private and public sectors, to address critical problems facing the community. Through a series of eleven seminars and workshops conducted over one year, the program sought specifically to channel the lifelong accumulated skills of the retirees into collaborative problem solving to implement new projects throughout the entire community.

By stressing the important role played by retirees in the decision-making process, the program promoted the retirees as real agents of change, while creating a deep sense of personal involvement and contribution to the community among the participants. So far, three sessions have been held. The last session, Staying-Power, asked the retirees to address issues affecting children and youth. In initiating action to help solve problems affecting children, the session also sought to build new bridges between the generations.

Many of those who have participated in these sessions praise the program's usefulness. Retired English professor Miriam Showalter said she felt "energized to go beyond what has felt safe. To plow new fields." Bette E. Flanders, a retired personal banking officer, said, "Retirees in Leadership has and will provide guidance as to where I can utilize my interests and talents without disappointment or burnout. It provided a challenge which retirees so need."

A few private foundations have become engaged in these issues. In 1992, the Commonwealth Fund released the results of a new study as part of its Americans Over 55 at Work program, begun in 1988 by Commonwealth President Margaret E. Mahoney. Its premise was that people over fifty-five are an underutilized resource with tremendous productive potential. The researchers in the study group chose fifty-five and over rather than sixty-five because they were interested in looking at people who had a ten-year window before turning sixty-five and who would offer a different perspective from those over sixty-five.

The 1992 study was the third in a series. The first study found some two million retirees aged fifty to sixty-four ready to return to work. The second part had examined the experiences of three companies, including Travelers, and found that hiring older workers makes good business sense. The most recent study, based on a survey conducted by Louis Harris and Associates with 2,999 Americans aged fifty-five and over, examined participants' organizational volunteer activities and their direct care of family and friends.

The survey results found that almost three-quarters of Americans over fifty-five are actively engaged in helping American society, in either full- or part-time work; as volunteers through organizations; or caring for sick or disabled relatives, neighbors, family, or friends. Furthermore, the results showed that over five million of those over fifty-five not working are willing and able to work. The study concluded that the contribution of older Americans to society has been severely underestimated and undervalued and that these people constitute our greatest unrecognized human resource.

SUMMARY

Whether we realize it or not, we will ultimately be forced to create more flexible rule systems governing retirement. "Each new generation," reflected Dr. John Riley, "has to invent things for itself, and it gets impatient with the old ways. They want to get the old ways out of there. That's the seed of the great human tragedy, I think: the inability to learn from past experience."

"We are living in an unprecedented time," Riley continued, "in which the number of competent, capable older people is increasing. And we can't imagine any kind of a social organization existing for very long in which those people don't have something valuable to do. Gradually, we'll see increasing opportunities for older people in educational institutions. Gradually, we'll see opportunities for them in jobs, in occupations—very gradually. Gradually, we'll see recognition of their wisdom in the political arena, religion, the arts, and so on."

Retirement policies are beginning to evolve into more flexible and subtle programs, which are better suited to adapt to a greater variety of interests and abilities. New opportunities for older people will increase gradually, as Riley suggests, as the younger members of our society learn the value of incorporating older people in organizations or institutions. But if, in spite of ageism, older people act now on their desire to remain at work or to develop new roles and occupations, they will be making a direct contribution to increasing the number and types of new opportunities available to future generations.

15

Staying in Good Health

If we could design our own future, probably most of us would prefer to follow the plateau model of aging: to stay in good health and keep a relatively normal level of activity throughout later life, regardless of how old we live to be. In thinking about growing older, it isn't so much the minor adjustments in lifestyle that are intimidating. Most of us don't object that much to having glasses changed periodically or gaining an extra five pounds here and there. It's the prospect of major catastrophe that is frightening—the fear of being ill and incapacitated. Good health is primary to the enjoyment of life. It enables us to maintain our relationships with friends and family and to keep doing the things we enjoy most.[1]

Based on information gathered for the Long Careers Study (interviews with expert participants, survey responses, and research done by participants themselves), several consistent factors emerged that are related to how these long-lived people have maintained their health and energy through such long productive lives.

STAYING ACTIVE, STAYING IN SHAPE

One of the biggest surprises in the study was the very high percentage of participants who told us that they exercised regularly—68.5 percent, more than two-thirds of all the participants. Furthermore, 61.6 percent said that they exercised every day. This was unexpected partly because of the high average age (seventy-nine) of the participants and partly because the current trend toward exercise didn't come into existence until very recently, in the 1970s and 1980s. The participants belonged to age cohorts that by and large didn't exercise very much once they became adults; women especially did not exercise on a regular basis. Yet these people do exercise.

The exercise routines they described were varied, with walking and swimming as the most popular choices. Eighty-one-year-old Dr. Lawrence Wylie rides a bicycle eight miles a day along the river near his home in Cambridge, Massachusetts. Norman Cousins and former diplomat Franklin Williams played tennis regularly, and Cousins also played golf. Among the female participants, the most strenuous exercise was performed by Julia Walsh, who swims daily for thirty to forty-five minutes. She recently had her swimming pool "winterized" so she could swim all year round. Françoise Gilot has done yoga exercises every day since she was nineteen. Daily stretching exercises and calisthenics were popular, especially among the women; for example, Elizabeth Janeway adopted an Elizabeth Arden exercise routine, which she performs daily for forty minutes or more. Indoor biking and cross-country ski machines were also popular. Dr. Jonas Salk alternates between walking and riding a stationary bicycle. Both Warren Robbins and Felice Schwartz exercise for twenty minutes or more daily on exercise machines. However, Millicent Fenwick's simple regimen of a daily walk for a half-hour to one hour was typical of most participants, who found it easier to exercise while carrying out other activities such as gardening or shopping.

There is confirmation from recent research in human physiology of the importance of exercise in maintaining good health. At Tufts University, the U.S. Department of Agriculture–funded Human Nutrition Research Center on Aging has been studying the effect of exercise on older adults since 1986. The results are quite striking. They show that most of the previous pessimistic conclusions about physical aging were based either on studies of animals or on projections from research with young human subjects. As with all such projections, there is the possibility that real life may prove you wrong. When the Tufts scientists began their own research, with older human subjects, the results were very different from most of the popular ideas about the effects of old age.

What the Tufts experiments have shown is that many of the characteristics people believe to be the inevitable results of aging are instead the products of disuse and inactivity. Without adequate exercise, people gain weight more easily; their joints become stiff; they lose muscle mass and strength, and add fat; their metabolism slows down; and they feel less energetic. The result is a vicious cycle in which lack of exercise causes them to feel less energetic and get even less exercise as a result.

The Tufts team has concluded that exercise is the single most important factor in maintaining healthy functioning in later life. The researchers created a scale of the ten most important biological processes within the human body, and they evaluated the effect of exercise on each one compared with other factors. In every case, exercise turned out to be crucial in keeping functions within a normal range and preventing damage from disease. Exercise maintained muscle strength, prevented weight gain by keeping muscle mass higher and body fat percentage lower, and improved the aerobic capacity of the heart, lungs, and circulatory system. It normalized the body's blood-sugar curve and helped reduce the chances of getting diabetes. It helped regulate blood pressure, maintained a more favorable cholesterol ratio, improved the body's internal temperature-regulating mechanism, and increased bone density.

Moreover, the Tufts studies show that it is never too late to start. People can reverse, or at the very least retard, many of the physiological declines associated with aging, even at very old ages and when they are in poor condition. One member of the Tufts team, Dr. Maria Fiatarone, designed an experiment to see whether frail older people could be strengthened by regular exercise. The results were astonishing: weight-bearing exercise increased muscle mass at about the same rate as in younger people—20–30 percent over a six-week period. Non-weight-bearing exercise improved flexibility but did not increase muscle mass.

In summary, the message behind these research results is that the time-worn colloquial phrase "Use it or lose it" has been scientifically validated. Many of the symptoms we have thought of as part of the inevitable deterioration of aging are not inevitable at all: they are just the result of inactivity.

To date, one book on this research has been published for the general reader: *Biomarkers,* by the laboratory's overall director, Dr. Irwin Rosenberg, and the director of its human physiology laboratory, Dr. William Evans, who designed many of the experiments undertaken in this area. There will undoubtedly be much more valuable information emerging from this research group in the future.

The Tufts project's research suggests that the high exercise rate among the Long Careers Study participants may be an important factor in keeping them healthy. Note that exercise is different from athletic competition, and that its purpose is to keep your body healthy, not to try out for the Olympic team. Over time there is a very slight decrease in athletic ability that can show up, which sometimes frustrates serious athletes. "Playing tennis, I find my reaction time is not what it used to be," said the late ambassador Franklin Williams, president of the Phelps-Stokes Fund. "When I used to see a ball coming, if I'm playing doubles— which is all I play now—my head says I can reach that ball, but the body doesn't react as rapidly, and I make the move and frequently don't get there. And then you're embarrassed because your partner thinks you're going to get it and you don't." But if you exercise regularly, these changes are minor ones, unless you have the standards of an Olympic athlete.

There was one participant who was a particularly interesting late bloomer as far as exercise is concerned. Former representative Orval Hansen, an Idaho native who served three terms in Congress, took up running in his early fifties to prepare himself for a physically demanding trip to Nepal, and he entered his first marathon at age fifty-three. Now in his late sixties, Hansen still runs twenty miles a week, entering one marathon annually. "To do that when you are no spring chicken convinces you that you can do whatever you want to," Hansen said. "It becomes part of the whole process of looking at and seeking new challenges and opportunities." He added, "I'm in better physical shape now than when I was in college."

THE IMPORTANCE OF GOOD NUTRITION

The subject of nutrition—how much and how well we eat—has been a topic of frequent controversy in recent years. As scientists have mounted large research efforts to discover the causes of the three major killers of adults (heart disease, cancer, and stroke), news bulletins have periodically cautioned Americans about the dangers of eating too much cholesterol or too much saturated fat. Undoubtedly, millions of people have changed their diets to conform to these admonitions.

At times, the public has been confused by reversals of some of these pronouncements. After years of regarding cholesterol as "bad" and eliminating cholesterol-containing foods from our diets, for example, American consumers were recently told that there are different kinds of cholesterol, and that some of them are good. Moreover, it is not so much the quantity of cholesterol in your bloodstream but the ratio of "good" cholesterol to "bad" cholesterol that is significant. Although it can be confusing and unsettling for the consumer, this shift in perspective is part of a normal process of advancing knowledge, as researchers have gained a clearer and more detailed picture of extremely complex biological processes. In the past such research took decades, so the about-face seemed less sudden; now progress is accomplished so rapidly that barely a few years fall between the pronouncement and its refutation.

The topic of vitamins is another nutritional area in which early categorical pronouncements have subsequently been modified or reversed. For many years nutritional authorities called the taking of vitamin supplements, beyond a certain minimal amount, a pointless waste of money, or worse. Consumers were told that no one needed more vitamins than are provided by a normal diet and that in any case vitamins have no impact on any of the major diseases.

But recent research on a variety of illnesses indicates that certain vitamins do tend to protect against particular diseases—for example, reducing the incidence of cardiovascular disease or inhibiting the development of cancer. One study participant, Dr. Alan Cott, a psychoanalyst who specialized in orthomolecular medicine, began prescribing megavitamins in 1965 to treat patients with childhood schizophrenia and autism. "When I began treating patients at the hospital with vitamins," Cott explained, "the other doctors were laughing at first. Then they began to see how many more of my patients improved than the patients they were treating, and some of them came around." As more research is completed and the results released, it seems likely that nutrition will be given greater importance.

TAKE VITAMINS AND MINERALS

One of the participants in the Long Careers Study has been a pioneer in the understanding of nutrition. Dr. Linus Pauling, a biochemist who has won two Nobel Prizes and was nominated for a third, may know more about nutrition than any other human being alive; he has spent the past thirty years reading extensively in nutrition-related scientific research and experimenting with his own nutritional regimen.

In his early nineties, apple-cheeked and fresh-faced, Pauling is a remarkable figure. He has the pleasantly weathered look of someone who has spent a lot of time outdoors. His home on the Big Sur coast is filled with the signs of his perpetual curiosity—books, periodic tables of the elements, reprints of his more than eight hundred published scientific papers, a sprawling mineral collection, and on the deck just outside his office a rainfall gauge and weather instruments. Pauling is a walking encyclopedia of twentieth-century scientific research, and he is constantly trying to push the limits of knowledge.

Pauling grew up in a small town in Oregon. He became fascinated with chemical reactions from experiments done by his father, a pharmacist, and by a childhood friend who had learned how to produce flashy effects by mixing chemicals, liberating heat and light and turning one substance into another. As a result, Pauling shifted his interest from engineering to chemistry and enrolled in Oregon Agricultural College, the only type of institution in that era where one could study subjects like chemistry and plant genetics.

Pauling received his first Nobel Prize in 1954 for work on the chemical bond between molecules. He also did path-breaking research on the hemoglobin molecule and discovered the whole family of diseases that are caused by a malformation or malfunction of the red blood cell molecules (sickle-cell anemia is probably the best known among these). He was nominated for a Nobel Prize in medicine for this work but did not receive it. During this time, Pauling also became interested in world peace; at the instigation of his wife, he decided to take some time off to pursue this cause. He spent fifteen years traveling widely, making speeches and trying to persuade influential figures that peace was attainable. In 1963 he was awarded the Nobel Prize for Peace for these efforts.

In the late 1960s Pauling became interested in the biochemistry of nutrition. He had read two papers by Dr. Abram Hoffer and Dr. Humphrey Osmund about their discovery that large doses of vitamin B-3 (niacin) and vitamin C could markedly improve the condition of some schizophrenics. At the time, no word existed for the treatment of illness by substances normally present in the body itself, such as vitamins and minerals, and Pauling coined the term *orthomolecular medicine* to describe this process. He then began reading in depth the scientific literature on nutrition.

To Pauling's surprise, he found that there was a huge quantity of research literature on nutrition, and that an enormous amount of research ("thousands and thousands of papers") had already been published showing that vitamin C has substantial positive effects on health in a number of respects. In particular, it had been shown that vitamin C reduced the frequency and duration of colds, and that it is centrally involved in the manufacture of the basic building blocks of the body, collagen and elastin, so it is important in keeping the walls of the veins and arteries strong. The research literature was so impressive that in 1971 Pauling decided to publish a book on it: *Vitamin C and the Common Cold*.

He was completely unprepared for the torrent of criticism unleashed by this book. "I was sort of surprised," he said. "I thought, everybody will be happy that I've written this book. The doctors will be happy that they're not pestered so much with patients with colds; and the people with colds will be happy that they don't suffer so much." Instead it seemed that the entire medical profession was up in arms, and Pauling was called a wide range of names, including a quack—a novel experience for a Nobel Prize winner.

Pauling continued his work, taking on the additional task of trying to encourage more research on the subject of nutrition. Meanwhile, using his extensive knowledge of biochemistry, he worked out a basic nutritional regimen for himself.

Pauling believes that while it is important to eat a sound and balanced diet, it is also important for older people to take nutritional supplements of vitamins and minerals. The principle reason, he says, is that research shows that the vitamin and mineral intake of older people tends to be low. Moreover, as we age we absorb nutrients less efficiently, so older people actually need a larger nutrient intake just to maintain the same nutritional level. Finally, it is impossible to know exactly how much of any nutrient is present in any particular food item. Studies have shown, for example, an enormous variation in the amount of vitamin C in oranges plucked from supermarket shelves, ranging from zero to three hundred milligrams—with the majority on the low side. Vitamin C is especially important because of its key role in the cardiovascular system and in strengthening the immune system. But vitamin C is the only nutrient that human beings cannot synthesize internally, so we must get it from external sources. In his 1986 book, *How to Live Longer and Feel Better,* Pauling discusses in detail his own nutritional regimen and the scientific reasoning behind it.

Pauling's list of supplements is simple, but the suggested amounts are far larger than those ordinarily sanctioned by conventional medical authorities: vitamin C, six thousand to twelve thousand units daily; vitamin B, one or two high-potency B-complex tablets; vitamin A, one twenty-five-thousand-unit capsule; vitamin E, one eight-hundred-unit capsule; and one mineral supplement.

His rationale for the larger amounts, in addition to the reasons given above, is that there is a very clear distinction between the amount of a nutrient needed to prevent deficiency disease, and the amount needed for the highest possible level of functioning. When government-approved levels for daily vitamin intake (now called the RDAs, recommended dietary allowances) were established in the 1940s, the amounts selected were those that research had shown were enough to prevent a deficiency disease.

But the amounts needed for the highest possible level of functioning are far larger that the amounts sufficient to prevent disease. Moreover, because every person is biochemically individual, what is ample for one person may be completely inadequate for another. Pauling described this in detail in a speech that he gave in November 1991 at the Gerontological Society of America:

What astonished me was this. You need only a pinch of these vitamins every day—17 milligrams is the RDA for vitamin B-3, niacin—just a little bit, to keep you from developing pellagra. Here are these patients of Hoffer and Osmund: some of them are getting 17,000 milligrams a day. Five milligrams per day of vitamin C is probably enough to keep most people from developing scurvy. The RDA is about sixty milligrams a day for an adult. But some of these patients were being given 5,000 or 10,000, or 20,000 milligrams a day.

Pauling discovered that there were no guidelines for the optimum daily amount of vitamin C for human beings. However, he found that there were guidelines for all sorts of animals used in laboratory experiments, including some fairly large mammals such as the goat. He used the animal guidelines to calculate the optimal amount for an average-sized human being based on weight and came up with 12,000 milligrams daily (if one wanted to keep human beings as healthy as lab animals, he added).

He elicited gasps of astonishment from his audience of experts in aging when he mentioned that he himself takes 18,000 milligrams of vitamin C each day, an amount so large that most physicians would turn pale at the thought if it were suggested. He went on to say that he had upped his dosage with advancing years; for a long time he took only 10,000 milligrams a day (still an immense quantity measured by the RDA standards).

Pauling recalled that some years back, a skeptical fellow scientist who heard this comment sniped that Pauling probably excreted all 10,000 units, so his vitamin intake was just producing expensive urine. "I decided to do a little experiment," Pauling said, smiling archly. "After all, I'm a biochemist; I can do these things!" He measured "everything that went in and everything that came out" for one week, and found that he was absorbing about 8,500 milligrams of the vitamin C. He felt that the remaining 1,500 milligrams was an adequate cushion in case of additional stress, and he left his dosage as it was for the time being.

Pauling's intake of 18,000 milligrams should not be imitated without consulting a physician, or unless you have scientific training. But Pauling's intake is undoubtedly right for him, because at ninety-two he is still thriving.

In November 1992, the medical journal *Lancet* published results of a Canadian study that provide interesting validation for Pauling's contention that older people generally would benefit from taking vitamin and mineral supplements. The study, designed by a physician at the Memorial Hospital of Newfoundland, Dr. Ranjit Kumar Chandra, showed that the control group of upper-class and upper-middle-class Canadians (who had standard diets for their age and economic group, adequate blood levels of nutrients, and no known serious or chronic illnesses) had the amount of infection-related illness they experienced reduced by more than 50 percent as a result of taking a daily supplement composed of eighteen vitamins and minerals. During the year of the study, the group that received the supplements had twenty-three days of infection-related illness; the control group that received no supplements had forty-eight days of infection-related illness. In addition, there was a statistically significant improvement in the immune systems of those who received the supplements.

These results were obtained with supplements that contained fairly modest quantities of the vitamins and minerals, on a study group of upper-income, well-nourished, healthy people. The study outcome underscores Pauling's view that absorption difficulties and the unpredictable quantities of nutrients available in food make it prudent for all older people to take vitamin and mineral supplements of some kind.

AVOID SMOKING

Four of the medical expert participants in the study had emphatic views about the long-term disadvantages of smoking. The first was the oldest participant, biochemist Dr. Michael Heidelberger, who began his interview by recalling that when he was in public school around 1900 his class was told point-blank that cigarettes were very dangerous.

"They called them 'coffin nails,'" he said. "It is really strange that it didn't make more of an impression on people. The advertising, I suppose, has kept it going. I was just reading an account of an autopsy that took place in 1909 of lung cancer. It was so rare that they called everybody in to see it. But they warned us about it in school before that."

During most of his career, Dr. William Cahan, a thoracic surgeon, has been centrally involved with the relationship between smoking and lung cancer. In the 1950s he designed an experiment that became famous because it ended up on the cover of *Life* magazine: utilizing a device that allowed dogs to smoke. It was the first experiment to establish clearly the connection between smoking and lung cancer. At the end of the study when the dogs were sacrificed, their lungs were black with tar and they were already beginning to suffer from heart problems and lung cancer. Cahan played a significant role in the passage of the legislation that placed the surgeon general's warning on cigarette packages; a decade later he helped rally support for passive-smoking legislation, which banned smoking in many restaurants, elevators, and airliners.

Dr. Alvar Svanborg's studies found that smoking had more of a negative impact on physical health than did abuse of alcohol—to the astonishment of the researchers, who anticipated the opposite. Dr. Linus Pauling contends that there is plentiful evidence in the medical research literature that smoking shortens the life span. "Scores of careful studies have been made in which the death rate of a population of cigarette smokers is compared with that of a similar population of nonsmokers," he writes. "The smokers die faster than the nonsmokers, at every age and with every larger number of cigarettes smoked, and they die at a greater rate from every disease. Their natural protective mechanisms are damaged to such an extent as to make them vulnerable to every assault." Pauling goes on to say that even the nonsmoking wives and husbands of smokers have a decreased life expectancy as a result of breathing their spouse's smoke.

Two out of the three study participants who died at the youngest age (sixty-seven) were former heavy smokers who had emphysema; and one lung cancer victim who died in his early seventies was a former heavy smoker. This means that three (14 percent) of the twenty-one study participants who had died by the time this book was written had illnesses directly derived from smoking. John Crystal was in a wheelchair most of the time when I interviewed him in Bend, Oregon, in August 1988. He died barely a month later, on September 10, after he returned to his Long Island home and the heavy, humid, smoggy air of a hot East Coast summer. Japan expert Robert Christopher, secretary of the Pulitzer Prize Committee at Columbia University, had been a journalist for three decades and smoked heavily for many years. In the fall of 1991, just after a celebration for the Pulitzer Prize's twenty-fifth anniversary, Christopher contracted pneumonia. It progressed rapidly because of his emphysema and his condition became critical. After six months of illness, he died in June 1992. Finally, former Peace Corps official and ambassador Franklin Williams developed lung cancer suddenly and died of it after a brief illness.

EXERCISE MODERATION IN DRINKING

Numerous studies have shown a slight longevity advantage in moderate alcohol consumption and a great disadvantage in heavy drinking. Dr. Linus Pauling cites a study (by Chope and Breslow) in San Mateo County, California, which found that moderate drinkers are healthier than teetotalers. People who take more than four drinks a day, however, are less healthy than either moderate drinkers or teetotalers.

CUT DOWN ON SUGAR

Another piece of precautionary advice from scientific studies is to reduce your intake of sugar. Research has shown that there is a high correlation between sugar intake and heart disease—a higher correlation, in fact, than there is between saturated fat consumption and heart disease.

Pauling cites two scientists whose work is particularly important on this subject. First, there is an extremely well-designed study by Milton Winitz that shows that cholesterol levels in the bloodstream rise significantly when sugar is added to the diet and decrease when sugar is removed. As sugar is broken down by the body, one of its components is turned into a chemical (acetate), which is used to synthesize cholesterol by the liver cells. Thus, whenever you eat sugar, you are increasing the amount of cholesterol in your bloodstream.

Second, English physiologist Dr. John Yudkin traced the original research showing a relationship between animal fat intake and heart attacks.[2] He discovered that in the populations included in that study, there was a much higher correlation between their sugar intake and their heart disease ratio than there was between saturated fat consumption and heart disease. In other words, sugar intake seemed to have a much closer relationship to coronary disease than did fat intake. The original research team was focusing on fat consumption, so they did not take sugar consumption into consideration and missed the even stronger link between sugar intake and heart disease.

KEEP COPIES OF YOUR MEDICAL RECORDS

Form the habit of getting copies of all your medical records from your physician and dentist as you go along. If you live eighty or a hundred years, you may outlive several different sets of physicians and dentists. For at least the first thirty years of your life, your doctors and dentists are likely to be considerably older than you are, and therefore may retire from practice or die long before you do. If you have copies of the records, you won't have to waste time and energy trying to remember thirty or forty years after the fact when a particular health event happened or what was done about it by whom.

BE AWARE OF HEREDITY

Take account of your genetic heritage. If there's a history of a particular condition in your family, like heart disease, stroke, or breast or ovarian cancer, find out what the early symptoms are so that you'll recognize them if they occur. When there are reasonable preventive measures you can take, take them.

BE CAUTIOUS ABOUT MAJOR CHANGES IN ROUTINE

Study participants stressed the importance of being very careful about abrupt or drastic changes in their routine as they got older, particularly in their nutrition regimen or activity level. If it's working, they said, don't tinker with it—at least not without carefully considering what the negative consequences might be.

To give one example of a change that had negative consequences: At eighty-five, Travelers Job Bank employee Elizabeth Burns was told by her personal physician that her cholesterol level was a trifle high and that she should stop drinking her daily two-to-three glasses of milk. She complied—and during the following year her height shrank two and a half inches. Her doctor had neglected to suggest an alternative source of calcium; so, deprived of the regular dose of calcium she had been accustomed to for many decades, her skeleton demineralized.

Dr. Linus Pauling cautions that if you are accustomed to a particular intake of nutrients—from any source, whether from food or from supplements—you should continue them or, if you do stop, taper off gradually. If you stop your intake suddenly, immediately afterward your body will actually deteriorate more rapidly than normal, as it struggles to adapt to the sudden change.

MANAGING STRESS EFFECTIVELY

A number of participants in the Long Careers Study said that in unusually stressful periods, especially major transitions such as completing an important project, leaving a primary job, or losing a relationship, they consciously tried to compensate for the stress by doing things that they enjoyed or being with people they liked.

When we began thinking about the deaths in the participant group, we realized that many of them had come in the wake of a significant life change or a major event of some kind. Five of the six cancer victims and three of the six heart disease victims had just finished a major project, stepped down from a primary job, or made plans to retire. Or they had a major professional or personal cause of stress in the two-year period before the onset of illness. In other words, seven out of thirteen (more than 50 percent) had life stresses whose presence indicated the possibility of a relationship among stress, the onset of illness, and the occurrence of death.

Several participants experienced a trauma that caused a change in their health. Alberta Jacoby, a filmmaker who taught at Yale University, was in an automobile accident in February 1992 that was extremely traumatic; she suffered injuries herself and the driver of the car, a younger woman who was a close friend, was killed. Within a few months Jacoby developed cancer, and she died in June 1992.

Another participant was working in a city office building that had a sudden blackout during the summer months. Since there was no electricity, this woman and others on her floor were forced to walk down a darkened stairwell four or five stories to the street. The experience was so traumatic that the woman's personality and functioning were changed by it. She was no longer able to function professionally as she had done up until then, and she found it necessary to give up most of her responsibilities shortly afterward. In effect, quite literally overnight, she went from being a well-functioning adult to being identifiably elderly, incapable of leading the relatively normal life she had maintained until that point.

Scientists have been aware for some time that there is a connection between life stress and illness, although there is still a certain degree of controversy about the subject. Certainly, there is enough evidence implicating life stress in the onset of many illnesses to warrant concerted attention. The feelings that are most likely to cause physical illness are the negative emotions that often remain buried; because they are suppressed, they can have a powerful effect on the immune and nervous system.

We do not know what changes in brain chemistry and functioning may be made when the brain is flooded with the powerful hormones stimulated by negative experiences such as terror, grief, and despair. It may be that a particularly powerful experience of that kind can cause permanent changes in brain chemistry or in cell functioning. The experiences of these two individuals, along with those of other members of the study, suggest that there is a great deal yet to be learned about the relationship among the mind, the emotions, and physical health.

Evidence suggests that there are a number of concrete things we can do to offset the impact of negative stress. One of the milestones in our understanding of the connection between mental states and physical health occurred in August 1964. After a month-long trip to the Soviet Union, *Saturday Review* editor Norman Cousins flew home to Connecticut, accompanied by his wife, Ellen; he was feeling exhausted and was running a slight fever. Cousins was hospitalized, but within a week his condition inexplicably worsened.

Doctors diagnosed his problem as ankylosing spondylitis, a disease of the body's collagen and connective tissue in which it literally falls apart. He was given one chance in five hundred to survive. The hospital staff tried to dull his excruciating pain by giving him large doses of aspirin and other medications.

Since medical science offered little help, Cousins decided to tackle the problem himself, based on the considerable knowledge about physical health he had accumulated through a lifetime of interest in the subject. First he decided not to accept the doctors' verdict that he was going to die. Then he began mentally examining the Soviet trip to try to decipher the reasons for his illness. He had been exposed to large doses of hydrocarbons from diesel and jet plane exhaust on the trip, and he had been extremely tired by a driver's mistake that took him five hours out of his way on his last night in Moscow. He concluded that the hydrocarbons in the exhaust had overstrained his immune system and that fatigue from the unwanted detour had imposed further stress, exhausting his adrenal glands. He also concluded that the aspirin and other drugs administered in the hospital were overstressing his system more, even while they reduced his pain.

Cousins knew that adrenal exhaustion involved vitamin C deficiency, that vitamin C supports the immune system as well as a host of other body functions. He was also familiar with research on placebos, which showed that positive emotions themselves can sometimes be a factor in restoring physical health. With the cooperation of his physician, Dr. William Hitzig, he reasoned that an intravenous drip of vitamin C to replenish the adrenal glands, along with a positive atmosphere (for example, watching reruns of "Candid Camera"), might help his condition.

After the first "Candid Camera" session, Cousins was able to get two hours of pain-free sleep, and he knew he was on the right track. But his laughter at the funny shows was disturbing the other patients, and the hospital's routines made demands on him that added to the stress of his illness. When four different technicians from four different labs visited him in one day, each demanding a blood sample, Cousins "had a fast-growing conviction that a hospital is no place for a person who is seriously ill," and he decided to check out. With Dr. Hitzig's help he moved to a hotel, where he could at least control his own environment. He improved steadily and eventually regained his full health.

Cousins was well known, and the story of his recovery got around. The editor of the *New England Journal of Medicine*, Franz Inglefinger (the same man who asked Lewis Thomas to start writing essays), asked whether he would be willing to write a piece for the *Journal*, and Cousins agreed. Its publication led to the suggestion that he write a book about the experience. *Anatomy of an Illness* was published in 1979 and quickly became a best-seller. Cousins's experience led many researchers to begin investigating the power of laughter and positive emotions in maintaining and restoring health. [3]

Cousins hoped that his book could communicate to people that they need to become more involved in their recovery from illness, and more responsible for participating in their own health care in general. He believed not that people should deny their diagnosis but that they should defy the verdict. He felt especially strongly that medical personnel should not discuss negative outcomes of a patient's case within the patient's hearing, even if the person is unconscious.

Like a number of participants in the Long Careers Study, Cousins believed that the solution to many problems people encounter in caring for their health is to learn as much as they can about their bodies and become, in a very real sense, their own health care consultants. Sometimes that might mean being "difficult": pushing their doctors to do additional tests if the symptom can't be explained; finding a different doctor if the one they're dealing with can't give satisfactory answers. But being difficult, he said, is better than being a mortality statistic.

In Cousins's ten years as an adjunct professor of medicine at UCLA's medical school, he played a key role in designing and directing research on the relationship of the mind and emotions to physical health. At the conclusion of the decade, Cousins and the UCLA scientists had shown that the mind has a significant impact upon the body. In one experiment, for example, Cousins had a blood sample drawn from his arm in a normal resting state and then spent five minutes thinking about the most positive things he could imagine. Then another sample was taken and compared with the first. In the second sample, there was an average increase of 53 percent in the various components of his immune system.

SUMMARY

The message that flows from this research is simple. Your emotions have an impact on your physical health: the brain and nervous system form one of the most widely distributed organ systems in the body. What happens in your brain affects the rest of your body. Because of this, positive emotions have a constructive effect on the entire physical body. If your life is satisfying, filled with positive events and good relationships, you are much more likely to stay in good shape. Happiness is good for your health.

The opposite conclusion follows: if you do not like your work and you are unhappy, you may be at risk. The most life-enhancing thing you can do for yourself is to change the situations that are causing your unhappiness, regardless of your age.

The Road Not Yet Traveled

MANAGING YOUR OWN CAREER

Originally I intended to subtitle this chapter, "Planning Your Own Career," but I decided against it for one reason: virtually none of the people in the Long Careers Study planned their careers, in the way we normally think of as career planning. In fact, more than half (51 percent) of the study participants said they had done little or no planning in developing their careers. Instead, chance or luck were cited by the participants far more often as having played an important role in the development of their careers: 78 percent said that luck was a major factor.

Moreover, it appears that this is not exceptional. When I mentioned this absence of planning among the interviewees to one career expert I know, she replied, "Oh, that's not unusual. Most people don't really plan their careers, even the most successful ones." While I was still digesting this, she added, "Of course, you can't *tell* people that!"

Later I asked another career expert about this. Richard Gummere had been for many years the innovative and widely respected head of admissions and career planning at Columbia University. He confirmed that most people don't plan, and that it's well known that they don't. In the 1960s, Gummere said, a long-term, multimillion-dollar, government-funded research project was mounted to analyze how people made successful career changes. "The only thing they found out," he commented ruefully, "was the tremendous importance of chance."

If most people—even the most successful ones—don't plan, and if chance is so important, then why do we bother? Why are we told we should engage in career planning? Why not just spend our time getting ice cream sodas and waiting to be discovered at the soda fountain, like the old story about Hollywood star Lana Turner? What's going on, anyway?

What's going on is this: career counselors know that planning is important as a failsafe in case luck doesn't materialize when you want it to. The trouble with luck is that you can't produce it at will, you can only be ready to grasp it when it appears. The rest of the time, you're on your own.

It is true that by and large the Long Careers Study participants didn't plan their careers. But this wasn't done as a matter of principle; they didn't consciously decide not to plan their careers. Rather, they seemed to depend much of the time on *process* instead of *planning*.

Most of us don't really know what career planning is or how to do it. We spend more time working than in any other single activity except sleep, yet our actual knowledge about how to find the right work, what makes one kind of work ideal for one person and torture for the next, how to assess our ongoing relationship to our work, and how to manage change in our work life, is probably less developed than our knowledge of any other practical area of everyday life.

But the fact that most people don't plan their careers and don't know how to doesn't mean that planning isn't a good thing, or that it doesn't work. "Nearly all of the planning we've been taught has been organizationally related," says Nella Barkley, cofounder of the Crystal-Barkley Center. "A lot of people view planning as a straitjacket. I don't; I view it as a very flexible tool. When it's done well, it allows lots of room for serendipitous things to happen, but it gives you a template that is accurate for moving ahead."

Barkley sees personal planning as a smaller-scale version of organizational planning. "People don't see the language of management planning as applicable to their personal dilemmas," she said. "But it is, and it *does* work. Any good planning is the same thing: a strategic way to look at your future and make things turn out the way you want them to."

What this means is that developing your career is a two-level process. Because there are so many chance elements in life, a tightly structured, abstract plan can't take all of them into account, so you can't just put together a career plan in your head and have it work out exactly that way in reality. Career development is a combination of inner desires and traits (who you are, what you're good at, what you want to do) and external factors (the job market in your community, whether your company is growing or shrinking, the state of the national economy, whether the nation is at war or at peace, the current development of manufacturing and technology, and so on).

So you need to plan while simultaneously adjusting the plan constantly as you live with it. Career or life-work planning is a mixture of the theoretical and the practical, because it has to be.

FINDING THE WORK YOU LOVE

Regardless of your age, your occupation, or your level of responsibility, a long lifetime provides a lot of time for unhappiness if you don't like your work. Perhaps the most often repeated phrase in the Long Careers Studies interviews was, "I love what I do"—and the most common advice the participants gave was, "Find work you love." Noted career expert Richard Bolles quoted Joseph Campbell's famous admonition to "follow your bliss." Psychotherapist Dr. Lawrence LeShan gave similar advice: "Find something that would make you glad to get up in the morning and glad to go to bed at night. And settle for nothing less."

The participants in the Long Careers Study told me over and over how much they loved what they did. "What I work with is the most important thing in the world," said ninety-one-year-old Sayra Lebenthal of her role as chairman of the bond company she and her husband founded in 1926. "Money is what enables people to keep living and to keep paying the bills. There's nothing more meaningful to me than helping people to take intelligent care of their money." Frances Etter, eighty-year-old Memphis real estate broker, said the same thing, in almost exactly the same words: "I love real estate. There's nothing more important than helping people to find a home. What I do is just the most important thing I can think of." And the participants who stopped liking their work, or began liking it less, went out and found something else.

Loving your work is not only important and valuable in maintaining a long career, it may be vital in staying healthy as well. Dr. Lawrence LeShan earned his widest fame as a psychological researcher and a therapist. He was the first scientist to identify and document the role of negative emotional factors—loss, grief, and hopelessness—in the onset of cancer. As part of this research, for many years LeShan served as a therapist for cancer patients, many of whom were terminally ill. He discovered that a number of these patients were deeply unhappy with their work. As an experiment, LeShan devised his own method of teaching them how to find out what they wanted to do. Since they had nothing to lose, many of them went along with it. Using this strategy for career change in conjunction with ongoing therapy, LeShan was eventually able to achieve a 50 percent long-term remission rate in people with terminal cancer.

The implications of this remarkable result have not been followed up very widely by psychologists in general. But it bears repeating: LeShan's research indicates that doing work that you love is not just good for your day-to-day happiness, it is good for your health. And in the long run, it is a positive factor in survival. The message is very clear: if you don't like what you're doing now, don't just sit there. Get busy and find something you like better.

CAREER ADVICE FROM THREE EXPERTS

Three Long Careers Study participants had significant skills in helping people to plan or restructure their work lives. John Crystal, Richard Bolles, and Dr. Lawrence LeShan each had developed a system for finding the right work and for changing careers. In addition, the organization Operation Able runs extremely useful career planning services at each of its offices.

JOHN CRYSTAL: THE CRYSTAL-BARKLEY METHOD

John Crystal, the late cofounder of the Crystal-Barkley Center, invented what has become one of the most popular job search methods used today. He developed it in the course of seeking a job for himself just after the World War II. It utilizes personal assessment and survey techniques to target a particular company or job. In addition to interviewing Crystal before his death, I also interviewed his partner at the Crystal-Barkley Center, Nella Barkley.

During World War II, John Crystal had served in intelligence in North Africa and Europe. "In other words," he said, "I was a spy." He had had tremendously challenging and difficult assignments, which he enjoyed to the hilt. When Crystal returned to the United States and began looking for a civilian job, he realized that he was being stereotyped and that he was sometimes given short shrift by placement agencies because he had been a spy. "A spy can do some really amazing things," Crystal noted, "but he can't prove that he can do them. He has no pieces of paper." When you're a spy, of course, all that matters is having the skills; if you don't have them you won't be around very long to look for another job anyway.

But the placement agencies seemed to care more about the pieces of paper than the skills themselves, and Crystal's lack of credentials was a real handicap. When he visited employment agencies he was constantly being asked to prove his abilities by submitting diplomas or transcripts, neither of which existed for his on-the-job "spook" training. One job listing, for example, said that fluent spoken Italian would be an advantage. Crystal could speak Italian fluently; he had learned to do so in Italy. But it wasn't enough for the placement agencies that he could actually speak fluent Italian; they wanted to be presented with some kind of formal certification. To add to his irritation, the employment agencies' staff couldn't speak any foreign language at all and couldn't recognize spoken Italian when they heard it!

Frustrated by the mindlessness and bureaucracy of the job hunt, Crystal decided to attack the problem as if it were an intelligence assignment, and figure out how to solve it himself. He started by asking himself a series of questions. Where did he want to be? What kind of abilities did he want to use the most? And what effect did he want his work to have?

First, he realized that he wanted to be in Europe. He had found the reentry to the United States difficult after the challenge and excitement of his war experience. He had spent four years in Europe and wanted to go back, partly because he knew that there was an enormous amount of rebuilding to be done there, and he wanted to help.

Second, Crystal wanted a position where he could exercise his leadership and problem-solving skills and where he could be his own boss. "Ex-spies are very bad at being supervised," he commented wryly.

Third, he wanted to help people. People in various European countries were having difficulty in getting just the bare necessities of life after the war—pots and pans, blankets and sweaters and shoes. He had seen this repeatedly and wanted to be able to help change it.

Once Crystal had thought this through, the next step seemed clear to him: he needed a company that dealt with everyday necessities of life, did not already have a European operation, and might be interested in starting one. He went to a business school office and asked whether they knew of a company like that. The answer was immediate: Sears, Roebuck.

Through his network of friends Crystal found a college classmate whose uncle had gone to school with the chairman of Sears, Roebuck. Crystal asked the classmate to call his uncle and set up an appointment with the chairman for him, and then he got on a train and went to Chicago, where Sears, Roebuck was headquartered. The visit was a success. "Fifteen minutes after I got there," Crystal recalled, "the chairman said, 'It's a wonderful idea, young man. I've been thinking about this for a long time. How would you like to start as our first manager?'"

In today's job market, this story may sound too fantastic to be believed, but it is true. Crystal worked for Sears, Roebuck as head of its European operations for twelve years, until the chairman who hired him stepped down. Then he returned to the United States. Eventually he began using what he knew about work and career change to help others, founding the Crystal-Barkley Center with Nella Barkley.

Using Crystal's technique, your first step is to decide what is most important to you, regardless of what that might be. The next step is to evaluate your priorities in terms of your present work. In many cases it is possible to restructure your current job or to propose a change in position to your company, which will give you work closer to what you want. If you decide to move to a different field or opportunity, you then enter an information-gathering phase to pinpoint the type of work you prefer and the kind of company you might approach.

Although John Crystal died in September 1988, his work is being carried on by his charismatic partner, Nella Barkley. The Crystal-Barkley Center offers a five-day course at its New York City headquarters. In addition, it has developed a software package that puts a self-directed version of the five-day course at your fingertips, if you prefer to reassess your life at home and on your own timetable.

Crystal-Barkley's materials are extremely useful if you are dissatisfied with what you do but don't know how to get to the next step. The center does not provide leads on particular jobs or other immediate and specific help if day-to-day survival is an issue, but its programs offer an exercise in self-exploration that can lead you eventually to a far more satisfying career.

RICHARD BOLLES: THE PARACHUTE METHOD

Richard Bolles is a Midlife Transformer whose unexpected career change ultimately has influenced millions of people because it led to the creation of the best-selling career change manual of all time, *What Color Is Your Parachute?*[1]

Bolles began his career as a minister in the Episcopal church in 1953. After seminary and service in several New Jersey parishes, he was called to Grace Cathedral in San Francisco, where he was one of a staff of four clergy working under the bishop and dean. In 1968 there was an unexpected budget crunch, and to Bolles's surprise, he was laid off, after only two years there.

The experience proved to be life changing. In one sense Bolles landed on his feet: he got a job within six months, this time with a church-related organization, the United Ministries in Higher Education, a coalition of ten denominations. But the experience of suddenly being jobless made a profound impression on him. In this new job, one of his functions was to oversee campus ministries in nine western states. Many of the people he was supervising and visiting were also about to lose their jobs; the "religious revival" of the 1950s and early 1960s was coming to an end. They were finding themselves out of work, just as Bolles had. And they asked him what they should do.

So Bolles set out on a quest: he wanted to pull together a helpful little manual on career change for these campus ministers, telling them what to do and what pitfalls to avoid. He read every book on job hunting he could find (there were eight of them at the time). In his new job he traveled a great deal around the United States, and he made it his business to find career experts in each city to which his job carried him.

In early 1970, Bolles encountered John Crystal, who at that time was living near Washington, D.C., and was little known.

Crystal and Bolles liked each other immediately, so when Bolles told him of his quest, Crystal responded by sending Bolles, week in and week out, envelopes stuffed with notes and clippings he had saved about the whole career change process. With this added material, Bolles's little manual for campus ministers turned out to be 160 pages long; it was self-published December 1, 1970.

The unusual name of the manual came about in an interesting way. At an area staff meeting of United Ministries in 1969, members were calling out proposed agenda items, which Bolles, who was nearest the blackboard, was writing out for them. One staff member said, "Remember, we need to talk about these guys who have to bail out of campus ministry." Bolles wrote on the blackboard, "What color is your parachute?" The others were much amused. More than a year later, when Bolles put his little manual together, he remembered the laughter and made that phrase the title of his book.

Two years after Bolles first self-published *What Color Is Your Parachute,* Berkeley, California, publisher Phil Wood of Ten-Speed Press sought him out and offered to publish the book commercially. Bolles rewrote the book for a larger audience, and it first appeared with the Ten-Speed imprimatur in November 1972. It has since sold well over four and a half million copies and is currently available in eight languages throughout the world.

Bolles's life was completely changed by *Parachute*'s popularity. It gave him a whole new career, and freedom from worrying about how to support himself. I should add that he probably works much harder in this new ministry than the church would ever have asked him to. Since 1976, he has revised *Parachute* every year, a task that consumes an enormous amount of time, sometimes involving, as in 1992, completely rewriting the book for a new era.

For some twenty years Bolles had lectured extensively in the United States, Canada, and Great Britain. But now he restricts his teaching to one event a year, a two-week intensive workshop on life/work planning, taught with his European friend Daniel Porot each August in Bend, Oregon. People from all over the world attend the seminar. As part of my research for the Long Careers Study I participated in one of these workshops myself. It is an extraordinarily rich and thought-provoking experience, and it is also hard (but rewarding) work. Bolles is currently working on two new writing projects: a book on relationships and a book on practical spirituality.

One tool that Bolles recommends and uses in his workshop is a skills classification system developed by famed vocational psychologist John Holland. Holland has classified over twelve-thousand job titles (and eight thousand duplicate titles) according to the skills, personality traits, and people environments linked to each job. He has sorted these into six basic categories, or codes, which greatly simplifies the task of choosing a new career once you know what your present preferred skills, traits, and people environments are. Basic information on the Holland system, together with a listing of the various related resources, is included in *Parachute*. Resources of this kind are important because most of us know very little about the enormous variety of occupations that exist.

Richard Bolles's method took some of his friend John Crystal's processes as a starting point. But Bolles has multiplied and expanded his basic fund of information and techniques many times over in the twenty-two years since *Parachute* first appeared. The workshop has a heavy spiritual framework and emphasis, as do current editions of *Parachute*. When asked why he thinks the book has been so successful, Bolles told me, "I think it is a healing book masquerading as a job-hunting manual." He sees the search for a new job or career as inevitably a spiritual journey. The job hunt, he says, creates a pause in your life

in which you are given the chance to reexamine the fundamental principles that animate your life, along with your perceptions of your experience. What are the basic things you are trying to do with your life? What are the basic beliefs you have about your life and the world and God? During this process, you must choose the attitude you wish to have; and the attitude you choose about the job hunt will be the attitude you have about life. You can see it all as a possible series of problems, or as a possible series of opportunities. You will only use it well if you see the whole experience as basically a friend to your life, from which new growth and happiness will eventually come.

DR. LAWRENCE LESHAN: THE EXPERIENTIAL METHOD

The process of career exploration created by Dr. Lawrence LeShan in his therapeutic work is simple and relatively unstructured. But, like the Bolles and Crystal techniques, it requires a good deal of deep self-examination.

"The first thing," LeShan says, "is to make a commitment to yourself to find out what you want to do." Fundamentally that means making this process of discovery your central concern, for however long it takes to come up with the answer. Ask yourself, What do I enjoy when I watch myself during the day? Or if you don't particularly enjoy what you do, what *would* you enjoy doing?

To make room for this process, LeShan suggests setting aside specific time for it: take one afternoon a week just to do whatever you want to do. This means starting the process by focusing on what you would like to do in the present moment and in a non-work activity. As you experiment with finding out what you want to do with one afternoon of your time every week, you will make it possible for feelings about other parts of your life to surface as well.

LeShan says that at the beginning of this process, most people don't really know what they would best like to do. But what's important is to start. If you think you would like to take a walk in the park, then take a walk in the park. Or you may want to go to the theater. But then when you go, you may find that you don't really like the theater any more. Or you may think you want to play a musical instrument but discover when you try it that you hate practicing. Doing this will take time, LeShan adds, but the very act of working at it will make the inner voices that you've lost touch with slowly begin to speak louder.

LeShan believes that there should be certain restrictions to this process. His rules are that during the time you set aside, you can't do anything to get ready for the rest of the week, and you can't do chores you haven't yet had time to do, like your laundry or cleaning your apartment. The night before, you should spend an hour thinking about what you would like to do and making up your mind about the next day.

At first this process will not be easy. You may well spend one or several afternoons wandering around, still trying to come up with an answer to the question of what you want to do with your afternoon! But after a certain period of time, "you stop staring at the ceiling and you get new ideas," LeShan says, "because staring at the ceiling is boring. You may try something you wanted to do in childhood, or something totally new that you've never thought of before. But in any case, you will begin to get to know yourself in a different way. Some things will work, and some things won't, but gradually you'll come to a sense of what you would rather do than anything else."

Although he is a psychologist, LeShan does not believe that psychological testing services have much value in finding a new career choice. "Once in a while psychological tests are useful," he says. "What they are really useful for, it seems to me, is that these services usually have long lists of jobs. And you look these over and sometimes something catches your eye. Beyond that, I don't think they're the least bit useful. That isn't the way you do it. *You* happen to be the world's leading authority—nobody even comes close to second place—on how you feel, and what you enjoy, and what you don't enjoy."

"People aren't quantitative," LeShan says. "They don't fit quantitative scales. Anytime [you fit] into a quantitative scale, you're doing one of two things: either you're measuring a very unimportant aspect of [yourself], like how many times in an hour do you have a little puff of air, or take a drink, or blink. Really unimportant. Or else, you're dealing with a very damaged person. Nothing else gets onto a quantitative scale. People are unpredictable."

LeShan's approach describes the path taken by most of the study participants: do what you love, and if you don't know what that is, spend some time looking around.

BUILDING A LONG CAREER

The experiences of the Long Careers Study participants are extremely instructive when taken as a whole in suggesting many steps to take in building a long career. These steps are very useful for those making changes later in life as well as those starting out in their careers because the same elements should be included in the evolution of every career, no matter what age you are.

FOLLOWING (OR FINDING) AN ASPIRATION

At some point relatively early in their lives, all the participants formed an idea of the kind of work they thought they wanted to do. This process was usually spontaneous, even haphazard. Only about 10 percent of the participants had strong specific childhood

aspirations to which they remained committed as they grew
up, and this group consisted mainly of Homesteaders. Some
formed childhood aspirations that they then outgrew, like J. Peter
Grace's and Milton Petrie's desire to be baseball players. Others
formed aspirations as children that they would set aside and then
fulfill many years later in a second or third career, like John W.
Gardner, Lewis Thomas, Frances Lear, and Helen Breed. A number began their real careers late in life, like Evelyn Nef and Toy
Lasker, and in areas that they had never previously imagined
being engaged in.

Most participants, however, had a variety of childhood ambitions but formed their real career goals in their late teens and
early twenties. Many did a lot of looking around before they
found what they really wanted to do. Occasionally, friends, relatives, or teachers served as role models, or suggested a field that
the participant then decided to explore.

Some of these incidents were astonishingly serendipitous.
James B. Lewis, a highly successful tax lawyer at Paul Weiss
Rifkind in New York, began his career as a Treasury Department
employee in Washington; he enrolled in a night law school program quite literally to keep a friend company, because the friend
needed someone to talk to about the work. Shirley Brussell's
teacher in one of her University of Chicago undergraduate classes
sent everyone in the class to take a civil service exam one day, for
practice in exam taking. Knowing that it didn't matter whether
she passed or failed, Brussell was completely relaxed, and she
sailed through the questions. On the basis of that exam, Brussell
was one of two people from Illinois who were offered fellowship
appointments in Washington; it launched her on her first career as
a personnel officer.

Former secretary of labor Willard Wirtz ultimately found his
first job at the Department of Labor as a result of being bored
with the food in the cafeteria of the agency where he worked at
the time. He decided to go across the street for lunch one day, to
the Labor Department cafeteria. There he ran into a casual
acquaintance, Lloyd Garrison. The two had lunch together and
Garrison suggested that Wirtz apply for a job in the Labor
Department. He did; ultimately, after returning to the private
practice of law for a time, he became secretary of labor under
presidents Kennedy and Johnson.

In summary, a few people do decide what they want to be

very early in life—beginning as early as age two and a half. But they're the minority. If you didn't figure out what you wanted to do by the age of five, don't worry: it just means that you're like most of the rest of us. One thing that is reassuring about the study participants' experience is that they have been successful regardless of whether they knew what they wanted to do early or had to go through a long search process (like Marvin Bower, Oscar Dystel, and Studs Terkel). The people who had to work to find their careers are in the vast majority.

In addition, as we have seen, the Transformers and the Explorers reevaluated their career goals and changed courses at various points. Many of them who had pursued careers different from their childhood aspirations returned to those early aspirations to fulfill them much later in life. If you find your career to be less satisfying than you had hoped and are considering a change, think back to your early aspirations to see if they might lead you in a new direction.

There is also a message here for parents who want to encourage their children's career success. First of all, never belittle a child, no matter how young, who proclaims that he or she wants to be something specific when he or she grows up. The child could be right—and you could be guilty of squelching the ambition of a future Isaac Asimov, Will Barnet, Françoise Gilot, Celeste Holm, Linus Pauling, or Henny Youngman. The only way to know whether the child will maintain the interest is to respect it and support the child in following it. If the child does persist, you will always have the satisfaction of knowing that your encouragement helped make it possible. If he or she outgrows it, you will get to go through the process all over again with a different career objective, perhaps several times. But this testing process is important, it's how both children and adults find out whether a particular career really fits them—and almost everyone needs to do it.

Second, if your child has a lot of trouble figuring out exactly what he or she wants to do, don't give up; stick with it. If the formal paths to self-discovery peter out, then look at what the child gravitates to in his leisure time—what he does and enjoys naturally—and try to relate it to possible adult occupations. If, like comedian Henny Youngman, your child has a talent that you find unsettling, try to see if there's a positive spin to it somewhere—and keep on trying. In the long run, the most important quality in success may be simple persistence. To paraphrase Groucho Marx: 85 percent of finding the right career is just showing up.

GETTING TRAINED

The participants' next step was usually to seek training for the occupation selected. This could mean enrolling in an educational program—for example, law school or commercial school—or in a company training program of some kind. Occasionally, if the person was still in high school or college, he or she would get a summer job as a way of becoming familiar with the work and finding out whether he or she liked it.

In short, what they did at this point was to engage themselves in some way in their chosen work. In doing this, the participants didn't look at what they had selected as temporary. They didn't say to themselves, "I'll try this out and see if it works." They threw themselves into it. They assumed that it would work and that they were going to do it.

This real involvement in the new job or field was important. The new job didn't always turn out to be what they wanted or expected. But even if they didn't stay in this first line of work, their whole-hearted commitment was a key factor. Because they put everything they had into it, if it didn't appeal to them they knew it wasn't from a lack of zeal on their part. So they felt no qualms or hesitation about changing. In addition, sometimes their good performance in the first job led them to another job that was much better but which probably wouldn't have been offered if their performance had been mediocre in the original position.

For a number of people the first job turned into a stage in which they learned more about themselves—their likes and dislikes, their talents and blind spots. For others it turned out to be the path they would follow for the rest of their lives.

WHO YOU KNOW—CREATING AND USING PERSONAL NETWORKS

Most of the participants relied heavily on their personal networks in getting jobs and seeking career changes. By far the majority of their job changes were made as a result of contacts from the individual's network of personal and professional acquaintances. At times these contacts were close friends, but just as often they were more distant friends or casual acquaintances.

However, it's not just a matter of knowing the right people; most of the participants were not well connected at the beginning of their careers. They developed their networks as they went along, in school, in their jobs, through friends and family. Often the person who was instrumental was someone the participant never would have expected. Part of the reason for relying on personal networks is that there weren't very many career-change resources available during the lifetimes of the study participants.

Bolles, Barkley, and Crystal all agreed that personal networks are still a very effective way of trying to find new opportunities. Bolles says that often it is the people you *don't* see frequently (those who live far away from you or who are in a field of work different from yours) who are the most useful contacts in a job hunt. They can bounce you back into different networks in your own area. Your close friends are people you see often, and your network and theirs may overlap to a great extent. It's the people you don't see as often who may be able to put you in touch with opportunities you wouldn't otherwise have known about.

There seemed to be a basic intellectual assumption among people in the Long Careers group that personal networks are the most important source of job change information—that this was how things happened. That is something of a contrast with the attitudes widespread today, when the basic assumption seems to be that if you are looking for a job, you answer advertisements and send out hundreds of resumes. Bolles, Crystal, and Barkley say that, by and large, only relatively small numbers of people actually find jobs through résumé mailings and through reading the want ads. You may get lucky, and it's worth a try, if it doesn't distract you from other aspects of your search. But don't consider résumés and want ads to be the core of your job search efforts because the percentage of people who actually get jobs that way is fairly small.

TESTING YOUR DECISIONS

Many of the participants went through a long, conscious process of making decisions, observing the results, and adjusting their decision-making process based on feedback from events and from other people they trusted. They understood that *how* they did things was as important as *what* they did. They thought about the consequences of their actions and the possible outcomes depending on the choices they made. They used their own lives as a kind of learning laboratory, looking at results and evaluating them from various perspectives.

TRUSTING YOUR INTUITION

Several times participants told me about instances when their decision-making process seemed logically to lead in one direction, but their intuitive response was to go in another. John Loeb, for example, ran the risk of deeply disappointing his father when he decided to leave his father's metals company, but his instinctive attraction to the field of finance led him into a field where he was magnificently successful (and where his father went also).

Test your intuition and learn from your own experience when to trust it. Your intuitive sense of direction can be your most useful resource; it can steer you in directions that your mind alone might not be able to find because the necessary information is not available.

MAKING CHANGES

For the participants, the ability to make productive changes was one of the qualities most necessary to developing a long career. As we have seen in the Transformers and Explorers chapters, the majority of the participants—fully two-thirds of the group—changed careers at least once. Over and over in the interviews, the participants talked about the importance of making changes in their careers. The right kind of career change can bring a renewed sense of vitality and commitment to your work.

Because of the rapid growth of knowledge and the higher rate of turnover in the job market, more careers in the 1990s and the twenty-first century are likely to resemble those of the Explorers. Census Bureau estimates show that most adults change their line of work four or five times now; in the future, with added longevity and longer work lives, it is predicted that the average person will have eight different jobs throughout their work life.

It works best, therefore, to think of your career as a succession of stages, each leading into the next, and as a long-term enterprise. Don't assume that you will be ready to stop at any particular chronological age. Once you are in a job, don't be afraid to explore the possibility of change if the work turns out not to be what you expected, or if circumstances change so that the situation is no longer rewarding.

The participants changed jobs for a variety of reasons, which are useful to examine. Knowing when to make a change is crucial in making the right change. The following are several of the most prevalent reasons for career change that the participants mentioned:

• *They were dissatisfied with their present work or career.* Either the actual work turned out to be different from the way it appeared from the outside, or in practice it did not provide satisfactions that were important to them.

Then, as now, it is hard to tell what a job will really be like until you are actually in it. You may discover that it doesn't work the way you thought it would. It may look glamorous and be boring, like Studs Terkel's civil service job. Or it may just not be a good fit for your talents or personality.

• *They knew how to do everything their work required and they were restless.* Usually this took a certain amount of time to develop—sometimes three or four years, sometimes as long as forty years. (The Homesteaders, of course, never got to this point.)

• *Someone happened to offer them a different job.* These were almost all chance occurrences, most of which took place via their network of personal and professional acquaintances. For example, Franklin E. Williams, former ambassador to Ghana and one of the founding members of the Peace Corps, changed roles many times in his career, responding to new opportunities and unexpected offers. He commented: "It's hard for me to be objective [about change] because circumstances dictated my changing and I have found that both beneficial to me and satisfying."

• *Their financial needs changed.* A handful of participants changed careers, usually early in their work lives (but not in every case) because they realized they could not otherwise make enough money to do something they needed or wanted to do: have a family, send their children to college, help a relative in some way.

• *They or someone else in their family became seriously ill.* Two men changed their work so they could make more money, one to support a child who was born with serious birth defects and the other because his wife had developed a serious illness. Several people took time off from work temporarily to care for ill relatives—a parent, sister, brother, husband, or wife. Two participants became seriously ill at relatively young ages and found that their attitudes changed substantially afterward; when they went back to work both became much more involved in philanthropy and helping other people, outside their working hours.

So if you go into a particular kind of work and it doesn't measure up in practice, don't agonize—just marshal your energies to find something that's a better fit.

MOST IMPORTANT—FINDING MEANING IN YOUR WORK

In summary, it takes many different kinds of activity and effort to keep the world running. Your chance of making your maximum contribution is directly related to how meaningful your own work is to you. It doesn't matter so much what that work is; what matters is how you feel about it. In the long run it is worth spending a little time exploring in order to find a job that really makes your heart leap. When you've found it, Richard Bolles says, your work becomes a pleasure rather than a job or a chore.

GREENER PASTURES, GOLDEN PONDS:
MANAGING YOUR RETIREMENT

In the 1990s, when many people are still vigorous in their seventies and a good number remain so in their eighties, there is no reason to withdraw from anything if you are healthy, enjoy what you do, and are still getting good feedback from your environment. Whatever you do after the age of sixty-five is an opportunity to use and build on everything you have learned and experienced before.

If you are thinking seriously of leaving a primary job and taking a form of retirement, at whatever age, there are a few general principles that you should bear in mind, regardless of whether it is a retirement that you choose or one that you have thrust upon you.

IS YOUR WORK STILL THE CENTER OF YOUR LIFE?

This question has a different answer for each individual. Many of the people in the Long Careers Study would have answered it affirmatively, though not all. What matters is *your* answer, not that of anyone else.

If your work is still the center of your existence, if it is the thing you look forward to every morning when you get up, if your identity is built into what you do in such an intricate way that you and your work can't really be separated—then maybe you shouldn't retire, in the classic sense.

One participant, psychotherapist Penelope Russianoff, described this dilemma perfectly: "I think the notion of retiring makes people old. For example, a man who retires sits at home and wonders what's going on back at the office; he'd really like to make some of those good deals again, he'd like to strategize and so on. But it depends on the value of your job [to you]. If you're doing some job that is simply awful, then retirement looks great."

At the very least, you should think long and hard about how you would structure your time and what you would do in the absence of your current work. As Judge Simon Rifkind commented, "If somebody was considering retiring, I would say: What are your alternatives? Have you some alternative activity that you think you might be interested in?" People whose work is really part of their inner nature often have great difficulty leaving it, and sometimes never find an adequate substitute. Like Sam Goody, they may spend the rest of their lives mourning their lost role.

If you're still engaged in your work but would like to shift your priorities somewhat, there are ways of allowing more flexibility in your schedule and giving yourself the freedom to add other activities to your life. If you want to travel more, you can take more or longer vacations; if you want more free time, you can experiment with alternatives to full retirement, such as cutting back to a four-day week. Many people who retire simply because they think it's the thing to do are unhappy later because they cannot find a good replacement for the work they loved and gave up.

THE NEXT STEP

If you are ready to move on from what you are doing now, then retirement can free you for activities that are closer to the heart of your own interests, whatever they are. In that case your planning time should be devoted to identifying resources you can use and to building a new base for yourself in whatever activities you want to engage in. It's important to be realistic about interests you've never had the opportunity to develop before. If, for example, you've always dreamed of writing a novel, it may not be as easy as you think to begin. Former director of the American Ethical Union and currently head of the Humanist Institute in New York, Jean Kotkin explained this problem from her own experience: "All my life I've said to myself, 'If I only had time to write!' But the thought of doing nothing but writing is scary. Now, if I have to write on a certain subject, it's done fast. But to pull something out of my head and write about it—well, it's the fear of just sitting there with that word processor in front of me and having to produce something without a goal."

Many participants saw retirement as changing careers rather than ceasing to work. As Janet Sainer, the creator of the Retired Senior Volunteers Program, put it, "I think of retirement as retiring to the next step of what you plan to do in the next stage of your life." Psychologist Dr. Kenneth Clark described his own retirement from teaching as "changing focus."

If you approach your retirement in this manner, looking for the next step becomes very similar to the typical job search process. All the comments in the last chapter about how to find the right career can be applied to finding the right post-retirement work for you. In fact, your options are less limited now because you have one or several careers behind you that provide you with a base of financial security and experience.

MAKING PLANS

Although most of the study participants did not plan their careers in the sense that we normally understand as planning, the one exception to this was when the participant left a primary job at an age past sixty. In most cases, these transitions were planned to a greater or lesser degree. Pollster Florence Skelly feels that this planning is crucial, especially for people like herself whose main interest is their work. "I'm so work-centered that I don't have a tremendous amount of other interests. I wouldn't be able to go into other areas immediately," she explained. "You just don't retire and get involved in a big way in volunteer activity, for example. You have to start earlier."

The people who made the transitions most successfully invariably created a base for themselves somewhere else, while they were still in their primary job. When the time came for the transition, they moved from the primary job to the new base in a relatively seamless process. In other words, they made sure there was something to go to instead of just leaving their existing job.

Engineering this kind of shift takes time. There was a transition period of one to three years during which the person was looking for, finding, and building up the new base, while they were still operating from the primary base. Film producer David Brown, when asked what his advice would be to someone thinking of retirement, came up with a novel strategy. "First of all, I'd cut my standard of living by possibly moving to a less costly place, if I lived in a large city," he said. "Then I would look around and see what services are needed. Is there a messenger service required? Is there something in the community that is not being provided? Then I would go and try to raise money, a modest amount of capital, not putting my own money in (because I need it for the rest of my life!). I would try to sell someone on coming in and staking me to a business, after doing careful market research."

SLOW FADE-OUT: FROM EMPLOYEE TO CONSULTANT

In general, it does not seem to be reliable to expect a part-time or consulting relationship with the company where you had your primary job to last beyond one or two years. Several people in the group tried such arrangements; invariably they proved temporary, and the person felt less than fully satisfied with such a position.

If you have been deeply involved in your work and have held a position of some power or influence, being a part-time consultant can feel like being a football player who got sidelined in the middle of an exciting game. The organization will move on; someone else will take your old job; new projects will appear that will consume others' energies but in which you are not directly involved. As more time passes you are likely to feel more and more peripheral because the nature and degree of your participation has been massively diluted.

COMING TO TERMS WITH MANDATORY RETIREMENT

The decision to retire is not always one that an individual makes freely. Mandatory retirement rules were significantly reduced in their impact in 1978, when mandatory retirement was legally abolished. But in practice some companies have managed to keep the effect while calling it something else.

Early retirement offers have replaced mandatory retirement rules at many companies; the impact in the long run is very much the same, except that it moves people out of the work force even earlier than mandatory retirement did.

If you love your work but are in an organization that has an obligatory retirement policy, then you need to confront well before retirement the fact that you may have to find another kind of work when you reach that age. In this situation, anger, denial, and grief are common reactions that can keep you from coming to terms with the separation until it is too late to create another position conveniently. These are stages that must be worked through before you can move on to something else—ideally, before you leave—so that your feelings won't be obstacles in finding your next position.

DON'T JUST QUIT

If you do decide to retire, don't just stop working suddenly. Sudden, drastic changes in your activity level can trigger psychological or physiological problems in people of any age, but the reaction may be more marked in older people.

If you are accustomed to a certain level of activity and to the stimulation of work—being around other people, being involved in projects, learning new things, going from home to the office every day, visiting other organizations or traveling—then having nowhere in particular to go and nothing in particular to do can be an unsettling and even unpleasant experience.

Many retirees do not realize how different the pace of their lives will be after retirement, and they are both physically and psychologically unprepared for it, especially if they have been in a highly structured organization, surrounded by people and stimuli.

Medical research in recent years has shown that the causes of illness are not as simple as we once believed. The mind and the body are interconnected in ways our science has only begun to explore. Such phenomena as anniversary deaths (deaths that take place on a date associated with a tragic event) and illness resulting from a change in activity level (the weekend migraine and the vacation heart attack, which occur when a usually tense and active person slows down to a stop during a supposedly relaxing time) were identified only very recently.

Drastically and suddenly changing your activity level is stressful for your whole system, regardless of whether you have speeded up or slowed down. Everyone in the field of aging hears anecdotes about people who are in good health when they retire and who then become ill or die. Almost all the people I interviewed referred to one or two people they had known personally who were examples of this. Aging experts for many years rationalized these stories by saying that the person was already ill and retired because they weren't feeling well in the first place.

The real-life facts behind these stories are almost certainly more complex than the surface appearances. One thing is clear, however, from what we now know about the interrelationship of the mind and the body: loss and unhappiness can create a climate within the body that leads to illness, and a sudden change in activity level can upset the body's equilibrium.

GIVE YOURSELF SOME TIME

Retirement is a more definitive break than an ordinary job change. If anything, it needs more cautious planning than an ordinary career shift. It is seen as a move out of the working world altogether. As such, it is often considerably harder to undo if it doesn't work. If you've sold essential assets, for example, there is ordinarily no way to get them back.

If you have several options before you, some that are reversible and some that aren't, see if you can stage them so that you take the reversible steps first. Then test your reactions and the response of your environment at each step. If the process works well, then you can move on to the next step. If it doesn't, that's a sign that factors you didn't take into account are influencing the process, or that your plan is not complete. In that case, pull back until you have clarified the discrepancy and understand why your first plan didn't work.

SUDDEN MOVES TO SUNNY CLIMES

Part of the popular ideal of retirement is the couple who quits work, pulls up all their roots immediately, and moves to Florida to start a new life. In this idealized version, which we have all heard repeated for decades, there is a happy ending, with the couple arriving at their beach condo to lead a joyous, carefree life.

This myth proves tissue-paper thin in reality. Floridians tell a different version of this mythical story. In it, the stress of the move and of adjustment to a very different environment takes its toll on the couple's health, and one member—usually the man—falls ill within a year after the couple arrives. When he dies, the wife is left alone and bereaved in a strange place, with family and friends far away and financial resources reduced. The absence of family and friends is particularly painful; after a short time the surviving spouse moves back to the place they left, at an additional expenditure of time, energy, and money. Frequently the only option remaining is to move in with the children, a solution that may not be ideal for either side.

This advice doesn't apply just to couples. Widows and widowers are often frequently tempted to move away, start all over again, and find a retirement residence with a friend or where they'll be close to other people. Public relations expert Eleanor Lambert told how after her husband died, she went to visit a friend in Knoxville, Tennessee, thinking that perhaps she might move there and share her friend's house. "She had a beautiful apartment that she retired to, and had a big formal garden in the middle and a swimming pool, and all sorts of things. I went down twice and spent the weekend, and then I said to her, 'You know, it's all right—but if you should die first, I don't know anybody in this town, and I don't care about your relatives. What would I do?' And she said, 'Well, you're perfectly right.'" Lambert's intuition was working hard in her behalf in this instance, because her friend did die first, relatively soon after Lambert's visits. Lambert has never doubted that she made the right decision.

On the other hand, there are examples of radical moves being very successful, as was the move from New York to Los Angeles for Norman Cousins. It is important to emphasize that there is no general rule on this subject that works equally well for everyone. You must assess carefully your own feelings and situation, in order to know whether the move is right for you personally at that time. Moving may be the logical next step if you are genuinely ready for a change of scene. On the other hand, if you are moving just because you think you should, or because you think a resortlike environment will be nirvana, then you may be making a large-scale and possibly irreversible mistake.

Perhaps the best reality test is to ask yourself who you know and what you will do when you get to the new location. If you have no prior acquaintances, no particular plans, and don't know what kind of activity you might find in that geographic area, the chances are good that you may be moving on the basis of mythology instead of reality.

It is a good idea to postpone your move until you have spent some time in the new destination. Try to schedule a four- to six-week stay to give yourself time to explore the area thoroughly. You should do enough homework on the town and surrounding area to know exactly what the circumstances of life are, what is available that you might do, and what is not available that you may have hoped or expected to find. If one of a couple were to fall ill after the move, how would you feel about being isolated and away from your family and your community of friends? Only if you can answer questions like these concretely and knowledgeably can you be sure that the move has a realistic chance of success.

SUMMARY

In managing your own career, being open to unexpected opportunities and sheer luck are as important as careful planning. Flexibility, adaptability, and a refusal to stay too long at work they didn't enjoy are all trademark qualities of the Long Careers Study participants that worked to their advantage.

And, again, the single most important element to developing a long career or creating an active post-retirement life is to find meaningful and fulfilling work, whether paying or nonpaying, that keeps you active, engaged, and happy.

Epilogue

The Long Careers Study participants have been at the forefront of the longevity revolution in this century. Their experiences show all the range of possibilities now open to people in the decades beyond sixty-five. They are proving by example that, as more and more people live to be one hundred or older, it is not the crippling social problem we may have assumed. Instead, the extension of healthy, active adult life offers tremendous benefits to our society.

In a long-lived society, the range of experience in the second fifty years of life will be as diverse as that in any earlier period. As we have seen, there is not just one pattern of experience in a long career—there are endless variations. Just as there is not one single pattern of experience for the middle-aged, the young adult, and the adolescent, nor a single image for any of these stages, the image of the older years needs to be equally diverse. We need to discard our monolithic view of aging.

Acknowledging that there are positive aspects to the older years does not mean that we deny that there are negative aspects as well. Though more older people are remaining healthy well into their eighties and beyond, there are hundreds of thousands of older people who genuinely are ill, who require institutionalization, and whose old age we would not wish on ourselves nor on those we love. We must address the issues raised by the negative experiences of these older people and look for better ways to help them cope with their medical and social problems.

Nevertheless, I believe that we as a society have used these real problems to characterize many more older people than are affected by them. We have magnified our negative image of aging until it is far out of proportion with reality—until it fills the entire screen, as it were, leaving no room for any positive view. Becoming aware of the positive aspects and opportunities of aging gives us a more complex and even-handed view of this part of the life course.

This positive aspect of aging is not important just for our society as a whole but for each of us individually. Because "positive aging," as much as it depends on health and outside circumstances, is also a personal choice. No one wants to be lonely, alienated, bitter, fearful, and without friends in their later years. But the choice is not a simple one-time decision; it is a choice we must make every day, in a series of many activities—through the stance we take toward ourselves and others, the feelings we nurture, the continuing commitments and responsibilities we choose, and the beliefs we hold about our role in the world. Over a span of ten or twenty years, one's attitude, whether positive or negative, etches a clear image. A ball rolling on a smooth surface can be tapped lightly, and at first its change in direction will be barely visible. But by the time it has covered a substantial amount of ground, its course may have branched very far from where originally it would have gone.

All of us know people in their mature decades who are enthusiastic and energetic and who have continued to grow throughout their lives. We will have increasing opportunities in the years ahead to decide how we will define the time that has been added to our adult lives. It is useful to look at people like the Long Careers Study participants to see how they have sustained their pattern of growth and to ask what we can do in our own lives to build a life that continues to open new possibilities, to expand our minds and spirits, and to contribute to the world in which we live.

It may seem inconceivable to us now that in 1900, scientists, as well as the general public, believed that people over forty could not be productive and creative. In the early years of the twenty-first century, it may seem just as inconceivable that we did not believe that people over sixty-five have a wealth of talents to con-tribute to our lives.

ACHIEVEMENTS AFTER AGE SIXTY-FIVE

In looking ahead to the years after sixty-five, you should begin to see not only the possibility of continued, productive work, but also the potential for tremendous achievement. Many of the Long Careers Study participants have achieved remarkable goals and new heights in their years since age sixty-five. Everything they have learned, written, done, experienced, and contributed in the time beyond that is a net gain. We owe all of these accomplish-ments to the longevity factor, for without it, most of these people would not have had these bonus years to create.

The following list is a representative sample of the achieve-ments of some Long Careers Study participants since age sixty-five.

Isaac Asimov published approximately twenty books from age sixty-five to his death at seventy-two in 1992, bringing his total lifetime production close to five hundred.

Rena Bartos's fifth book, *Marketing to Women Around the World*, was published in 1989, and she has started her own very successful marketing research company.

Edward Bernays moved to Cambridge, Massachusetts, in his early sixties and published his autobiography; more than thirty-five years later, clients still seek his advice on public relations mat-ters, for a fee of $1,000 per hour.

Dr. James Birren moved from the University of Southern Cali-fornia, where he had founded the Andrus Center for Gerontology, and established the Borun Center for Gerontological Research at the University of California in Los Angeles at age seventy-one. He has also reissued a new four-volume edition of *The Handbook of Aging*.

Marvin Bower is still a director at the company he founded, McKinsey & Co., and was elected to the National Business Hall of Fame in 1989 at age eighty-six.

Virginia Boyd maintains her law practice in Connecticut. In 1989, at age seventy-seven, she was given a special award by the Connecticut Bar Association and the State of Connecticut for her contributions to the legal profession in that state.

Helen Breed began her acting career at age sixty-five. Now eighty-one, she has worked steadily on stage and in films, including *The Witches of Eastwick* with Cher and Jack Nicholson, *Who's That Girl?* with Madonna, and *Passed Away,* starring Maureen Stapleton.

David Brown has produced many Hollywood mega-hits, including *Neighbors, The Verdict, Target, Cocoon,* and *The Player,* as well as several Broadway plays. He was also Executive Producer of *Driving Miss Daisy.* He produced both the play and the movie of *A Few Good Men,* and has published three books, including his autobiography, *Let Me Entertain You* (1990). He is seventy-six.

Dr. William Cahan sued at the age of seventy to be allowed to continue performing cancer surgery, and won. He recently published his autobiography, *No Stranger to Tears.*

Liz Carpenter is working on her third book, giving speeches across the country, and raising her late brother's three youngest children, at age seventy-two.

Julia Child has given us countless hours of cooking instruction and television entertainment as well as her latest and most definitive cookbook, *How to Cook.* In 1992 Child turned eighty; her eightieth birthday was celebrated through the year in dinners and benefits to honor the American Institute of Food and Wine, which she founded.

Norman Cousins, during the last ten years of his life, conducted mind-body research at UCLA and wrote his last two books, *The Healing Heart* and *Head First: The Biology of Hope,* along with advising and working with the staff and patients of the UCLA Medical School. He died in 1990 at the age of seventy-five.

Hume Cronyn has starred in movies like *Cocoon* and on Broadway with his wife Jessica Tandy in the Pulitzer prize–winning play, "The Gin Game," among many other plays and movies.

Dr. W. Edwards Deming insists that the years between seventy and ninety have been his most productive ones: he has given seminars all over the world on management style and economic recovery, and continues to travel to two or three cities a week at age ninety-two. He has published one book, *Out of the Crisis,* and his second book will appear in 1993.

C. Douglas Dillon made many of his most brilliant contributions as Chairman of the Metropolitan Museum of Art between the ages of sixty-five and seventy-four, when he left the position. He is still a member of the Museum Board, and contributes in many ways, including his continuing interest in the Astor Court and Dillon Gallery.

Hugh Downs came out of "retirement" to host "20/20" at age fifty-five, and remains, at age seventy-one, the host of one of the highest rated news shows on television.

John Forsythe created his world-famous role as Blake Carrington, Denver oil magnate, on TV's mega-hit show, "Dynasty," which conveyed a sense of vigor, aliveness, excitement, fascination, and yes, sex appeal to the nation—age be damned. He and his fellow "Dynasty" cast members continue to sustain that image as they have moved into other roles.

John Gardner founded two organizations, Common Cause and Independent Sector, and then, at age seventy-nine, accepted a new position as Centennial Professor of Business at Stanford Business School. He has published three books: *Morale* (1978), *Quotations of Wit and Wisdom* (1980), and *On Leadership* (1991), and is working on another. A second edition of *Self-Renewal* was published in 1981 and a revised edition of *Excellence* appeared in 1984.

Francoise Gilot continues both to write and to paint, and is a highly respected lecturer on art. *Matisse and Picasso: A Friendship in Art* was published in 1991.

"Mother" Clara Hale, at age sixty-four, began to take in drug-addicted women and their children, which led her to establish "Hale House," the organization she still runs today at eighty-seven.

Louis Harris continues to conduct some of the most authoritative national and international polls in the world and most recently (at age sseventy-one) founded a new polling organization in Moscow.

Frances Lear created and developed *Lear's* magazine, heightening awareness about the value of women who weren't "born yesterday," and has given considerable support to research on incest and on manic depression. She has just published her autobiography, *The Second Seduction* (1992), and is working on plans for a television program.

Theresa Bergman Meyerowitz had a retrospective of her work called "Echoes of New York" at the Museum of the City of New York from November 1990 to March 1991; she was one hundred and one. She is about to publish her autobiography, *The Journal*.

Dr. Linus Pauling has conducted almost all of his three-year study of nutrition and has published three books on the subject: *Vitamin C and the Common Cold* (1970), *Cancer and Vitamin C* (1979) and *How to Live Longer and Feel Better* (1986). He is working on two other books. During his life he has published over eight hundred scientific papers. He is ninety-one.

Dr. Jonas Salk has been working since 1984 on a prototype AIDS vaccine. He has published several books: *World Population and Human Values* (1981) and *Anatomy of Reality* (1983). He is seventy-eight.

Arthur Schlesinger, Jr., has spent the ten years since his sixty-fifth birthday teaching history at the City University of New York. He has just published two books, *Cycles of American History* (1986) and *The Disuniting of America* (1992). He is currently writing the fourth volume of *The Age of Roosevelt*.

Jessica Tandy won the Academy Award for her performance in *Driving Miss Daisy* at age seventy-nine, and in 1991 received another Oscar nomination for her performance in *Fried Green Tomatoes*.

Dr. Lewis Thomas, who began his writing career at age fifty-seven and published *Lives of a Cell* in 1974, when he was sixty-one, has since published four other volumes of essays: *The Medusa and the Snail*, 1979; *The Youngest Science*, 1983; *Late Night Thoughts on Listening to Mahler's Ninth Symphony*, 1985; and *The Fragile Species*, 1992. He is seventy-nine.

Cyrus Vance has used his exceptional wisdom and political understanding to mediate international disputes and resolve the causes of contention, including an assignment to Yugoslavia as the Personal Envoy of the United Nations Secretary General.

Appendix

LONG CAREERS STUDY PARTICIPANTS

Name	1992 Age	Year of Birth
1. Issac Asimov	(d. April 6, 1992, age 72)	1920
2. Janet Jeppson Asimov	66	1926
3. Will Barnet	81	1911
4. Rena Bartos	74	1918
5. Dr. Robert Bell	74	1918
6. Edward L. Bernays	101	1891
7. Elizabeth Birren	75	1917
8. Dr. James Birren	74	1918
9. Richard Bolles	66	1926
10. Marvin Bower	89	1903
11. Virginia Boyd	74	1918
12. Helen Breed	81	1911
13. David Brown	76	1916
14. Louise Brown	80	1912
15. Shirley Brussell	72	1920
16. McGeorge Bundy	73	1919
17. Elizabeth Burns	89	1903
18. Thomas Cabot	95	1897
19. Dr. William Cahan	77	1915
20. Marjorie Cantor	71	1921
21. Liz Carpenter	72	1920
22. Julia Child	80	1912
23. Robert C. Christopher	(d. June 26,1992, age 68)	1924
24. Dr. Kenneth Clark	78	1914
25. Dr. Alan Cott	81	1911
26. Norman Cousins	(d. Nov. 30, 1990, age 75)	1915
27. Hume Cronyn	81	1911
28. Samuel S. Cross	73	1919
29. John C. Crystal	(d. Sept. 10, 1988, age 67)	1921
30. Evelyn Cunningham	74	1918

Name		1992 Age	Year of Birth
31. Maxwell Dane		86	1906
32. The Hon. Shelby Cullom Davis		83	1909
33. Kathryn Wasserman Davis		85	1907
34. Dr. W. Edwards Deming		91	1900
35. The Hon. C. Douglas Dillon		83	1909
36. Dr. Rose Dubrof		68	1924
37. Hugh Downs		71	1921
38. Peter Drucker		86	1906
39. Dr. James Dumpson		83	1909
40. Oscar Dystel		80	1912
41. Joan Erikson		89	1903
42. Frances Etter		81	1911
43. Nell Eurich		73	1919
44. Hon. Millicent Fenwick	(d. Sept. 16, 1992, age 82)		1910
45. Arthur Flemming		87	1905
46. Eileen Ford		72	1920
47. John Forsythe		74	1918
48. Margaret Fox	(d. Jan. 6, 1989, age 79)		1909
49. Sen. William Fulbright		87	1905
50. Betty Furness		76	1926
51. John Gardner		80	1912
52. Robert D. Gibson		73	1919
53. Francoise Gilot		71	1921
54. Roswell Gilpatrick		86	1906
55. Eli Ginzberg		81	1911
56. William Golden		83	1909
57. Sam Goody	(d. Aug. 8, 1991, age 87)		1904
58. Jane Gould		74	1918
59. J. Peter Grace		79	1913
60. Dr. William Greenough	(d. Dec. 14, 1989, age 73)		1914
61. Elinor Guggenheimer		80	1912
62. Richard "Buzz" Gummere		80	1912
63. Clara McBride "Mother" Hale	(d. Dec. 18, 1992, age 87)		1905
64.. The Hon. Orval Hansen		66	1926
65. Louis Harris		71	1921
66. Louis Hector		75	1917
67. Dr. Michael Heidelberger	(d. June 25, 1991, age 103)		1888
68. Celeste Holm		73	1919
69. The Hon. Lucy Somerville Howorth		96	1896
70. Alberta Jacoby	(d. July 8, 1992, age 81)		1911
71. Eliot Janeway	(d. Feb. 8, 1993, age 80)		1913
72. Elizabeth Janeway		79	1913
73. William Kirby	(d. Oct. 1, 1990, age 79)		1911
74. Jean Kotkin		70	1922
75. Maggie Kuhn		87	1905
76. Carol Laise	(d. July 25, 1991, age 73)		1918
77. Eleanor Lambert		75	1917
78. The Hon. Morris Lasker		75	1917
79. Toy Lasker		73	1919
80. Frances Lear		70	1922
81. Sayra Lebenthal		94	1898
82. Amy Freeman Lee		78	1914
83. Vassily Leontief		86	1906
84. Edna Lerner		79	1913
85. Max Lerner	(d. June 5, 1992, age 90)		1902
86. Eda LeShan		70	1922
87. Dr. Lawrence LeShan		72	1920

Name		1992 Age	Year of Birth
88. James B. Lewis		81	1911
89. John L. Loeb		90	1902
90. Dr. Rollo May		84	1908
91. Dr. Barbara McClintock	(d. Sept. 2, 1992, age 90)		1902
92. Elizabeth McCormack		70	1922
93. Robert McNamara		76	1916
94. Theresa Bergman Meyerowitz		102	1890
95. Elisabeth Luce Moore		90	1903
96. Evelyn Nef		79	1913
97. Dr. Bernice Neugarten		76	1916
98. David Ogilvy		81	1911
99. Mrs. Henry Parish II		82	1910
100. Dr. Linus Pauling		91	1901
101. Rev. Norman Vincent Peale		94	1898
102. Ruth Stafford Peale		86	1906
103. Esther Peterson		86	1906
104. Milton Petrie		90	1902
105. Eleanor Piel		72	1920
106. Gerard Piel		77	1915
107. Alan Pifer		71	1921
108. Robert Popper		84	1908
109. Dr. Harold Proshansky	(d. Dec. 13, 1990, age 70)		1920
110. Lt. Gen. Elwood R. Quesada	(d. Feb. 10, 1993, age 88)		1904
111. Judge Simon Rifkind		91	1901
112. Elizabeth Riley		85	1907
113. Dr. John Riley		84	1908
114. Dr. Matilda Riley		81	1911
115. Warren Robbins		69	1923
116. Penelope Russianoff		74	1918
117. Samuel Sadin		74	1918
118. Janet Sainer		74	1918
119. Dr. Jonas Salk		78	1914
120. Dr. Lee Salk	(d. May 3, 1992, age 65)		1926
121. Arthur Schlesinger, Jr.		75	1917
122. Felice Schwartz		67	1925
123. Robert Schwartz		71	1921
124. Lucy Scott		87	1905
125. Florence Skelly		68	1924
126. Sen. Margaret Chase Smith		95	1897
127. Dr. Frank Stanton		84	1908
128. Jessica Tandy		82	1909
129. Studs Terkel		80	1912
130. Dr. Lewis Thomas		79	1913
131. Ollie Thompson		78	1914
132. Molly Kimball Todd		88	1904
133. Pauline Trigere		80	1912
134. The Hon. Cyrus Vance		75	1917
135. Julia Walsh		69	1923
136. Arthur Wang		74	1918
137. Herbert West	(d. Jan. 14, 1990, age 73)		1916
138. Frances Whitney		80	1912
139. William H. Whyte		75	1917
140. Franklin Williams	(d. May 20, 1990, age 73)		1917
141. Samuel Allen Williams		93	1899
142. The Hon. Willard Wirtz		80	1912
143. Richard Witkin		73	1909
144. Dr. Irving Wright		92	1900

APPENDIX

Name	1992 Age	Year of Birth
145. Lawrence Wylie	82	1910
146. Dr. Rosalyn Yalow	71	1921
147. Dan Yankelovich	68	1924
148. Henny Youngman	86	1906
149. Frank Zachary	79	1913
150. Charlotte Zolotow	77	1915

Notes

All quotations from study participants and experts that are not otherwise identified are verbatim excerpts from interviews conducted personally with the individual quoted.

PROLOGUE

1. Information in this paragraph is from an interview with Dr. Robert Butler, author of the Pulitzer Prize–winning book *Why Survive? Being Old in America* (New York: Harper & Row, 1975), the first book to call to the nation's attention the blight of age prejudice.

2. Samuel Preston, "Children and the Elderly in the U.S.," *Scientific American* (December 1984), p. 44.

CHAPTER 1

1. I am deeply indebted to three expert demographers for the detailed statistical information included in this book: Dr. Jacob Siegel, who for many years was senior demographic statistician for research in special populations, U.S. Bureau of the Census; Cynthia Taueber, branch chief selective populations, U.S. Bureau of the Census and Arnold Goldstein, statistician, demography.

The correlations between state population size and the over-sixty-five population in the United States are my own. The figures are drawn from *The Information Please Almanac, Atlas & Yearbook 1992*, 45th ed. (Boston: Houghton Mifflin, 1992).

Population statistics for the three states mentioned:
- New York: 17,990,498
- New Jersey: 7,730,000
- Massachusetts: 6,016,425

2. Art Linkletter's famous book is entitled *Old Age Is Not for Sissies.*

3. *Passages,* Gail Sheehy's 1976 best-seller, was the first book to bring the results of the new study of adult development to public attention. It was a milestone in the revision of American awareness of adulthood as not just a dreary, constant state lasting from the age of twenty-one until death but as a life as rich in developmental changes as that from birth to age twenty-one. The book was surrounded by controversy about whether Sheehy obtained proper permission to quote the experts she had interviewed, but this did not lessen its public impact. It is worth remarking that at the time, publication for a popular audience was scorned by most professionals. The controversy around *Passages* stimulated a gradual change in that attitude, and more research-based information was brought directly to the reading public; professionals themselves took on the communication of their research to a general audience.

CHAPTER 2

1. Information about Bismarck and about average life expectancies in different historical time periods comes from personal interviews with Prof. W. Andrew Achenbaum, deputy director of the Institute of Gerontology, University of Michigan, and from his book, *Social Security: Visions and Revisions* (New York: Cambridge University Press, 1986).

2. The concepts of average life expectancy and average life expectancy at birth require some explanation, since they are demographic terms whose meaning is never fully conveyed to the general public in books and articles about aging. Indeed, their meaning cannot be accurately expressed in a brief statement.

Just as the ideas of what is "old" and where "old age" begins are astonishingly flexible, the concept of "average life expectancy" is not a fixed element but a point on a scale, determined by conditions in a particular time and place. Moreover, there is a different average life expectancy for every age from birth forward, a fact that few members of the public are familiar with.

The point for which average life expectancy is calculated is birth (thus "average life expectancy at birth"). This is the figure commonly seen in journalistic accounts and descriptions of the increase of life expectancy (e.g., forty-seven in 1900 versus seventy-four in 1990). This figure, however, includes deaths of infants, children, and young adults. An average life expectancy figure calculated for older ages (e.g., twenty-one, fifty, or sixty-five) inevitably will be longer in our society, since the fragility of infants and children is necessarily not included.

Average life expectancy-at-birth figures do not indicate that your total life expectancy increases as you live longer. A baby boomer born in the first year of the boom, 1946, had an average life expectancy at birth of 66.7 (this figure was cited to me by Dr. Mary Grace Kovar of the National Center for Health Statistics, in a telephone communication in August 1991). But when that boomer reached 25, he or she could expect to live for 46.1 more years, or to the age of 71.1 (that is, if he or she was in good health, was reasonably careful about avoiding accidents, and didn't smoke or drink excessively). At age 50, our boomer can look forward to 28.6 more years, or a life lasting 78.6 years. And at 75, our baby boomer will have a life expectancy that has expanded once again: to 10.2 more years, to age 85.2.

This is the forecast as things stand in the 1990s. Total remaining life expectancy will increase even more in the future, according to demographer Dr. Jacob Siegel, himself in his seventies. With every year that you live, your statistical chances of living longer will grow. Future scientific advances in controlling or preventing illness and in understanding the aging process will almost certainly lengthen average life expectancy more.

Average life expectancy figures can give a distorted impression, because there are factors that these figures do not express clearly. First, a trend expressed in averages is just that: some people will live shorter lives than the average, and some will live much longer lives. Many Americans will still die at younger ages than the average life expectancy at birth. Many others will live longer, and some will live a great deal longer.

Another qualifying factor is that the figures don't express directly that so many of today's older generation are living into the decades beyond average life expectancy—into the eighties, nineties, and beyond. During this century the probability of living into these later decades has increased even more than the average life expectancy at birth itself. Only 14 percent of the babies born in 1900 could expect to live to be eighty, but 45 percent of those born in the 1980s will reach that age (based on calculating only the average life expectancy at birth).

If we factor in the average years remaining as we did just above, it may be that more than half the baby boom generation will live to age eighty and beyond. Assuming that the current trends continue, these people are likely to stay physically young and active until very late in life.

Finally, despite the sophistication of our capacity to project large-scale population trends, it is still impossible to predict, using statistical or any other tools, how long a particular individual will live. All of the mathematical formulas used in predicting population growth deal with very large numbers of people. But, given these large-scale trends, the chances are very good that if you are healthy and take ordinary good care of your health, you will live longer than you probably expect. It is possible, however, to make an informed guess, based on particular risk factors that are known to increase or decrease life expectancy generally. For example, two of the biggest risk factors are smoking and drinking to excess; all the major causes of adult death (cardiovascular illness, cancer, and stroke), except AIDS and Alzheimer's, are linked to smoking, excess drinking, or both.

3. Information on Arthur Miller's play *Death of a Salesman* is quoted from a personal interview he gave for the study. Although he did not have time to serve as a full participant because he was overseeing the first American production of *The Ride Down Mount Morgan,* he generously spent over an hour talking about his concept of *Death of a Salesman* and the meaning for him both of the play and of its hero, Willy Loman. I found his interpretation of Willy astonishing; it is at variance with the interpretation of every drama expert and college or graduate school professor I have ever encountered. Willy is a hero, youthful and determined instead of old and beaten down, who ultimately beats the system even though the only way he can think of to do so involves sacrificing his own life.

4. The expression *middle age* seems to have entered the American vocabulary sometime after World War II, but I was unable to find documentation of who coined it and when. The only professional opinion I could find was the suggestion of Dr. Gilbert Brim, head of the MacArthur Foundation Research Network on Midlife, that it was Prof. Bernice Neugarten herself who first coined the term. Knowing Dr. Neugarten's facility for observing and naming new social trends and phenomena (she also coined the terms *young-old, old-old,* and *aging society*), I find this easy to believe. However, Dr. Neugarten herself would not admit to it.

It is clear, in any case, that middle age originally was considered to occupy the years between thirty-five and fifty. As longevity has increased and old age has slid gradually forward, middle age has crept forward, too, in the public mind.

5. Dr. Sagan's ideas were expressed in his book, *The Health of Nations* (New York: Basic Books, 1988), and also in a personal interview at the Gerontological Society of America annual meeting, San Francisco, California, 1989.

6. No general work has yet been published in the United States on the Svanborg studies, although hundreds of scientific papers have been pub-

lished by the team to date. Svanborg himself wrote a short pamphlet for the Swedish Ministry of Health, which was translated into English and republished for American and English readers as *Health and Vitality: Research on Aging* (Swedish Medical Research Council, 1988), but it is not easily available in this country. All information on the studies was communicated directly to me in a number of long detailed interviews with Dr. Svanborg and his wife, Dr. Marianne Svanborg, and by Dr. James E. Birren and Betty Birren, two American psychologists thoroughly familiar with the studies' structure and results.

7. The work of Drs. Rose and Johnson was reported by Tim McDonald in "New Studies Reveal Aging Process Can Be Slowed," *Chronicle of Higher Education* (March 4, 1992), p. A-9.

8. The work of Drs. Carey and Curtsinger was reported in "Study Challenges Longevity Theory," *New York Times* (October 16, 1992), p. A22. Out of their one million fruit flies, a few lived a lot longer than was predicted, once they reached old age.

CHAPTER 3

1. The career of Osler and the debacle of his valedictory speech are discussed in William Graebner, *A History of Retirement: The Meaning and Function of an American Institution, 1885–1978* (New Haven: Yale University Press, 1980); and in Thomas Cole, *The Journey of Life: A Cultural History of Aging in America* (New York: Cambridge University Press, 1992). Cole is more sympathetic to Osler than is Graebner, but reading direct quotations from the text places Cole's interpretation in some doubt, in this reader's mind at least. Cole is willing to believe that Osler meant his comments humorously. However, the text does not read as if it were so intended, to this author.

2. Lehman published substantially on his theories that there is a major decrement in performance as we age and that this decrement is significant. See Harvey Lehman, *Age and Achievement* (Princeton: Princeton University Press, 1953). See also "The Age Decrement in Outstanding Scientific Creativity," *American Psychologist* 15 (1960), pp. 128–134; and "The Creative Production Rates of Present versus Past Generations of Scientists," in Bernice Neugarten, ed., *Middle Age and Aging* (1968).

3. Information on McLeish's work comes from two telephone interviews with Professor McLeish and from *The Ulyssean Adult: Creativity in the Middle and Later Years* (Toronto: McGraw Hill-Ryerson, 1976).

4. Dennis published a number of articles on the debate on age and achievement. See "Age and Achievement: A Critique," *Journal of Gerontology* 11 (1956), pp. 331–333; "The Age Decrement in Outstanding Scientific

Contributions: Fact or Artifact?" *American Psychologist* 13 (1958), pp. 457–460; "Creative Productivity Between the Ages of 20 and 80 Years," in Bernice Neugarten, ed., *Middle Age and Aging* (1968); the University of Chicago Press, Chicago; and "Creative Productivity Between the Ages of 20 and 80 Years," *Journal of Gerontology* 21 (1966), pp. 1–8.

5. From lengthy telephone interviews with Harriet Zuckerman and from her book, *Scientific Elite: Nobel Laureates in the United States* (New York: Free Press, 1977). See also Harriet Zuckerman and Jonathan R. Cole, "The Sociology of Science," chap. 16 in Neil J. Smelzer, ed., *Handbook of Sociology* (Newbury Park, California: Sage Publications, 1988), pp. 511–574.

6. Psychologist Dean Keith Simonton has become an acknowledged expert on the historiometric study of aging (i.e., looking at the total life production of an individual and analyzing its patterns). Among his publications are "Age and Literary Creativity: A Cross-cultural and Transhistorical Survey," *Journal of Cross-cultural Psychology* 6 (1975), pp. 258–277; "Age and Outstanding Achievement: What Do We Know After a Century of Research?"; and "Creativity and Wisdom in Aging," in J. E. Birren and W. K. Schaie, eds., *Handbook of the Psychology of Aging,* 3d ed. (New York: Academic Press, 1990), pp. 321–329; "Creativity in the Later Years: Optimistic Prospects for Achievement," *Gerontologist* 30 (1990); *Genius, Creativity and Leadership: Historiometric Inquiries* (Cambridge, Mass.: Harvard University Press, 1984); and "The Swan-song Phenomenon: Last-Works Effects for 172 Classical Composers," *Psychology and Aging* 4 (1989), pp. 42–47.

7. Comments about the work of Robert Boyd are from material gained from interview with Dr. Harold Brody and with Arthur Downing, chief librarian at the New York Academy of Medicine's library. No publications of his were found.

8. Raymond Pearl, M.D., "Variation and Correlation on Brain Weight," in *Biometrika: A Journal for the Statistical Study of Biological Problems* 4 (June 1905–March 1906), pp. 50–57; and F. W. Appel and E. M. Appel, "Intracranial Variation in the Weight of the Human Brain," in *Human Biology: A Record of Research* (Baltimore: Johns Hopkins University Press, 1942).

9. Information on the work of Dr. Brody comes from tape-recorded telephone interviews with him, which were subsequently transcribed to ensure accuracy, and from additional interviews with Dr. James E. Birren, who as a psychologist and a trained observer watched the controversy around the brain-cell-loss issue develop.

For further information, see Harold Brody and N. Vijayashanbar, "Cell

Loss with Aging Brain," in K. Nandy and A. Sherwin, eds., *Aging Brain and Senile Dementia* (New York: Plenum Press, 1977).

10. Alex Comfort, *A Good Age* (New York: Crown, 1976).

11. Cell redundancy has been the subject of a good deal of research by Paul Coleman. See Paul D. Coleman and Stephen J. Buell, "Regulation of Dendritic Extent in Developing and Aging Brain," in *Synaptic Plasticity* (New York: Guilford Press, 1985), pp. 311–325; and Paul D. Coleman and Dorothy G. Flood, "Neuron Numbers and Dendritic Extent in Normal Aging and Alzheimer's Disease," *Neurobiology of Aging* 8 (1987), pp. 521–545.

12. Janet L. Hopson, "A Love Affair with the Brain" (conversation with Marian Diamond), *Psychology Today* 18 (November 1984), pp. 62–73.

13. K. Warner Schaie and Sherry Willis have published dozens of articles about their work on the Seattle Longitudinal Study. These include Schaie, K. Warner, "Intellectual Development in Adulthood," chap. 17 in *Handbook of the Psychology of Aging* (San Diego: Academic Press, 1990); Schaie, K. Warner, "Individual Differences in Rate of Cognitive Change in Adulthood," in *The Course of Later Life: Research and Reflections* (New York: Springer); Schaie, K. Warner, "Toward a Stage Theory of Adult Cognitive Development," *Journal of Aging and Human Development* 8 (1977), pp. 129–178; and Willis, L. Sherry, "Cognition and Everyday Competence," *Annual Review of Gerontology and Geriatrics* 11 (1991), pp. 80–109.

CHAPTER 4

1. Dr. Avorn's brilliant paradigm of cumulative decline was originally published in his article "Medicine: The Life and Death of Oliver Shay," in Alan Pifer and Lydia Brontë, eds., *Our Aging Society: Paradox and Promise* (New York: W. W. Norton and Company, 1986), pp. 283–296.

2. Elaine Cumming and William Henry, *Growing Old: The Process of Disengagement* (New York: Basic Books, 1961).

3. Nathan Shock, T. Franklin Williams, and James L. Fozard, *Older and Wiser,* National Institutes of Health pub. 89-2797 (Baltimore, Md., 1989).

4. Dr. Hayflick has published numerous books, articles, and papers about his research on the multiplication of cells in vitro. Among them are "Recent Advances in the Cell Biology of Aging," *Mechanisms of Ageing and Development* 14 (1980); "The Longevity of Cultured Human Cells," *Journal of the American Geriatrics Society* 22 (1974); "Cell Biology of Aging," *BioScience* (October 1975); and "Human Cells and Aging," *Scientific American* (March 1968).

5. Dr. James Fries, "Aging, Natural Death, and the Compression of Morbidity," *New England Journal of Medicine* 3 (1980), pp. 130–35. See also his "The Compression of Morbidity," *Milbank Memorial Fund Quarterly/Health and Society* 61 (1983), pp. 397–419; and *Gerontologist* (March 1983). For further information, see also R. R. Kohn, "Causes of Death in Very Old People," *Journal of the American Medical Association*, 247(20) (May 1982).

6. From personal interview with Prof. Mary Catherine Bateson.

CHAPTER 5

1. Drs. John and Matilda White Riley, "Longevity and Social Structure," in Alan Pifer and Lydia Brontë, eds., *Our Aging Society: Paradox and Promise* (W. W. Norton and Company, 1986).

2. From telephone conversation with representative of the AARP, 1989.

3. The Louis Harris studies for NCOA were published five years apart and had a great influence on our ability to see older people through the bias that had clouded our vision until then. See Louis Harris and Associates, *The Myth and Reality of Aging in America* (Washington, D.C.: NCOA, 1977); and Louis Harris and Associates, *Aging in the Eighties: America in Transition* (Washington, D.C.: NCOA, 1981).

CHAPTER 9

1. Dr. Brim's book, *Ambition: How We Manage Success and Failure Throughout Our Lives* (New York: Basic Books, 1992), the fruit of years of research and observation, was aimed at a general rather than a scientific audience.

CHAPTER 10

1. See Harvey Lehman, *Age and Achievement* (Princeton: Princeton University Press, 1953).

2. Dean Keith Simonton, presentation at the American Psychological Association meeting, August 1992.

CHAPTER 12

1. Susan Faludi, *Backlash: The Undeclared War against American Women* (New York: Crown, 1991).

CHAPTER 13

1. Dr. Birren's list of nine "commandments" for older people, "My Responsibilities for My Old Age," is found in his article "Abilities, Opportunities and Responsibilities in the Third Quarter of Life," in the Executive

Summary in *Resourceful Aging Today and Tomorrow,* conference report, AARP New Roles in Society, vol. 1, pp. 15–23.

CHAPTER 15

1. This chapter is based mainly on three path-breaking studies. The first is the massive decade of research conducted by Dr. William Evans and Dr. Irwin H. Rosenberg and written up with Jacqueline Thompson as *Biomarkers: The 10 Determinants of Aging You Can Control* (New York: Simon & Schuster, 1991). Their work was done at the U.S. Department of Agriculture Human Nutrition Research Center on Aging at Tufts University.

The second body of research is the work on vitamins and human health by Dr. Linus Pauling, who has written three books on the subject and is at work on a fourth with Dr. Abram Hoffer, a Canadian physician who codirected the first study of vitamins on human illness at Saskatchewan Hospital in 1952, and an American psychologist, Dr. Humphrey Osmund.

The third is the breakthrough work of Norman Cousins establishing a link between mental state and physical health, which is documented in his book, *Head First: The Biology of Hope* (New York: E. P. Dutton, 1989).

2. Dr. John Yudkin, ed., with I. Edelman and L. Hough, *Sugar: Chemical, Biological and Nutritional Aspects of Sucrose* (Hartford, Conn.: Daniel Davey Publishers, 1971). Yudkin was professor of physiology at Queen Elizabeth College of London University from 1945 to 1954 and then professor of nutrition and dietetics from 1954 to 1971. He also wrote a book for the educated general public, *Sweet and Dangerous* (New York: Peter H. Weiden and Company, 1972). This important study was reported by Milton Winitz and his associates in 1964 and 1970; the clinical trial conducted by Winitz and his collaborators strongly supports the conclusion reached by Yudkin that sugar (sucrose) is dangerous as well as sweet.

3. Norman Cousins, *Anatomy of an Illness, as Perceived by the Patient: Reflections on Healing and Regeneration* (New York: W. W. Norton and Company, 1979). See also Cousins, *Head First: The Biology of Hope* (New York: E. P. Dutton, 1989); and *The Healing Heart: Antidotes to Panic and Helplessness* (New York: W. W. Norton and Company, 1983).

CHAPTER 16

1. *What Color Is Your Parachute?* (Walnut Creek, California: Ten-Speed Press, 1992).

Index